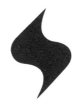

Stedman's

NEUROSURGERY
WORDS

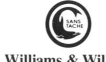

Williams & Wilkins

BALTIMORE • PHILADELPHIA • HONG KONG
LONDON • MUNICH • SYDNEY • TOKYO

A WAVERLY COMPANY

Series Editor: Elizabeth Randolph
Production Coordinators: Barbara Felton, Kim Nawrozki
Cover Design: Carla Frank

Copyright © 1993
Williams & Wilkins
428 East Preston Street
Baltimore, Maryland 21202, USA

Printed in the United States of America

Library of Congress Cataloging-in-Publication Data
Stedman's neurosurgery words
     p. cm.—(Stedman's word books)
    Developed from Stedman's medical dictionary, 25th ed. and supplemented by terminology found in the current medical literature.
    ISBN 0-683-07962-X
    1. Nervous system—Surgery—Terminology.   2. Neurology—Terminology.
I. Stedman, Thomas Lathrop, 1853–1938. Medical dictionary.   II. Title:
Neurosurgery words.   III. Series.
    [DNLM: 1. Nervous System—terminology.   2. Neurosurgery—terminology.
3. Nervous System Diseases—terminology.   WL 15 S812 1993]
   RD593.S73   1993
   617.4'8'003—dc20
   DNLM/DLC
   for Library of Congress   93-16861
                                  CIP

8 9 10

Contents

Acknowledgments

An important part of our editorial process is the involvement of medical transcriptionists—as advisors, reviewers and/or editors. Vicki Willms, CMT and Jenny Maggiore, CMT used their expertise to edit and proof the manuscript. Thanks go to Susan Grant, CMT, Averill Ring, CMT, Susan Eastwood and Mary Algiers Bellile, CMT, who perused texts, journals, and manufacturer's information to compile an accurate, up-to-date base of neurosurgery terms. We gratefully acknowledge Shawne Tubinis and the office of Don Long, MD at the Johns Hopkins Department of Neurosurgery, for assisting us in our word research.

Special thanks to Carol-Lynn Brown, who helped launch the project with research and finish it with her proofreading. Barbara Ferretti's corrections brought us from first draft to final pages.

Also, as with all our Stedman's word references, we have benefited from the suggestions and expertise of our many contacts in the medical transcriptionist community. Thanks to all our advisory board participants, reviewers and editors, AAMT meeting attendees, and others who have written in with requests and comments—keep talking, and we'll keep listening.

Explanatory Notes

Stedman's Neurosurgery Words offers an authoritative assurance of quality and exactness to the wordsmiths of the health care professions—medical transcriptionists, medical editors and copy editors, medical records personnel, and the many other users and producers of medical documentation. It can be used to validate both the spelling and accuracy of terminology in neurosurgery. This compilation of over 30,000 entries, fully cross-indexed for quick access, was built from a base vocabulary of 19,000 medical words, phrases, abbreviations and acronyms. The extensive A-Z list was developed from the database of **Stedman's Medical Dictionary, 25ed**. and supplemented by terminology found in the current medical literature.

Medical transcription is an art as well as a science. Both are needed to correctly interpret a physician's dictation, whose language is a product of education, training, and experience. This variety in medical language means that there are several acceptable ways to express certain terms, including jargon. **Stedman's Neurosurgery Words** provides variant spellings and phrasings for many terms. This, in addition to complete cross-indexing, makes **Stedman's Neurosurgery Words** a valuable resource for determining the validity of terms as they are encountered.

Stedman's Neurosurgery Words includes up-to-date terminology of neuroanatomy and neurology, general neurosurgery, neuroradiology, aneurysms/arteriovenous malformations, radiosurgery, stereotaxis, brain and skull-base tumors, cerebrovascular disease, epilepsy, pediatric neurosurgery, spinal cord injury and repair, pain and trauma. The user will find listed thousands of diseases and syndromes, abbreviations, eponymic terms and diagnostic tests and procedures. Drugs and equipment names (including neuroendoscopy and spinal instrumentation) related to neurosurgery are also included.

Alphabetical Organization

Alphabetization of entries is letter by letter as spelled, ignoring punctuation, spaces, prefixed numbers, Greek letters, or other characters. For example:

> **acid-fast staining methods**
> **acid formaldehyde hematin**
> **α_1-acid glycoprotein**
> **acid hematin**

In subentries, the abbreviated singular form or the spelled-out plural form of the noun main entry word is ignored in alphabetization.

Format and Style

All main entries are in **boldface** to speed up location of a sought-after entry, to enhance distinction between main entries and subentries, and to relieve the textual density of the pages.

Irregular plurals and variant spellings are shown on the same line as the singular or preferred form of the word. For example:

> **substantia**, pl. **substantiae**

> **fiber, fibre**
> A f.'s
> accelerator f.'s
> adrenergic f.'s

Possessive forms that occur in the medical literature are retained in this reference. To form the non-possessives advocated by the American Association for Medical Transcription and other groups, simply drop the apostrophe or apostrophe "s" from the end of the word. It should be noted that eponymic equipment and instrument names frequently appear in non-possessive form.

Cross-indexing

The word list is in an index-like main entry-subentry format that contains two combined alphabetical listings:

(1) A noun main entry-subentry organization typical of the A-Z section of medical dictionaries like **Stedman's**:

acid
acetylsalicylic a.
amino a.
aminocaproic a.
amoxicillin-clavulanic a.

nerve
abducent n.
accelerator n.'s
accessory n.
acoustic n.

(2) An adjective main entry-subentry organization, which lists words and phrases as you hear them. The main entries are the adjectives or modifiers descriptors in a multiword term. The subentries are the nouns around which the terms are constructed and to which the adjectives or descriptors pertain:

pituitary
p. abscess
p. adamantinoma
p. adenoma
p. apoplexy

neural
n. axis
n. canal
◄ n. crest
n. crest syndrome

This format provides the user with more than one way to locate and identify a multi-word term. For example:

forceps
McGill f.

McGill
M. forceps

degenerative
d. brain disease

disease
degenerative brain d.

It also allows the user to see together all terms that contain a particular modifier as well as all types, kinds, or variations of a noun entity. For example:

aneurysm
    clinoidal a.
    a. clip
    a. clipping
    congenital a.

field
    f. expansion
    f.'s of Forel
    fringing f.
    gradient f.

flow
    hypothalamic blood f.
    f. imaging
    intraarterial f.
    f. misregistration

line
    l. frequency noise dot
    Garrett l.
    Garrett orientation l.
    l. of Gennari

Abbreviations are defined and cross-referenced throughout. For example:

PICA
    posterior inferior cerebellar artery
posterior
    p. inferior cerebellar artery (PICA)
artery
    posterior inferior cerebellar a. (PICA)

References

American Journal of neuroradiology. Baltimore: Williams & Wilkins; 1991; 1992.

An HS, Cotler JM, eds. Spinal instrumentation. Baltimore: Williams & Wilkins, 1992.

Apuzzo, Brain surgery, Vols 1–2. New York: Churchill Livingstone; 1993.

Atlas, MRI of the brain and spine. New York: Raven; 1991.

Little JR, Awad IA, eds. Reoperative neurosurgery. Baltimore: Williams & Wilkins; 1992.

Journal of neurosurgery. Baltimore: Williams & Wilkins; 1992.

Miller, Walsh and Hoyt's clinical neuro-ophthalmology, 4ed. Vol 4. Baltimore: Williams & Wilkins; 1991.

Rengachary/AANS, Atlas of Neurosurgery, Vol 2. Baltimore: Williams & Wilkins; 1992.

Stedman's medical dictionary, 25ed. Baltimore: Williams & Wilkins; 1990.

Sundt, Surgical technique for saccular and giant aneurysms. Baltimore: Williams & Wilkins; 1990.

Wilkins RH, Rengachary SS, eds. Neurosurgery, Vol 3. New York: McGraw-Hill; 1985.

Wilkins RH, Rengachary SS, eds. Neurosurgery update I. New York: McGraw-Hill; 1990.

Wilkins RH, Rengachary SS, eds. Neurosurgery update II. New York: McGraw-Hill; 1991.

Wilson, Neurosurgical procedures. Baltimore: Williams & Wilkins; 1992.

Youmans, Youmans neurological surgery, 3rd ed. Vols 1–6. Philadelphia: W. B. Saunders; 1990.

Your Medical Word Resource Publisher

We strive to provide you with the most up-to-date and accurate word references available. Your use of this word book will prompt new editions, which will be published as often as justified by updates and revisions. We welcome your suggestions for improvements, changes, corrections, and additions—whatever will make this **Stedman's** product more useful to you. Please use the postpaid card at the back of this book and send your recommendations to the Reference Division at Williams & Wilkins.

AANS
   American Association of
      Neurological Surgeons
Abadie's sign of tabes dorsalis
abarognosis
abasia
   atactic a., ataxic a.
   choreic a.
   spastic a.
   a. trepidans
abasia-astasia
abasic, abatic
abbau
Abbokinase
Abbreviated Injury Score (AIS)
abdominal
   a. brain
   a. discomfort
   a. migraine
   a. pain
   a. reflexes
   a. trauma
abducens
   a. nucleus
   a. palsy
abducent
   a. nerve
abduction weakness
aberrant
   a. bundles
   a. ganglion
   a. regeneration
ablation
   stereotactic surgical a.
ablative procedure
abnerval
abneural
abnormality
   convergence a.
   cytoskeletal a.
   gait a.
   migration a.'s
   pupillary a.
   saccadic a.
   spinal cord injury without
      radiological a. (SCIWORA)
   transient signal a.
ABO antigen compatibility
aboiement
abortive neurofibromatosis

aboulia
ABR
   auditory brain stem response
abrin
abscess
   brain a.
   cerebral a.
   cranial epidural a.
   epidural a.
   intracranial a.
   otic a.
   parasitic brain a.
   periapical a.
   pituitary a.
   Pott's a.
   psoas a.
   retropharyngeal a.
   spinal epidural a.
   sterile a.
   subdural a.
   tuberculous a.
absence
   atonic a.
   atypical a.
   automatic a.
   complex a.
   enuretic a.
   epileptic a.
   hypertonic a.
   myoclonic a.
   pure a.
   retrocursive a.
   a. seizure
   simple a.
   sternutatory a.
   subclinical a.
   tussive a.
   typical a.
   vasomotor a.
absent
   a. spinous process
   a. state
absentia epileptica
Absidia infection
absolute
   a. agraphia
   a. refractory period
   a. terminal innervation ratio
   a. threshold

absorbable
    a. gelatin film
    a. gelatin sponge
abterminal
abulia
abulic
abuse
    cocaine a.
    drug a.
    methamphetamine a.
acalculia
acanthamebiasis
acanthesthesia
acatamathesia
acataphasia
accelerans
acceleration injury
accelerator
    a. fibers
    linear a. (LINAC)
    a. nerves
    Philips linear a.
access
    arterial a.
accessorius
    a. willisii
accessory
    a. cramp
    a. cuneate nucleus
    a. flocculus
    Isola spinal implant
      system a.
    a. middle cerebral artery
    a. nerve
    a. nerve paresis
    a. olivary nuclei
accident
    cerebrovascular a. (CVA)
    a. neurosis
accidental image
accommodation
    a. curve
    a. disorder
    a. of nerve
accommodative
accoucheur's hand
Ace
    A. halo-cast assembly
    A. halo pelvic girdle
    A. Hershey halo jig
    A. low profile MR halo
    A. Mark III halo

    A. Trippi-Wells tong
      cervical traction
    A. universal tong cervical
      traction
acenesthesia
acephalgic migraine
acervuline
acervulus
acetaldehyde
acetaminophen
    chlorzoxazone and a.
    oxycodone and a.
    propoxyphene napsylate
      and a.
acetate
    cortisone a.
    Cortone a.
    desmopressin a. (DDAVP)
    desoxycorticosterone a.
    methylprednisolone a.
acetazolamide
acetohexamide
acetonide
    triamcinolone a.
***N*-acetylaspartate (NAA)**
acetylcholine
acetylsalicylic acid
acetyltransferase
    choline a.
achalasia
    esophageal a.
acheiria, achiria
Achilles
    A. reflex
    A. tendon reflex
achondroplasia
acid
    acetylsalicylic a.
    amino a.
    aminocaproic a.
    amoxicillin-clavulanic a.
    arachidonic a.
    carbonic a.
    clavulanic a.
    deoxyribonucleic a. (DNA)
    diethylene triamine penta-
      acetic a. (DTPA)
    docosahexanoic a.
    eicosapentaenoic a.
    epsilon-aminocaproic a.
    ethacrynic a.

gadolinium
  diethylenetriamine
  pentaacetic a. (Gd-DTPA)
glutaric a.
kynurenic a.
a. lipase
oxolinic a.
palmitic a.
polyanhydroglucuronic a.
tolfenamic a.
tranexamic a.
uric a.
valproic a.
acid-base imbalance
acidemia
  methylmalonic a.
acidophil adenoma
acidosis
  hypokalemic metabolic a.
  lactic a.
  metabolic a.
  respiratory a.
Acinetobacter
acmesthesia
acnes
  Propionibacterium a.
ACNU
  nimustine
acoustic
  a. agraphia
  a. aphasia
  a. area
  a. bone window
  a. crest
  a. lemniscus
  a. nerve
  a. nerve sheath tumor
  a. neurilemoma
  a. neurinoma
  a. neuroma
  a. noise

a. papilla
a. radiation
a. reflex
a. schwannoma
a. striae
a. tubercle
Acoustic Neuroma Registry
acousticofacial
  a. crest
  a. ganglion
acousticopalpebral reflex
AC-PC
  anterior commissure-posterior
  commissure
AC-PC line
  anterior commissure-posterior
  commissure line
acquired
  a. epileptic aphasia
  a. hepatocerebral
  degeneration
  a. hepatocerebral syndrome
  a. immunodeficiency
  syndrome (AIDS)
  a. reflex
acquisition
  target a.
acral
Acremonium alabamensis
acroagnosis
acroanesthesia
acroataxia
acrobrachycephaly
acrocephalia
acrocephalic
acrocephalous
acrocephaly
acrodynia
acrodysesthesia
acroedema
acroesthesia

NOTES

3

acrognosis
acromegaly
acromelalgia
acromial reflex
acroneurosis
acroparesthesia
   a. syndrome
acrosclerosis
acrotrophodynia
acrotrophoneurosis
acrylic prosthesis
ACTH
   adrenocorticotropic hormone
   ACTH-producing adenoma
Acthar
actinic keratosis
actinomycin D
actinomycosis
actinoneuritis
action
   a. potential
   a. tremor
activated epilepsy
activation
   EEG a.
activator
   recombinant tissue
    plasminogen a.
   tissue plasminogen a.
   tissue-plasminogen a.
active surface electrode
activity
   blocking a.
acuology
acusticus
   porus a.
acute
   a. African sleeping sickness
   a. angular kyphosis
   a. anterior poliomyelitis
   a. ascending paralysis
   a. ataxia
   a. atrophic paralysis
   a. brachial radiculitis
   a. bulbar poliomyelitis
   a. burst injury
   a. decubitus ulcer
   a. delirium
   a. disconnection syndrome
   a. disseminated
   encephalomyelitis
   a. epidemic
   leukoencephalitis

   a. fracture
   a. hemorrhagic encephalitis
   a. idiopathic polyneuritis
   a. intermittent porphyria
   a. necrotizing encephalitis
   a. porphyria
   a. posterior multifocal
   placoid pigment
   a. primary hemorrhagic
   meningoencephalitis
   a. reflex bone atrophy
   a. subdural hematoma
   a. transverse myelitis
   a. trypanosomiasis
   a. tubular necrosis
Acute Physiology Score
acyclovir
adamantinoma
   pituitary a.
Adamkiewicz
   artery of A.
Adams-Stokes
   A.-S. disease
   A.-S. syndrome
Adapin
adaptation diseases
adaptor
   Brown-Roberts-Wells ring a.
Addison's disease
adduction weakness
adductor reflex
adendric
adendritic
adenine arabinoside
adenocarcinoma
   mucin-secreting a.
adenohypophyseal compromise
adenohypophysial
adenohypophysis
adenohypophysitis
   lymphocytic a.
adenoma
   acidophil a.
   ACTH-producing a.
   basophil a.
   choroid plexus a.
   chromophil a.
   chromophobe a.
   endocrine-inactive
   pituitary a.
   eosinophil a.
   fetal a.
   gonadotropin-producing a.

growth hormone-
producing a.
growth hormone-secreting a.
hypersecretory a.
null-cell a.
pituitary a.
prolactin-producing a.
sebaceous a.
thyrotropin-producing a.
undifferentiated cell a.
adenomatoid
adenomectomy
adenoneural
adenosine
a. triphosphatase (ATPase)
a. triphosphate (ATP)
adequate stimulus
ADH
antidiuretic hormone
adhesio, pl. **adhesiones**
a. interthalamica
a. interthalamica tumor
adhesion
arachnoid a.
interthalamic a.
adhesive arachnoiditis
adiadochokinesia, adiadochocinesia
adiadochokinesis, adiadochocinesis
adiaphoria
Adie's
A. pupil
A. syndrome
A. tonic pupil syndrome
adiposalgia
adipose graft
adiposis
a. cerebralis
adiposogenital
a. degeneration

a. dystrophy
a. syndrome
aditus, pl. **aditus**
a. ad aqueductum cerebri
a. ad infundibulum
adjoining pedicle
adjunctive
a. fixation
a. screw fixation
adjustability
3-D positional a.
adjustable
a. connector
a. pedicle connector
adjuvant
a. therapy
a. whole-brain radiation
therapy
adnerval, adneural
adrenal
a. crisis
a. gland
a. insufficiency
a. medulla transplantation
adrenergic
a. fibers
a. hyperstimulation
a. innervation
a. receptor
adrenocortical insufficiency
adrenocorticotropic
a. compromise
a. hormone (ACTH)
adrenoleukodystrophy (ALD)
adrenoleukodystrophy-
adrenomyeloneuropathy (ALD-
AMN)
adrenoleukomyeloneuropathy
adrenomyeloneuropathy (AMN)
Adriamycin
adromia

NOTES

Adson
    A. forceps
    A. rongeur
    A. scalp clip
    A. suction tube
Adson-Brown forceps
adterminal
adult
    a. pseudohypertrophic
    muscular dystrophy
    a. respiratory distress
    syndrome (ARDS)
    a. scoliosis
    a. scoliosis patient
    a. scoliosis surgery
advancement
    monobloc a.
adventitial neuritis
adverse side effect
adynamia
    a. episodica hereditaria
adynamic
aerophilus
    Haemophilus a.
aeruginosa
    Pseudomonas a.
affect disorder
affected pain
affective disorder
affectomotor
afferent
    a. fibers
    a. nerve
    a. pupillary defect
A fibers
African
    A. sleeping sickness
    A. trypanosomiasis
afterdischarge
afterhearing
afterimage
afterimpression
afterloading catheter
aftermovement
afterperception
afterpotential
aftersensation
aftersound
aftertaste
aftertouch
agarose gel electrophoresis
agastroneuria

agenesis
    callosal a.
    corpus callosum a.
agent
    alpha-adrenergic blocking a.
    antibradycardiac a.
    antifibrinolytic a.
    beta blocking a.
    calcium channel blocking a.
    cerebral vasodilating a.
    contrast a.
    ganglionic blocking a.
    neuromuscular blocking a.
    susceptibility a.
ageusia, ageustia
aggregation
    familial a.
aging
    brain a.
agitans
    paralysis a.
agitolalia
agitophasia
agnea
agnosia
    associative visual a.
    auditory a.
    finger a.
    ideational a.
    localization a.
    optic a.
    position a.
    tactile a.
    visual a.
    visual-spatial a.
agrammatica
agrammatism
agrammatologia
agranular cortex
agraphia
    absolute a.
    acoustic a.
    amnemonic a.
    atactic a.
    cerebral a.
    literal a.
    mental a.
    motor a.
    musical a.
    verbal a.
agraphic
agyria
ahylognosia

AICA
anterior inferior cerebellar artery
Aicardi's syndrome
AIDS
acquired immunodeficiency
syndrome
AIDS-related myelopathy
air
a. conduction test
a. drill
a. embolism
a. embolus
a. ventriculography
air-powered drill
airway
artificial a.
a. control
a. edema
esophageal a.
a. protection
AIS
Abbreviated Injury Score
akatama
akatamathesia
akathisia
akinesia
a. algera
a. amnestica
akinesic
akinesis
akinesthesia
akinetic
a. epilepsy
a. mutism
Akureyri disease
ala, gen. and pl. **alae**
a. cerebelli
a. cinerea
alae lingulae cerebelli
a. lobuli centralis

alabamensis
Acremonium a.
alalia
alalic
alanine
alar
a. lamina of neural tube
a. plate of neural tube
a. screw
alarm
ventilator a.
alba
albocinereous
albumin
a. transfusion
albuminocytologic dissociation
albuterol
Alcock's test
alcohol
a. amnestic syndrome
isopropyl a.
polyvinyl a. (PVA)
alcoholic deterioration
ALD
adrenoleukodystrophy
Aldactone
ALD-AMN
adrenoleukodystrophy-
adrenomyeloneuropathy
ALD-AMN complex
Aldomet
aldosterone deficiency
alemmal
Alexander's disease
alexia
incomplete a.
motor a.
musical a.
optical a.
sensory a.
visual a.

NOTES

7

alexic
alfentanil
algesia
algesic
algesichronometer
algesiogenic, algogenic
algesiometer
algesthesia
algesthesis
algetic
algogenesia
algogenesis
algogenic (*var. of* algesiogenic)
algometer
algometry
algorithms
     bone a.
algospasm
aliasing
     frequency a.
Alice in Wonderland syndrome
alien hand sign
alignment
     sagittal anatomic a.
alimentation
     enteral a.
     parenteral a.
aliquot
alkalosis
     metabolic a.
     respiratory a.
alkaptonuria
Alksne's iron suspension
allachesthesia
Allen pictures
Allen's test
allergic
     a. angiitis
     a. reaction
allesthesia, alloesthesia
     visual a.
allied reflexes
alligator
     a. cup forceps
     a. MacCarty scissors
     a. scissors
allocheiria, allochiria
allocortex
allodynia
alloesthesia (*var. of* allesthesia)
allograft
     a. bone grafting
     fibular a.

     a. iliac bone
     Tutoplast a.
allokinesis
allolalia
allomeric function
allonomous
allophasis
alloplastic material
allopurinol
allotriosmia
almond nucleus
Alnico
alogia
alopecia
Alpers' disease
alpha
     a. blocking
     a. fibers
     a. motor neuron
     a. rhythm
     a. wave
alpha-adrenergic
     a.-a. blocking agent
     a.-a. receptor
dl-alpha-difluoromethylornithine
(DFMO)
alpha-fetoprotein
ALS
     amyotrophic lateral sclerosis
     antilymphocyte serum
alternate hemianesthesia
alternating
     a. hemiplegia
     a. hypoglossal hemiplegia
     a. mydriasis
     a. skew deviation
     a. tremor
alternative
     graft material a.
althesin
aluminum
     a. contouring template set
     a. cranioplasty
     a. hydroxide and
     magnesium hydroxide
     a. hydroxide with
     magnesium hydroxide and
     simethicone
     a. master rod
Alupent
alveolus, pl. alveoli
alveus, pl. alvei
     a. hippocampi

Alzheimer's
    A. dementia
    A. disease
    A. sclerosis
amacrine cell
amantadine
    a. hydrochloride
amaurosis
    a. fugax
amaurotic familial idiocy
ambageusia
ambidexterity
ambidextrism
ambidextrous
ambient cisterna
ambiguous
    a. nucleus
ambiguus
    nucleus a.
ambilevous
ambisinister
ambisinistrous
amblyaphia
amblygeustia
ambulation
amebiasis
ameboid
    a. astrocyte
    a. cell
ameboidism
amelioration
amenorrhea
amentia
    nevoid a.
AME PinSite shield
American
    A. silk sutures
    A. Sterilizer operating room
      table
    A. Sterilizer operating table

American Association of
  Neurological Surgeons (AANS)
American Society of
  Anesthesiology (ASA)
American Society for Testing and
  Materials (ASTM)
AMI25
Amicar
Amidate
amikacin
    a. sulfate
Amikin
amiloride
amimia
amine
    biogenic a.
amino
    a. acid
    a. acid neurotransmitter
aminocaproic acid
aminoglutethimide
aminoglycoside
aminopenicillin
aminophylline
21-aminosteroid U74006F
aminotransferase
amitriptyline
    a. hydrochloride
    a. hydrochloride and
      chlordiazepoxide
ammonium chloride
Ammon's horn
AMN
    adrenomyeloneuropathy
amnemonic agraphia
amnesia
    global a.
amnesic aphasia
amnestic
    a. aphasia

NOTES

amnestic *(continued)*
    a. psychosis
    a. syndrome
amobarbital
amoebic aneurysm
amorphagnosia
amoxicillin
amoxicillin-clavulanic acid
amphetamine
amphicrania
amphotericin B
amphotonia, amphotony
ampicillin
    a. sodium
ampicillin-sulbactam
amplification
amplifier
    gradient a.
    power a.
amplitude
ampullary
    a. crest
    a. limbs of semicircular
      ducts
amputation neuroma
Amsler grid testing
amusia
    sensory a.
    vocal a.
amyelia
amyelic
amyelinated
amyelination
amyelinic
amyeloic, amyelonic
amyelous
amygdala, gen. and pl. **amygdalae**
    a. cerebelli
amygdaline
amygdalohippocampectomy
amygdaloid
    a. complex
    a. nucleus
    a. tubercle
amygdalotomy
amyl nitrite
amyloid
    a. angiopathy
    a. deposit
amyloidosis
    familial a.
amyoesthesia, amyoesthesis

amyotonia
    a. congenita
amyotrophia
amyotrophic lateral sclerosis (ALS)
amyotrophy
    diabetic a.
    hemiplegic a.
    juvenile a.
    monomelic a.
    neuralgic a.
    progressive spinal a.
Amytal
amytrophy
    benign focal a.
anacamptometer
anacatesthesia
anal
    a. reflex
    a. sphincter
    a. sphincter manometry
analeptic
analgesia
    a. algera
    a. dolorosa
    intrathecal morphine a.
    pentazocine a.
analgesic
    a. cuirass
analgesimeter
analgetic
analog
    a. domain
    a. filter
analysis
    biomechanical a.
    deformity a.
    Densitometric a.
    linkage a.
    SPECT a.
    three-dimensional a.
analyzer, analyzor
    fast Fourier transformation
      spectrum a.
    immunoturbidimetry a.
    wave a.
ananastasia
anapeiratic
anaphia
anaphylactoid reaction
anaphylaxis
anaplasia
anaplastic astrocytoma
anaptic

anarithmia
anarthria
anastomosing fibers
anastomosis, pl. **anastomoses**
    carotid-basilar a.
    carotid-vertebral a.
    cross-facial nerve graft a.
    end-to-end a.
    Galen's a.
    grafting a.
    hypoglossal-facial nerve a.
    Martin-Gruber a.
    microneurovascular a.
    microvascular a.
    primary end-to-end a.
    spinal accessory nerve-facial
      nerve a.
    STA-MCA a.
    temporal-cerebral arterial a.
anastomotic fibers
anatomical
    a. midline
    a. snuffbox
    a. variant
anatomic hook
anatomy
    cervicothoracic pedicle a.
    pedicle a.
    surgical a.
anaudia
anaxon, anaxone
anchor
    Isola spinal implant
      system a.
    traction a.
anchoring point
ancyroid
Andersch's ganglion
André
    A. anatomical hook
    A. hook

Andrews frame
anelectrotonic
anelectrotonus
Anel's method
anemia
    aplastic a.
    Cooley's a.
    drug-induced a.
    familial splenic a.
    hemolytic a.
    iron deficiency a.
    megaloblastic a.
    postoperative a.
    sickle cell a.
anencephalia
anencephalic
anencephalous
anencephaly
anepia
anergasia
anergastic
anesthekinesia, anesthecinesia
anesthesia
    barbiturate burst-
      suppression a.
    compression a.
    conduction a.
    corneal a.
    crossed a.
    diagnostic a.
    dissociated a.
    dissociative a.
    a. dolorosa
    girdle a.
    glove a.
    gustatory a.
    halothane a.
    hysterical a.
    isoflurane a.
    local a.
    muscular a.

NOTES

11

anesthesia *(continued)*
>olfactory a.
>painful a.
>perineural a.
>pharyngeal a.
>pressure a.
>segmental a.
>spinal a.
>splanchnic a.
>stocking a.
>tactile a.
>thermal a., thermic a.
>traumatic a.
>unilateral a.
>visceral a.

anesthetic
>a. leprosy
>a. monitoring

Aneuroid chest bellows
aneurolemmic
aneurysm
>amoebic a.
>anterior communicating artery a.
>atherosclerotic a.
>bacterial a.
>basilar bifurcation a.
>basilar tip a.
>berry a.
>carotid a.
>cavernous a.
>cavernous-carotid a.
>Charcot-Bouchard a.
>clinoidal a.
>a. clip
>a. clipping
>congenital a.
>congenital cerebral a.
>dissecting a.
>dissecting basilar artery a.
>distal anterior cerebral artery a.
>fusiform a.
>giant a.
>giant cavernous a.
>hypophyseal a.
>incidental a.
>infectious a.
>infraclinoid a.
>intracavernous a.
>intracavernous carotid a.
>intracranial a.
>lower basilar a.

>luetic a.
>miliary a.
>mycotic a.
>ophthalmic artery a.
>ophthalmic segment a.
>paraclinoidal a.
>ruptured a.
>saccular a.
>sellar a.
>serpentine a.
>spirochetal a.
>superior hypophyseal artery a.
>supraclinoid a.
>thrombosed giant vertebral artery a.
>traumatic a.
>unruptured a.
>unspecified a.
>vein of Galen a.
>venous a.
>vertebrobasilar a.

aneurysmal
>a. bleeding
>a. bone cyst
>a. hemorrhage
>a. rupture

aneurysmectomy
aneurysmoplasty
aneurysmorrhaphy
aneurysmotomy
angel dust
Angelucci's syndrome
angiitis
>allergic a.
>granulomatous a.
>isolated a.
>necrotizing a.

angina
>Prinzmetal's a.

angioblastic meningioma
angioblastoma
angiodysgenetic myelomalacia
angioedema
angioendotheliosis
>neoplastic a.

angiofibroma
>juvenile a.

angiogenesis
angioglioma
angiogliomatosis
angiogliosis

angiogram
cerebral digital a.
digital subtraction a.
vertebral a.
angiographic
a. reference system (ARS)
a. road-mapping technique
a. targetry
a. vasospasm
angiographically occult intracranial vascular malformation (AOIVM)
angiography
baseline a.
cerebral a.
closed a.
contrast a.
2DFT time-of-flight MR a.
digital a.
digital intravenous a.
digital subtraction a. (DSA)
intracranial MR a.
intraoperative a.
magnetic resonance a.
open a.
orthogonal a.
preoperative a.
spinal a.
stereomagnification a.
stereotactic a.
superselective a.
vertebral a.
angioid streaks
angiokeratoma corporis diffusum
angiokinetic
angiolipoma
epidural a.
spinal epidural a.
angiolithic sarcoma
angioma
capillary a.
cavernous a.

encephalic a.
extracerebral cavernous a.
venous a.
angiomatosis
cephalotrigeminal a.
congenital dysplastic a.
cutaneomeningospinal a.
encephalotrigeminal a.
meningeal a.
mesencephalo-oculofacial a.
neurocutaneous a.
neuroretinal a.
oculoencephalic a.
Rendu-Osler a.
retinocerebral a.
telangiectatic a.
angioneurectomy
angioneuredema
angioneurosis
angioneurotic
a. edema
angioneurotomy
angioparalytic neurasthenia
angiopathic neurasthenia
angiopathy
amyloid a.
cerebral amyloid a.
congenital dysplastic a.
congophilic a.
radiation a.
angiophacomatosis, angiophakomatosis
angioplasty
percutaneous transluminal a.
transluminal a.
angioreticuloma
angiosarcoma
angiostrongyliasis
angiotensin
angle
cephalomedullary a.

NOTES

13

angle *(continued)*
    cerebellopontine a.
    cervicothoracic pedicle a.
    Citelli's a.
    flip a.
    a. meningioma
    pedicle a.
    pedicle axis a.
    pontine a.
    pulse flip a.
    Rolando's a.
    sagittal pedicle a.
    Schmidt-Fischer a.
    sinodural a.
    sylvian a.
    tentorial a.
    transverse pedicle a.
    venous a.
angle-closure glaucoma
angled needle
angular
    a. convolution
    a. gyrus
    a. position
angulation
    radius of a., pl. radii of a.
    screw a.
anhaphia
ani (*gen. of* anus)
anile
anility
animal study
anisocoria
anisotrophy
    chemical shift a.
anisotropic 3DFT
ankle
    a. clonus
    a. jerk
    a. reflex
ankylosing spondylitis
ankylostoma
ankyroid
annectent gyrus
annulospiral
    a. ending
    a. organ
annulus
    a. fibrosus
    a. tendineus
anochlesia
anociassociation
anodal block

anode
anomalous
    a. branching
    a. origin
anomaly
    Aristotle's a.
    congenital a.
    duplication a.
    megadolichovertebrobasilar a.
anomia
    color a.
    tactile a.
anomic aphasia
anorectal
    a. atresia
    a. spasm
anorexia
    a. nervosa
anorthography
anosmia
    essential a.
    functional a.
    mechanical a.
    reflex a.
    respiratory a.
    true a.
anosmic
anosodiaphoria
anosognosia
anosognosic
    a. epilepsy
    a. seizure
anospinal
    a. center
anoxemia
anoxia
ansa, gen. and pl. **ansae**
    a. cervicalis
    Haller's a.
    lenticular a.
    a. lenticularis
    ansae nervorum spinalium
    peduncular a.
    a. peduncularis
    Reil's a.
    a. sacralis
    a. subclavia
    Vieussens' a.
ansiform lobule
ansotomy
Anspach
    A. drill
    A. 65K drill

A. 65K instrument systems
A. 65K neuro system
antagonistic reflexes
antebrachial cutaneous nerve
anterior
    anterior commissure-posterior commissure (AC-PC)
    a. approach
    a. basal encephalocele
    a. bulb syndrome
    a. C1-C2 fixation
    a. C1-C2 screw approach
    a. C1-C2 screw fixation
    a. central convolution
    a. central gyrus
    a. cerebral artery
    a. cerebral vein
    a. cervical discectomy and fusion
    a. cervical spine surgery
    a. cervical surgery
    a. cervical surgery vocal cord damage
    a. cervicothoracic junction surgery
    a. cervicothoracic surgery
    a. chiasmal syndrome
    a. choroidal artery
    a. clinoid process
    a. column disruption
    a. column of medulla oblongata
    a. column osteosynthesis
    a. column of spinal cord
    a. commissure
    a. commissure-posterior commissure line (AC-PC line, AC-PC line)
    a. communicating artery
    a. communicating artery aneurysm
    a. compartment syndrome
    a. construct
    a. cord impingement
    a. corpectomy
    a. correction
    a. cortex penetration
    a. corticospinal tract
    a. cranial base
    a. decompression
    a. discectomy
    a. distraction instrumentation
    a. extradural clinoidectomy
    a. extremity of caudate nucleus
    a. fixation device
    a. funiculus
    a. ground bundle
    a. horn
    a. inferior cerebellar artery (AICA)
    a. interbody fusion
    a. intermediate groove
    a. internal fixation device
    a. internal stabilization
    a. interosseous nerve
    a. jugular vein
    a. Kostuik-Harrington distraction system
    a. limb of internal capsule
    a. lobe of hypophysis
    a. lower cervical spine surgery
    a. lumbar spine interbody fusion
    a. lunate lobule
    a. median fissure of medulla oblongata

NOTES

anterior *(continued)*
    a. median fissure of spinal cord
    a. medullary velum
    a. meningeal artery
    a. metallic fixation
    a. neutralization
    a. notch of cerebellum
    a. nuclei of thalamus
    a. parolfactory sulcus
    a. part
    a. part of pons
    a. perforated substance
    a. pillar of fornix
    a. piriform gyrus
    a. plate fixation
    a. plating
    a. plexus
    a. pyramid
    a. pyramidal tract
    a. rhizotomy
    a. root
    a. screw fixation
    a. serratus muscle
    a. short-segment stabilization
    a. spinal artery
    a. spinal artery syndrome
    a. spinal fixation
    a. spinal plating
    a. spinocerebellar tract
    a. spinothalamic tract
    a. stabilization
    a. stabilization procedure
    a. surgical exposure
    a. temporal lobectomy
    a. tubercle of thalamus
    a. vein of septum pellucidum
    a. white commissure
anterior-posterior fusion with SSI
anterodorsal thalamic nucleus
anterograde memory
anterolateral
    a. column of spinal cord
    a. cordotomy
    a. groove
    a. sulcus
    a. tractotomy
anteromedial
    a. approach
    a. retropharyngeal approach
    a. thalamic nucleus
anteromedian groove

anteromesial temporal lobectomy
anteroposterior projection
anteroventral thalamic nucleus
anthrax
    cerebral a.
anthropometrics
antiadrenergic
antialias filtering
antiarrhythmic
antibiotic
    intrathecal a.
    a. penetration
    a. powder
antibody
    anti-BUdR monoclonal a.
    anticardiolipin a.
    antinuclear a.
    antiphospholipid a.
    antiretinal a.
    monoclonal a.
antibradycardiac agent
anti-BUdR monoclonal antibody
anticardiolipin antibody
anticephalalgic
anticholinergic
anticoagulant
    lupus a.
anticoagulation
    a. therapy
anticonvulsant
    a. prophylaxis
    a. therapy
anticonvulsive
anticus
    scalenus a.
antidepressant
    tricyclic a.
antidiuretic
    a. hormone (ADH)
antidromic
antiemetic
antiepileptic
antiferromagnetism
antifibrinolytic
    a. agent
    a. therapy
antiganglioside
antigen-antibody complex
antihemophilic
    a. factor A
    a. factor C
anti-human transferrin
antihypertensive

antihypnotic
antilymphocyte serum (ALS)
antimigraine therapy
antimyasthenic
antineuralgic
antineuritic
antinoise
antinuclear antibody
antioncogene
antiphospholipid
    a. antibody
    a. syndrome
antiplatelet therapy
antiretinal antibody
antisiphon device (ASD)
antispasmodic
antitetanic
antithrombin
    a. III
    a. III deficiency
antitonic
antitrismus
Antoni
    A. type A neurilemoma
    A. type A pattern
    A. type B neurilemoma
    A. type B pattern
Anton's syndrome
antra (*pl. of* antrum)
antrophose
antrostomy
antrum, pl. antra
    maxillary a.
Anturane
Antyllus' method
anuria
anus, gen. ani, pl. anus
    Bartholin's a.
    a. cerebri
anxiety state
anxious delirium

AO
    AO dynamic compression
    plate
    AO dynamic compression
    plate construct
    AO fixateur interne
    AO fixateur interne
    instrumentation
    AO gouge
    AO group
    AO guidepin
    AO internal fixator
    AO notched instrumentation
    AO reconstruction plate
    AO-stopped drill guide
AO/ASIF fixateur interne
AOIVM
    angiographically occult
    intracranial vascular
    malformation
aortic
    a. arch syndrome
    a. body
    a. body tumor
    a. coarctation
    a. insufficiency
    a. nerve
aorticorenal ganglia
aortocranial disease
apallesthesia
apallic
    a. state
    a. syndrome
aparalytic
apathetic
apathism
apathy
ape fissure
aperta
    spina bifida a.

NOTES

Apert's syndrome
apertura, pl. **aperturae**
  a. lateralis ventriculi quarti
  a. mediana ventriculi quarti
aperture
  lateral a. of the fourth
    ventricle
  median a. of the fourth
    ventricle
apex, gen. **apicis**, pl. **apices**
  a. cornus posterioris
  petrous a.
aphasia
  acoustic a.
  acquired epileptic a.
  amnestic a., amnesic a.
  anomic a.
  associative a.
  ataxic a.
  auditory a.
  Broca's a.
  conduction a.
  expressive a.
  functional a.
  global a.
  graphic a., graphomotor a.
  impressive a.
  jargon a.
  Kussmaul's a.
  mixed a.
  motor a.
  nominal a.
  optic a.
  pathematic a.
  psychosensory a.
  pure a.'s
  receptive a.
  semantic a.
  sensory a.
  syntactical a.
  thalamic a.
  total a.
  transcortical a.
  transcortical sensory a.
  visual a.
  Wernicke's a.
aphasiac, aphasic
aphasiologist
aphasiology
aphemesthesia
aphemia
aphemic

aphonia
  a. paralytica
  spastic a.
aphonic
aphonogelia
aphonous
aphrasia
aphthongia
aphthous stomatitis
apical
  a. dendrite
  a. distraction
  a. process
apices (*pl. of* apex)
apicis (*gen. of* apex)
apiospermum
  Scedosporium a.
aplasia cutis congenita
aplastic anemia
APLD
  automated percutaneous lumbar
    discectomy
apnea
  central a.
  episodic a.
  obstructive a., peripheral a.
  obstructive sleep a.
  sleep a.
  sleep-induced a.
apneic pause
apneusis
apneustic breathing
apocrine
  a. cystadenoma
  a. gland
apoferritin
apolar cell
aponeurotica
  galea a.
aponeurotic reflex
apophysary point
apophysial point
apoplectic cyst
apoplectiform
apoplectoid
apoplexy
  bulbar a.
  embolic a.
  functional a.
  ingravescent a.
  neonatal a.
  pituitary a.
  pontile a.

Raymond type of a.
serous a.
spasmodic a.
spinal a.
thrombotic a.
apparatus, pl. **apparatus**
C-arm fluoroscopic a.
halo a.
Kandel stereotactic a.
Mayfield-Kees skull
fixation a.
Wells stereotaxic a.
apparent origin
appearance
beaten-metal a.
ping-pong a.
thumbprinting a.
appestat
application
clip a.
force a.
Harrington rod
instrumentation force a.
Isola spinal implant
system a.
paraspinal rod a.
transverse fixator a.
vertebral plate a.
applier
Liga clip a.
Olivecrona clip a.
Raney scalp clip a.
approach
anterior a.
anterior C1-C2 screw a.
anteromedial a.
anteromedial
retropharyngeal a.
basal subfrontal a.
buccopharyngeal a.
cerebellopontine angle a.

combined anterior and
posterior a.
combined low cervical and
transthoracic a.
combined presigmoid-
transtransversarium
intradural a.
combined transsylvian and
middle fossa a.
extended subfrontal a.
extreme lateral
transcondylar a.
far lateral inferior
suboccipital a.
foraminal a.
frontotemporal a.
inferior extradural a.
inferior-lateral endonasal
transsphenoidal a.
inferior transvermian a.
infratentorial a.
infratentorial
supracerebellar a.
interfascial a.
interforniceal a.
interhemispheric a.
intradural a.
intratentorial
supracerebellar a.
labioglossomandibular a.
labiomandibular a.
lateral a.
lateral extracavitary a.
lateral intradural a.
low cervical a.
medial extradural a.
middle fossa a.
midline spinal a.
operative a.
orbitozygomatic
temporopolar a.

NOTES

approach *(continued)*
  petrosal a.
  posterior a.
  posterior occipitocervical a.
  posterolateral a.
  presigmoid-
    transtransversarium
    intradural a.
  pterional a.
  retrolabyrinthine
    presigmoid a.
  retroperitoneal a.
  retropharyngeal a.
  rhinoseptal a.
  sacral foraminal a.
  screw plate a.
  stabilization a.
  standard retroperitoneal
    flank a.
  sternum-splitting a.
  subchoroidal a.
  subfrontal a.
  subfrontal-transbasal a.
  sublabial midline
    rhinoseptal a.
  suboccipital a.
  suboccipital subtemporal a.
  suboccipital transmeatal a.
  subtemporal a.
  subtemporal intradural a.
  superior intradural a.
  supracerebellar a.
  supraclavicular a.
  supraorbital-pterional a.
  supratentorial a.
  sylvian a.
  thoracoabdominal a.
  thoracolumbar
    retroperitoneal a.
  transantral ethmoidal a.
  transcallosal
    transventricular a.
  transcavernous a.
  transcavernous transpetrous
    apex a.
  transcerebellar
    hemispheric a.
  transcochlear a.
  transcortical a.
  transcortical
    transventricular a.
  transcranial a.
  transcranial frontal-temporal-
    orbital a.
  transcranial supraorbital a.
  transcubital a.
  transfrontal a.
  translabyrinthine a.
  translabyrinthine and
    suboccipital a.
  transmandibular-
    glossopharyngeal a.
  transoral a.
  transpalatal a.
  transpedicular a.
  transperitoneal a.
  transsinus a.
  transsphenoidal a.
  transsylvian a.
  transtentorial a.
  transthoracic a.
  transtorcular a.
  transvenous a.
apractagnosia
apractic
apraxia
  a. algera
  cortical a.
  diagnostic a.
  ideational a.
  ideatory a.
  ideokinetic a.
  ideomotor a.
  innervation a.
  limb-kinetic a.
  motor a.
  ocular motor a.
  transcortical a.
apraxic
Apresoline
aprophoria
aprosexia
aprotinin
apyretic tetanus
aqueduct
  a. of cerebrum
  cochlear a.
  Cotunnius' a.
  sylvian a.
  a. of Sylvius
  a. veil
  a. of vestibule

aqueductal
  a. intubation
  a. stenosis
aqueductus, pl. aqueductus
  a. cerebri
  a. cochleae
  a. cotunnii
  a. sylvii
  a. vestibuli
aqueous
  a. humor deficiency
  a. povidone-iodine
ara-A
arabinoside
  adenine a.
arachidonic acid
arachnoid
  a. adhesion
  a. cyst
  a. foramen
  a. membrane
  a. villi
  a. villus
arachnoidal
  a. gliomatosis
  a. granulations
  a. hyperplasia
arachnoidea, arachnoides
  a. encephali
  a. spinalis
arachnoiditis
  adhesive a.
  chiasmal a.
  neoplastic a.
  obliterative a.
  ossifying a.
  spinal cord a.
Aramine
Aran-Duchenne disease
Arantius' ventricle

araphia
arbor, pl. arbores
  a. vitae
arborescent
arborization
arc
  a. radius system
  reflex a.
  Sceratti a.
  spinal reflex a.
arcade of Frohse
arc-centered guidance system
archeokinetic
archicerebellum
archicortex
archipallium
architectonics
arc-quadrant stereotactic system
arcuate
  a. fasciculus
  a. fibers
  a. nuclei
  a. nucleus
ardanesthesia
ARDS
  adult respiratory distress
  syndrome
area, pl. areae
  acoustic a.
  a. acustica
  association areas
  auditory a.
  Broca's a.
  Broca's parolfactory a.
  Brodmann's areas
  a. centralis
  cross-sectional a. (CSA)
  entorhinal a.
  excitable a.
  a. of facial nerve
  Flechsig's areas

NOTES

area *(continued)*
  frontal a.
  fronto-orbital a.
  Gasserian ganglion a.
  inferior vestibular a.
  insular a.
  motor a.
  a. nervi facialis
  olfactory a.
  oval a. of Flechsig
  parastriate a.
  a. parolfactoria, a.
   parolfactoria Brocae
  parolfactory a.
  peristriate a.
  piriform a.
  Pitres' a.
  postcentral a.
  a. postrema
  precentral a.
  precommissural septal a.
  prefrontal a.
  premotor a.
  preoptic a.
  prestriate a.
  pretectal a.
  primary visual a.
  Rolando's a.
  secondary visual a.
  sensorial areas, sensory areas
  sensorimotor a.
  septal a.
  silent a.
  somesthetic a.
  striate a.
  a. subcallosa
  subcallosal a.
  superior vestibular a.
  trigger a.
  vagus a.
  vestibular a.
  a. vestibularis inferior
  a. vestibularis superior
  visual a.
  Wernicke's a.
areflexia
  detrusor a.
argon
  a. laser
argyle trocar catheter
Argyll Robertson pupil
Aristocort Forte
Aristotle's anomaly

arm
  a. phenomenon
  a. weakness
Arnold
  canal of A.
Arnold-Chiari
  A.-C. deformity
  A.-C. malformation
  A.-C. syndrome
Arnold's
  A. bundle
  A. ganglion
  A. tract
arousal
  a. function
  a. reaction
array
  compressed spectral a.
  percutaneous electrode a.
  a. processor
  surface coil a.
arrhigosis
arrhinencephaly, arrhinencephalia
ARS
  angiographic reference system
arsenical
  a. tremor
Artane
arteria, gen. and pl. **arteriae**
  a. basilaris
  a. calcarina
  a. cerebelli inferior anterior
  a. cerebelli inferior posterior
  a. cerebelli superior
  a. cerebri anterior
  a. cerebri media
  a. cerebri posterior
  a. choroidea anterior
  a. choroidea posterior
arterial
  a. access
  a. bruit
  a. circle of cerebrum
  a. hemorrhage
  a. occlusive disease
  a. oxygen saturation
  a. vasospasm
arterialization
arteriography
  cerebral a.
  spinal a.
arteriolopathy
  retinocochleocerebral a.

arteriolosclerosis
arteriopathy
arteriosclerosis
hyaline a.
arteriosclerotic psychosis
arteriovenous
a. fistula
a. malformation (AVM)
arteritis
cranial a.
giant cell a.
granulomatous a.
Horton's a.
obliterative a.
rheumatoid a.
spinal a.
Takayasu's a.
temporal a.
artery
accessory middle cerebral a.
a. of Adamkiewicz
anterior cerebral a.
anterior choroidal a.
anterior communicating a.
anterior inferior
cerebellar a. (AICA)
anterior meningeal a.
anterior spinal a.
auditory a.
axillary a.
basal cerebral a.
basilar a.
calcarine a.
caroticotympanic a.
carotid a.
cerebellar a.'s
cerebral a.'s
a. of cerebral hemorrhage
Charcot's a.
choroidal a.
common carotid a. (CCA)

dolichoectatic a.
external carotid a. (ECA)
extradural vertebral a.
facial a.
frontal a.
great anterior medullary a.
innominate a.
internal carotid a. (ICA)
left common carotid a.
lenticulostriate a.'s
maxillary a.
maxillomandibular a.
medial striate a.'s
medullary a.
medullary a.'s of brain
meningeal a.
middle cerebral a. (MCA)
ophthalmic a.
parent a.
pial a.
polar a.
popliteal a.
posterior cerebellar a.
posterior cerebral a. (PCA)
posterior choroidal a.
posterior communicating a.
posterior inferior
cerebellar a. (PICA)
posterior inferior
communicating a. (PICA)
posterior spinal a.
primitive otic a.
primitive trigeminal a.
radial a.
radiculospinal a.
recurrent perforating a.
spinal a.
stapedial a.
subclavian a.
sulcocommissural a.

NOTES

23

artery *(continued)*
    superficial temporal a. (STA)
    superficial temporal artery to middle cerebral a. (STA-MCA)
    superficial temporal artery-posterior cerebral a. (STA-PCA)
    superficial temporal artery-superior cerebellar a. (STA-SCA)
    superior cerebellar a.
    superior hypophyseal a. (SupHypArt)
    superior laryngeal a.
    superior thyroid a.
    telencephalic ventriculofugal a.
    temporal a.
    ventriculofugal a.
    vertebral a.
    vertebrobasilar a.
artery-to-artery embolism
arthralgia
arthresthesia
arthritic general pseudoparalysis
arthritis, pl. **arthritides**
    cervical spine a.
    degenerative a.
    enteropathic a.
    gouty a.
    hypertrophic a.
    juvenile rheumatoid a.
    neuropathic a.
    psoriatic a.
    rheumatoid a.
arthrodesis
    atlantoaxial a.
    Brooks atlantoaxial a.
    C1-C2 posterior a.
    cervical a.
    extension injury posterior atlantoaxial a.
    flexion injury posterior atlantoaxial a.
    posterior a.
    posterior atlantoaxial a.
arthropathy
    Charcot's a.
    diabetic a.
    neuropathic a.
    tabetic a.

articular
    a. corpuscles
    a. leprosy
    a. mass separation
    a. mass separation fracture
    a. sensibility
articulation
    atlantoaxial a.
    Vermont spinal fixator a.
artifact
    beam hardening a.
    chemical shift a.
    ferromagnetic a.
    Gibbs a.
    line a.
    magnetic susceptibility a.
    motion a.
    tissue magnetic susceptibility a.
    truncation a.
artificial
    a. airway
    a. vertebral body
aryepiglottic fold neurofibroma
ASA
    American Society of Anesthesiology
    ASA score
ascending
    a. degeneration
    a. frontal convolution
    a. frontal gyrus
    a. myelitis
    a. neuritis
    a. paralysis
    a. parietal convolution
    a. parietal gyrus
ASD
    antisiphon device
Aseculap skull perforator
asemasia, asemia
asepsis
aseptic
    a. meningitis
    a. necrosis
ashen
    a. tuber
    a. tubercle
    a. wing
Ashworth scale

ASIF
A. broad dynamic compression bone plate
A. T plate
aspartame
aspartylglycosaminuria
aspect
laminar cortex posterior a.
aspergillosis
Aspergillus
A. *fumigatus*
aspiration
needle a.
stereotactic a.
ultrasonic a.
aspirator
Cavitron ultrasonic a.
Cavitron ultrasonic surgical a. (CUSA)
Sharplan Ultra ultrasonic a.
ultrasonic a.
ultrasonic surgical a.
aspirin
oxycodone and a.
a. with butalbital, phenacetin, and caffeine
assay
B_2-TFn a.
enzyme-linked immunosorbent a. (ELISA)
assembly
Ace halo-cast a.
Brown-Roberts-Wells arc-ring a.
multiple hook a.
assessment
videotape a.
in vivo stereological a.
assimilation
assisted ventilation
associated movement

association
a. areas
a. cortex
a. fibers
a. mechanism
a. system
a. tract
Association for Brain Tumor Research
associative
a. aphasia
a. visual agnosia
astasia
astasia-abasia
astatic
astereognosis
asterion
asterixis
asteroides
Nocardia a.
asthenia
neurocirculatory a.
asthenic
ASTM
American Society for Testing and Materials
astroblastoma
astrocyte
ameboid a.
fibrous a., fibrillary a.
gemistocytic a.
protoplasmic a.
reactive a.
astrocytoma
anaplastic a.
brainstem a.
chiasmatic-hypothalamic pilocytic a.
diencephalic a.
fibrillary a.
gemistocytic a.

NOTES

25

astrocytoma *(continued)*
  giant cell a.
  grade I a.
  grade II a.
  grade III a.
  grade IV a.
  hypothalamic a.
  juvenile pilocytic a.
  low-grade a.
  malignant a.
  optic nerve a.
  pilocytic a.
  piloid a.
  protoplasmic a.
  subependymal a.
  subependymal giant cell a.
  thalamic a.
astrocytosis
  a. cerebri
astroependymoma
astroglia
  a. cell
asyllabia
asymbolia
asymmetric motor neuropathy
asymmetry
atactic
  a. abasia
  a. agraphia
atactilia
ataxia
  acute a.
  Briquet's a.
  Bruns' a.
  cerebellar a.
  Friedreich's a.
  hand a.
  hereditary a.
  hereditary cerebellar a.
  hereditary posterior
    column a.
  hereditary spinal a.
  infantile X-linked a.
  kinetic a.
  Leyden's a.
  locomotor a.
  Marie's a.
  motor a.
  optic a.
  spinal a.
  spinocerebellar a.
  static a.
  a. telangiectasia

  vasomotor a.
  vestibulocerebellar a.
ataxiadynamia
ataxiagram
ataxiagraph
ataxiameter
ataxiaphasia
ataxia-telangiectasia
ataxic
  a. abasia
  a. aphasia
  a. breathing
  a. gait
  a. hemiparesis
  a. paramyotonia
  a. paraplegia
ataxiophemia
ataxy
atheroembolism
  diffuse disseminated a.
atheromatous disease
atherosclerosis
atherosclerotic
  a. aneurysm
  a. disease
athetoid
athetosic, athetotic
athetosis
  double a.
  double congenital a.
  posthemiplegic a.
Ativan
atlantal fracture
atlantoaxial
  a. arthrodesis
  a. articulation
  a. fusion
  a. instability
  a. joint
  a. stabilization
  a. subluxation
atlantodental
atlanto-occipital
  a.-o. joint
  a.-o. separation
  a.-o. stabilization
atlas
  a. fracture
  Schaltenbrand-Wahren
    stereotactic a.
  stereotactic a.
  a. vertebra
atlas-axis combination fracture

atonic
    a. absence
    a. bladder
    a. epilepsy
    a. impotence
atopognosia, atopognosis
ATP
    adenosine triphosphate
ATPase
    adenosine triphosphatase
atracurium
atresia
    anorectal a.
atrial
    a. fibrillation
    a. myxoma
atrium
atrophedema
atrophoderma
    a. neuriticum
atrophy
    acute reflex bone a.
    cerebellar a.
    cerebellar vermian a.
    circumscribed cerebral a.
    cortical a.
    diffuse a.
    diffuse cerebral a.
    Erb's a.
    facioscapulohumeral a.
    familial spinal muscular a.
    hippocampal a.
    Hoffmann's muscular a.
    Hunt's a.
    idiopathic muscular a.
    infantile muscular a.
    infantile progressive spinal muscular a.
    ischemic muscular a.
    juvenile muscular a.

    lobar a.
    muscular a.
    myopathic a.
    neuritic a.
    neurogenic a.
    neurotrophic a.
    nutritional-type cerebellar a.
    olivopontocerebellar a.
    optic a.
    peroneal muscular a.
    Pick's a.
    progressive muscular a.
    progressive spinal muscular a.
    pseudohypertrophic muscular a.
    scapulohumeral a.
    spinal a.
    Sudeck's a.
    transneuronal a.
    trophoneurotic a.
    vermian a.
    Vulpian's a.
atropine
attached
    a. cranial section
    a. craniotomy
attachment
    Hardy a.
    Mayfield-Kees table a.
    a. versatility
attack
    crescendo transient ischemic a.
    drop a.
    salaam a.
    transient ischemic a. (TIA)
    uncinate a.
    vagal a.
    vasovagal a.

NOTES

attention
    a. deficit
    a. deficit disorder
attitudinal
    a. reflexes
atypical
    a. absence
    a. facial neuralgia
    a. trigeminal neuralgia
audiofrequency eddy current
audiogenic epilepsy
audiogram
    pure tone a.
audiometry
    impedance a.
audition
    chromatic a.
    gustatory a.
auditory
    a. agnosia
    a. aphasia
    a. area
    a. artery
    a. brain stem response (ABR)
    a. canal
    a. compound actional potential
    a. cortex
    a. evoked potential
    a. ganglion
    a. hyperalgesia
    a. hyperesthesia
    a. lemniscus
    a. nerve
    a. nucleus
    a. oculogyric reflex
    a. pathway
    a. receptor cells
    a. reflex
    a. striae
    a. synesthesia
    a. tract
    a. transfer deficit
Auerbach's
    A. ganglia
    A. plexus
augmentor
    a. fibers
    a. nerves
aura, pl. **aurae**
    intellectual a.

    kinesthetic a.
    reminiscent a.
aural
aureus
    Staphylococcus a.
auricular ganglion
auriculopalpebral reflex
auriculotemporal nerve syndrome
auropalpebral reflex
Australian
    A. X disease
    A. X encephalitis
autocerebral cooling
autoclaving
autogenous
    a. bone graft
    a. cable graft interposition VII-VII neuroanastomosis
    a. iliac bone
autograft
    a. bone grafting
autoimmune disorder
autokinesia, autokinesis
autokinetic
autologous
    a. blood transfusion
    a. fat graft
    a. transfusion
automated percutaneous lumbar discectomy (APLD)
automatic
    a. absence
    a. chorea
    a. epilepsy
automatism
    immediate posttraumatic a.
autonomic
    a. disorder
    a. dysfunction
    a. epilepsy
    a. ganglia
    a. imbalance
    a. motor neuron
    a. nerve
    a. nervous system
    a. neurogenic bladder
    a. part
autonomotropic
autoradiography
autoregulation
autosomal
    a. dominant inheritance
    a. recessive inheritance

autosomatognosis
autosomatognostic
Autotechnicon
autotopagnosia
Avellis' syndrome
average
    pure tone a. (PTA)
    a. velocity
Avitene
    A. microfibrillar collagen hemostat
    A. packing
AVM
    arteriovenous malformation
avulsion
    brachial plexus a.
    cauda equina a.
    conus a.
    conus medullaris root a.
    a. injury
    nerve a.
    nerve root a.
    sacral plexus a.
    third nerve a.
awl
    T-handled bone a.
axes (*pl. of* axis)
axial
    a. compression
    a. gripping strength
    a. load
    a. loading
    a. loading fracture
    a. myopia
    a. neuritis
    a. pattern scalp flap
    a. plane angular deformity biomechanics
    a. projection
    a. spin-echo image

    a. stiffness
    a. traction
axial-occipital ligament
axifugal
axile corpuscle
axilla
axillary
    a. artery
    a. nerve
axion
axioplasm
axiramificate
axis, pl. axes
    cerebrospinal a.
    a. corpuscle
    a. cylinder
    encephalomyelonic a.
    neural a.
    a. vertebra
axis-atlas combination fracture
axoaxonic
    a. synapse
axodendritic
    a. synapse
axofugal
axolemma
axolysis
axon
    a. hillock
    a. reflex
    a. response
    a. terminals
axonal
    a. process
    a. regeneration
    a. terminal boutons
axonapraxis
axonography
axonopathy
axonotmesis
axopetal

NOTES

axoplasm
axoplasmic transport
axosomatic
    a. synapse
axotomy
Axsain
Ayala's disease
azathioprine

azidothymidine
aziridinylbenzoquinone (AZQ)
azlocillin
Azorean disease
AZQ
    aziridinylbenzoquinone
aztreonam

B

B$_{12}$
   vitamin B.
Babinski-Nageotte syndrome
Babinski reflex
Babinski's
   B. phenomenon
   B. sign
bacampicillin
bacillary layer
bacitracin
back
   b. of foot reflex
   b. pain
   poker b.
   rigid round b.
backache
Backlund's stereotactic instrument
backout
   screw b.
baclofen
bacterial
   b. aneurysm
   b. endocarditis
   b. meningitis
BAEP
   brainstem auditory evoked
      potential
BAER
   brainstem auditory evoked
      response
bag
   nuclear b.
bahnung
Baillarger's
   B. bands
   B. lines
Bailliart ophthalmodynamometer
balance
   b. disorder
   fluid b.
Balint's syndrome
Ballet's disease
ball-in-cone valve
ballism
ballismus
ballistic materials
balloon
   b. catheter
   detachable b.

   detachable silicone b.
   electrodetachable b.
   latex b.
   nondetachable b.
   nondetachable
      endovascular b.
   nondetachable occlusive b.
   b. occlusion
   b. occlusion test
   silicone b.
   b. test occlusion
balls
   Cajal's axonal retraction b.
Ball's operation
ball tip nerve hook
Baló's disease
Bamberger's
   B. disease
   B. sign
bamboo spine
band
   Baillarger's b.'s
   Bechterew's b.
   Broca's diagonal b.
   Essick's cell b.'s
   Gennari's b.
   b. of Giacomini
   b. heterotopia
   b. of Kaes-Bechterew
   b. keratopathy
   oligoclonal b.'s
   Reil's b.
   uncus b. of Giacomini
bandage
   hammock b.
bandwidth
   data acquisition b.
   receiver b.
Bannayan syndrome
Bannister's disease
Banthine
bar
   distraction b.
   Greenberg-type b.
   Leyla self-retaining
      tractor b.
   longitudinal spinal b.
   screw alignment b.
baragnosis

barbiturate
  b. burst-suppression
    anesthesia
  b. coma
Barbour technique
Bardet-Biedl syndrome
baresthesia
baresthesiometer
barium ferrite
Barkman's reflex
Barlow's syndrome
Barnes' dystrophy
baroceptor
baroreceptor
  b. nerve
baroreflex
barostat
barotrauma
Barré's sign
barrier
  blood-brain b. (BBB)
  blood-cerebrospinal fluid b.,
    blood-CSF b.
Bartel criteria
Bartholin's anus
basal
  b. cell nevus
  b. cell nevus syndrome
  b. cerebral artery
  b. ganglia
  b. ganglionic lesion
  b. joint reflex
  b. lamina of neural tube
  b. line
  b. meningitis
  b. plate of neural tube
  b. skull fracture
  b. subfrontal approach
  b. vein of Rosenthal
base
  anterior cranial b.
  b. of brain
  Brown-Roberts-Wells
    phantom b. (BRW-PB)
  skull b.
Basedow's pseudoparaplegia
baseline
  b. angiography
  Reid's b.
basicranial flexure
basilar
  b. artery
  b. artery migraine

  b. artery thrombosis
    syndrome
  b. bifurcation
  b. bifurcation aneurysm
  b. crest of cochlear duct
  b. impression
  b. invagination
  b. lamina
  b. leptomeningitis
  b. membrane
  b. meningitis
  b. part of pons
  b. skull fracture
  b. sulcus
  b. tip aneurysm
basis
  b. cerebri
  b. pedunculi
basket
  b. cell
basolateral
basophil
  b. adenoma
  b. substance
basophilia
  pituitary b.
basophilism
  Cushing's b., pituitary b.
bathmotropic
  negatively b.
  positively b.
bathyanesthesia
bathyesthesia
bathyhyperesthesia
bathyhypesthesia
Batten-Mayou disease
Batten's disease
battered infant syndrome
Battle's sign
Baxter's disease
Bayle's disease
bayonet
  b. clip
  b. forceps
  b. handle
BBB
  blood-brain barrier
BCNU
  carmustine
BEAM
  brain electrical activity mapping
beam hardening artifact
beaten-metal appearance

Bechterew-Mendel reflex
Bechterew's
    B. band
    B. disease
    B. nucleus
    B. sign
Becker's muscular dystrophy
Becker-type tardive muscular
   dystrophy
Beckman retractor
bed
    dynamic b.
    tumor b.
bed-wetting
Beevor's sign
Begbie's disease
behavioral
    b. disorder
    b. manifestation
behavior reflex
Behçet's disease
Bell-Magendie law
bellows
    Aneuroid chest b.
Bell's
    B. law
    B. palsy
    B. phenomenon
    B. spasm
Benadryl
bender
    French rod b.
bending
    rod b.
    b. strength
beneceptor
Benedek's reflex
Benedikt's syndrome
Benemid
benign
    b. essential tremor

    b. focal amytrophy
    b. lymphoepithelial parotid
     tumor
    b. myalgic encephalomyelitis
    b. paroxysmal torticollis
    b. paroxysmal vertigo
    b. stupor
    b. tetanus
benserazide
benzathine penicillin
benzilate
    quinuclidinyl b.
benzodiazepine
benztropine
    b. mesylate
Berger rhythm
Berger's paresthesia
Bergmann's
    B. cords
    B. fibers
beriberi
    dry b.
    wet b.
Bernard-Horner syndrome
Bernard-Soulier disease
Bernard's puncture
Bernhardt-Roth syndrome
Bernhardt's disease
berry aneurysm
beta
    b. blocker
    b. blocking agent
    b. fibers
    b. rhythm
    transforming growth
     factor b.
    b. wave
Betadine
beta-human chorionic gonadotropin
betahydroxybutyrate
betamethasone

NOTES

beta₂-microglobulin
bethanechol
Betz cells
Beuren syndrome
Bevan-Lewis cells
bevel
Beyer
 B. laminectomy rongeur
 B. rongeur
Bezold-Jarisch reflex
Bezold's ganglion
B fibers
bicaudate ratio
biceps
 b. femoris reflex
 b. reflex
Bichat's
 B. canal
 B. fissure
 B. foramen
Bicillin
BiCNU
Bielschowsky head tilt test
Bielschowsky's
 B. disease
 B. maneuver
Biemond's disease
Biemond syndrome
Bier block
Biernacki's sign
bifida
 spina b.
bifid cranium
bifrontal craniotomy
bifurcation
 basilar b.
 carotid b.
bigeminal bodies
bilateral
 b. arachnoid cyst
 b. choroid plexus cyst
 b. synchrony
 b. temporary tarsorrhaphy
 b. variable screw placement
 system
 b. ventral rhizotomy
biliary dyskinesia
bilious headache
bilirachia
bilirubin
 b. encephalopathy
bimanual coordination deficit
bimastoid line

Binet test
Bing's reflex
Binswanger's
 B. disease
 B. encephalopathy
Biobond
bioceramic
 calcium phosphate b.
biochemical
 b. pathway
 b. tumor markers
bioenergetic deficiency
biofeedback
 EMG b.
biogenic amine
biological response modifier
biologic time
biomechanical
 b. analysis
 b. factor
 b. testing
biomechanics
 axial plane angular
 deformity b.
 distraction
 instrumentation b.
 Dwyer instrumentation b.
 posterior fixation system b.
 Roy-Camille posterior screw
 plate fixation b.
biometal
bionic
biopercular syndrome
bioplastic
biopsy
 CT-guided b.
 endoscopic sphenoidal b.
 image-guided stereotactic
 brain b.
 lumbar spine b.
 PET-guided b.
 stereotactic b.
 thoracic spine b.
Biosol
Biot's
 B. breathing
 B. respiration
biphasic
biplane roentgenogram
bipolar
 b. bayonet forceps
 b. cell
 b. coagulating forceps

b. coagulation
b. electrocautery forceps
b. forceps
b. gradient
b. long-shaft forceps
b. neuron
b. vertebral traction
Birbeck granule
birdcage resonator
birth palsy
Bischof's myelotomy
bis-**guanylhydrazone**
methylglyoxal -g. (MGBG)
Bishop's putty
bitartrate
metaraminol b.
biundulant meningoencephalitis
bivalved speculum
biventral lobule
blackout
bladder
atonic b.
autonomic neurogenic b.
cord b.
nervous b.
neurogenic b.
b. reflex
reflex neurogenic b.
uninhibited neurogenic b.
blade
double-vector b.
retractor b.
ribbon b.
tapered b.
Blair-Ivy loop
Blake's pouch
blanket
thermal b.
blast effect
Blastomyces

blastomycosis
nasopharyngeal b.
bleeding
aneurysmal b.
b. disorder
b. time
blennorrhagicum
keratoderma b.
Blenoxane
bleomycin
b. sulfate
blepharophimosis
blepharospasm, blepharospasmus
blind headache
blindness
cerebral b.
cortical b.
letter b.
mind b.
music b.
note b.
object b.
sign b.
smell b.
taste b.
text b.
word b.
blink reflex
Bloch equation
block
anodal b.
Bier b.
cervical steroid epidural nerve b.
diagnostic b.
epidural b.
methylmethacrylate b.
nerve b.
nerve root b.
spinal b.
b. vertebra

NOTES

35

blockage
    shunt b.
blocker
    beta b.
    calcium channel b.
blocking
    b. activity
    alpha b.
Blocq's disease
blood
    b. flow
    b. flow measurement
    b. gas exchange
    b. loss
    b. test
    b. and thunder retina
    b. urea nitrogen (BUN)
    b. velocity
    b. vessel
    b. viscosity
    b. volume
blood-brain
    b.-b. barrier (BBB)
    b.-b. barrier disruption
    chemotherapy
blood-cerebrospinal fluid barrier
blood-CSF barrier
bloodless decerebration
blotting
    Southern b.
Blount spreader
blow-out fracture
blue
    b. edema
    b. nevus
Blumenau's nucleus
Blumenbach's clivus
blunt
    b. nerve hook
    b. suction tube
blunt-ring curette
blurring
    visual b.
blush
    choroidal b.
B-mode
    B-m. image
    B-m. ultrasonography
bobbing
    inverse ocular b.
    ocular b.
    reverse ocular b.
Bobechko's sliding barrel hook

Bochdalek's ganglion
Bock's ganglion
body
    aortic b.
    artificial vertebral b.
    bigeminal b.'s
    carotid b.
    b. coil
    cytoid b.'s
    foreign b.
    b. of fornix
    geniculate b.
    glomus b.
    Herring b.'s
    Hirano b.
    Hookean b.
    hyaline b.'s of pituitary
    b. image
    juxtarestiform b.
    Kelvin b.
    Lafora b.
    lateral geniculate b.
    Lewy b.'s
    Luys' b.
    mamillary b.
    medial geniculate b.
    metallic foreign b.
    myelin b.
    nerve cell b.
    newtonian b.
    Nissl b.'s
    olivary b.
    pacchionian b.'s
    paraterminal b.
    Pick's b.'s
    pineal b.
    psammoma b.'s
    quadrigeminal b.'s
    restiform b.
    b. righting reflexes
    sand b.'s
    b. schema
    striate b.
    tigroid b.'s
    trapezoid b.
    Verocay b.'s
    Wolf-Orton b.'s
Bohr effect
Bolt
    Philly B.
bolt
    Camino b.
    Camino micro ventricular b.

bone

Camino ventricular b.
Richmond b.

b. algorithms
allograft iliac b.
autogenous iliac b.
calvarial b.
b. conduction
b. curette
b. dissection
b. dust
b. exposure
b. flap
b. graft
b. graft collapse
b. graft decompression
b. graft extrusion
b. grafting
b. graft placement
hyoid b.
b. marrow suppression
b. mineral density
b. plate
b. plate selection
b. punch
b. reflex
b. screw
b. sensibility
b. stock
temporal b.
b. tumor
b. wax
bone-biting rongeur
bone/ligament dissection
bone-screw interface strength
bone-window CT scan
Bonhoeffer's sign
Bonnel
Bonnet-Dechaume-Blanc syndrome
Bonnier's syndrome

bony
b. canal
b. dissection
b. dysplasia
b. element destruction
b. exposure
b. overhang
b. purchase
booster clip
boots
thigh-high alternating
compression air b.
border cells
borderzone infarction
borreliosis
Lyme b.
Böttcher's
B. cells
B. ganglion
botulinum
b. A toxin
Clostridium b.
botulism
bouche de tapir
Bourneville-Pringle disease
Bourneville's disease
bouton
axonal terminal b.'s
b.'s en passage
synaptic b.'s
terminal b.'s, b. terminaux
bowel disease
brace
halo b.
Hudson b.
Milwaukee b.
SOMI b.
Yale b.
brachia (*pl. of* brachium)
brachial
b. birth palsy

NOTES

brachial *(continued)*
    b. neuritis
    b. plexus
    b. plexus avulsion
    b. plexus avulsion injury
    b. plexus neuropathy
brachial-basilar insufficiency
    syndrome
brachiocephalic vein
brachiocephaly
brachiofacial cortical hypesthesia
brachioradialis
brachioradial reflex
brachium, pl. brachia
    b. colliculi inferioris
    b. colliculi superioris
    b. conjunctivum cerebelli
    b. of the inferior colliculus
    inferior quadrigeminal b.
    .b. pontis
    b. quadrigeminum inferius
    b. quadrigeminum superius
    b. of superior colliculus
    superior quadrigeminal b.
brachybasia
brachycephalia
brachycephalic
brachycephalism
brachycephalous
brachycephaly
brachycranic
brachytherapy
    interstitial b.
    stereotactic b.
bracing
    external b.
    postoperative b.
Brackmann suction-irrigator
bradyarthria
bradycardia
    central b.
bradyesthesia
bradyglossia
bradykinesia
bradykinin
bradylalia
bradylexia
bradylogia
bradyphagia
bradyphasia
bradyphemia
bradypnea
bradypragia

bradypsychia
bradyteleokinesis, bradyteleocinesia
Bragg
    B. peak
    B. peak proton beam
    therapy
brain
    abdominal b.
    b. abscess
    b. aging
    b. biopsy needle
    b. cicatrix
    b. concussion
    b. congestion
    b. contusion
    b. cooling
    b. cyst
    b. death
    b. disease
    b. edema
    b. electrical activity
    mapping (BEAM)
    b. herniation
    b. infarction
    b. injury
    b. laceration
    b. mantle
    b. mapping
    b. metastasis
    b. murmur
    b. potential
    b. puncture
    respirator b.
    b. retention
    b. retraction
    b. retractor
    b. revascularization
    b. sand
    b. shift
    b. spatula
    split b.
    b. stem
    b. stimulation
    supratentorial b.
    b. swelling
    b. target
    tight b.
    b. transplantation
    b. tumor
    visceral b.
    b. wave
    b. wave complex
    b. wave cycle

braincase
Brain's reflex
brainstem, brain stem
    b. astrocytoma
    b. auditory evoked potential
    (BAEP)
    b. auditory evoked response
    (BAER)
    b. compression
    b. diencephalic mapping
    b. edema
    b. hemorrhage
Brain Tumor Registry
branch
    superior laryngeal nerve
    external b.
branchial efferent column
branching
    anomalous b.
branchiomotor nuclei
Brasdor's method
Brattleboro rat
breakage
    pedicle screw b.
    screw b.
break shock
breakthrough
    normal perfusion
      pressure b. (NPPB)
    perfusion pressure b.
    b. phenomenon
breath-holding
breathing
    apneustic b.
    ataxic b.
    Biot's b.
    Cheyne-Stokes b.
    b. disorder
bredouillement
bregmocardiac reflex

Bremer
    B. AirFlo vest
    B. halo crown
    B. halo crown traction set
    B. torque limiting cap
Brevital
Briquet's
    B. ataxia
    B. syndrome
Brissaud's
    B. disease
    B. reflex
    B. syndrome
broad AO dynamic compression
  plate
Broadbent's law
Broca's
    B. aphasia
    B. area
    B. center
    B. diagonal band
    B. dysphasia
    B. field
    B. fissure
    B. parolfactory area
Brodie's disease
Brodmann's
    B. areas
broken existing implant
bromide
    pancuronium b.
    b. psychosis
    vecuronium b.
bromocriptine
    b. test
bromodeoxyuridine (BUdR)
bronchodilatation
bronchodilation
bronchoscope
Bronkosol

NOTES

Brooks
- B. atlantoaxial arthrodesis
- B. technique
- B. type fusion

brow lift
Brown-Adson forceps
brownian motion
Browning's vein
Brown-Roberts-Wells
- B.-R.-W. arc-ring assembly
- B.-R.-W. arc system
- B.-R.-W. base ring
- B.-R.-W. computer
- B.-R.-W. floor stand
- B.-R.-W. head frame
- B.-R.-W. phantom base (BRW-PB)
- B.-R.-W. ring adaptor

Brown-Séquard's
- B.-S. paralysis
- B.-S. syndrome

Brown's syndrome
brucellosis
Bruch's membrane discontinuity
Brudzinski's sign
bruit
- arterial b.

Bruker Biospec system
Bruns' ataxia
Brushfield-Wyatt disease
BRW-PB
- Brown-Roberts-Wells phantom base

B₂-TFn
- B₂-transferrin
- B₂-TFn assay

B₂-transferrin (B₂-TFn)
bubble echocardiogram
buccopharyngeal approach
buckthorn polyneuropathy
Bucrylate
Budde
- B. halo retractor system
- B. halo ring
- B. halo ring retractor
- B. surgical system

Budge's center
BUdR
- bromodeoxyuridine

buffalo neck
bulb
- end b.
- jugular b.

Krause's end b.'s
- b. of lateral ventricle
- olfactory b.

bulbar
- b. apoplexy
- b. cephalic pain tractotomy
- b. myelitis
- b. palsy
- b. paralysis
- b. tractotomy

bulbi (*gen. and pl. of* bulbus)
- phthisis b.

bulbocavernosus reflex
bulboid corpuscles
bulbomimic reflex
bulbonuclear
bulbopontine
bulbosacral
- b. system

bulbospinal
bulbus, gen. and pl. **bulbi**
- b. olfactorius

bulk
- tumor b.

BUN
- blood urea nitrogen

bundle
- aberrant b.'s
- anterior ground b.
- Arnold's b.
- cingulum b.
- comma b. of Schultze
- Flechsig's ground b.'s
- Gierke's respiratory b.
- ground b.'s
- Held's b.
- Helweg's b.
- Hoche's b.
- hooked b. of Russell
- Krause's respiratory b.
- lateral ground b.
- Lissauer's b.
- Loewenthal's b.
- longitudinal pontine b.'s
- medial forebrain b.
- medial longitudinal b.
- Meynert's retroflex b.
- Monakow's b.
- oblique b. of pons
- olfactory b.
- olivocochlear b.
- Pick's b.
- posterior longitudinal b.

precommissural b.
predorsal b.
Schütz' b.
solitary b.
Türck's b.
uncinate b. of Russell
Vicq d'Azyr's b.
bunyavirus encephalitis
buphthalmos
bupivacaine
Burdach's
    B. column
    B. fasciculus
    B. nucleus
    B. tract
Burford retractor
Burn and Rand theory
burr
    diamond b.
    b. hole
    b. hole drainage
    Hudson brace b.
burst
    b. fracture
    b. injury

burst-suppression
    electroencephalographic b.-s.
Buschke's disease
Busse-Buschke disease
butterfly
    b. distribution
    b. needle
    b. rash
    b. vertebra
butterfly-shaped monoblock
  vertebral plate
butyrophenone
Buzzard's maneuver
bypass
    extracranial-intracranial b.
    extraintracranial b.
    Fukushima's cavernous b.
    b. graft
    STA-PCA b.
    STA-SCA b.
    superficial temporal artery
      to posterior cerebral
      artery b.

NOTES

C

C1-C2 posterior arthrodesis
C2-C3 cervical disk excision
C6-C7 dislocation
cable
    coaxial c.
    c. graft
    Songer c.
cabling
    percutaneous c.
cachexia
    c. hypophyseopriva
    hypophysial c.
    pituitary c.
cacosmia
café au lait spots
Cafergot
caffeine
    aspirin with butalbital,
      phenacetin, and c.
    ergotamine tartrate and c.
Cajal's
    C. axonal retraction balls
    C. cell
calamus
    c. scriptorius
calcar
    c. avis
calcarine
    c. artery
    c. cortex infarction
    c. fasciculus
    c. fissure
    c. sulcus
calcification
    gyriform c.
calcinosis
    c. intervertebralis
calcinosis, Raynaud's phenomenon,
  esophageal dysmotility,
  sclerodactyly, and telangiectasia
  (CREST)
calcium
    c. channel blocker
    c. channel blocking agent
    c. embolus
    fenoprofen c.
    c. phosphate bioceramic
calculus, gen. and pl. calculi
    cerebral c.
Caldwell-Luc incision

Caldwell projection
caliciform ending
caliculus, pl. caliculi
    c. ophthalmicus
California
    C. encephalitis
    C. Verbal Learning Test
callosal
    c. agenesis
    c. convolution
    c. gyrus
    c. splenium
    c. sulcus
callosomarginal
    c. fissure
callosotomy
    corpus c.
callostomy
callosum
    corpus c.
    hypogenetic corpus c.
caloric
    c. expenditure
    c. test
calorimetry
calvarial
    c. bone
    c. hemangioma
    c. hook
calvarium
calyciform ending
camera
    scintillation c.
Camino
    C. bolt
    C. catheter
    C. intraparenchymal
      fiberoptic device
    C. micro ventricular bolt
    C. transducer catheter
    C. ventricular bolt
campi foreli
campotomy
camptospasm
Camurati-Engelmann disease
canal
    c. of Arnold
    auditory c.
    Bichat's c.
    bony c.

canal *(continued)*
    caudal c.
    central c.
    Cotunnius' c.
    Dorello's c.
    Guyon's c.
    Hensen's c.
    internal auditory c.
    c. knife
    Löwenberg's c.
    neural c.
    optic c.
    semicircular c.
    spinal c.
    uniting c.
    c. of Vesalius
canaliculus, pl. **canaliculi**
    c. reuniens
canalis, pl. **canales**
    c. centralis
    c. reuniens
canals
    Haversian c.
Canavan's
    C. disease
    C. sclerosis
cancellation
    fat-water signal c.
cancellous screw
cancer
    metastatic breast c.
Candida
    C. infection
candidiasis
canine spasm
cannula
    Scott c.
    Sedan c.
    side-cutting c.
cannulation
    unilateral pedicle c.
Cantelli's sign
cap
    c. of the ampullary crest
    Bremer torque limiting c.
capacity
    cranial c.
capillariomotor
capillary
    c. angioma
    c. fracture
    c. telangiectasia
capita (*pl. of* caput)

capitis (*gen. of* caput)
capitium
capnography
capnometer
capsaicin
capsula, gen. and pl. **capsulae**
    c. externa
    c. extrema
    c. interna
capsulatum
    Histoplasma c.
capsule
    external c.
    extreme c.
    internal c.
    otic c.
capsulotomy
captopril
caput, gen. **capitis,** pl. **capita**
    c. cornus
    c. nuclei caudati
    c. succedaneum
carbamazepine
carbapenem
carbenicillin
    c. disodium
carbidopa/levodopa
carbon
    c. dioxide laser
    c. monoxide poisoning
carbonic acid
carboxypenicillin
carcinoma, pl. **carcinomas,**
  carcinomata
    leptomeningeal c.
    meningeal c.
carcinomatosis
    leptomeningeal c.
    meningeal c.
carcinomatous
    c. encephalomyelopathy
    c. myelopathy
    c. neuromyopathy
cardex
    medication c.
cardiac
    c. disease
    c. embolism
    c. function test
    c. ganglia
    c. gating
    c. glycoside
    c. index

c. output
c. risk index
cardiogenic shock
cardioneural
CardioSearch sensor
cardiospasm
care
postoperative c.
carebaria
carina, pl. **carinae**
c. fornicis
carisoprodol
C-arm
C-a. fluoroscopic apparatus
C-a. fluoroscopy
reversible C-a.
carmustine (BCNU)
carotic
caroticotympanic artery
caroticum
rete mirabile c.
carotid
c. ablative procedure
c. aneurysm
c. artery
c. artery dissection
c. artery occlusion
c. bifurcation
c. body
c. body tumor
c. contents
distal c.
c. endarterectomy
c. ganglion
c. occlusion
c. preservation
c. preservation technique
c. pulsation
c. rings
c. sheath
c. sinus massage

c. sinus nerve
c. sinus reflex
c. sinus syncope
c. sinus syndrome
c. vein
carotid-basilar anastomosis
carotid-cavernous
c.-c. fistula (CCF)
c.-c. sinus fistula
carotid-dural fistula
carotid-vertebral
c.-v. anastomosis
c.-v. vein bypass graft
carotodynia
carpal tunnel syndrome
carpopedal
c. contraction
c. spasm
carpoptosis, carpoptosia
carre-four sensitif
Cartesian coordinate representation
cartilage
c. inflammation
c. plates
thyroid c.
cartilaginous
c. end plate
c. plate
c. tumor
cascade
coagulation c.
Caspar
C. anterior plate fixation
C. cervical retractor
C. cervical screw
C. disk space spreader
C. drill
C. plate
C. plating
C. retraction posts

NOTES

Caspar *(continued)*
    C. retractor
    C. screw
CASS
    computer-assisted stereotactic
    surgery
       CASS whole brain mapping
       system
cast
    hinged c.
    Risser-Cotrel body c.
Castellani-Low sign
casting
    postoperative c.
Castroviejo eye suture forceps
catalepsy
cataleptic
cataleptoid
cataphasia
cataphora
cataplectic
cataplexy
cataract
cataract-oligophrenia syndrome
catastrophic migraine
catatonic rigidity
catecholamine
catelectrotonus
catheter
    afterloading c.
    argyle trocar c.
    balloon c.
    Camino c.
    Camino transducer c.
    cisterna magna c.
    Codman ventricular
      silicon c.
    cup c.
    delivery c.
    distal c.
    double-lumen Swan-Ganz c.
    e-PTFE ventricular c.
    e-PTFE ventricular shunt c.
    Foley c.
    French c.
    Hickman c.
    intraventricular c.
    Lapras c.
    lumbar c.
    1505 NDSB occlusion
      balloon c.
    nondetachable silicone
      balloon c.

    peritoneal c.
    Phoenix Anti-Blok
      ventricular c.
    Pudenz ventricular c.
    Raimondi peritoneal c.
    red rubber c.
    Shiley c.
    Silastic c.
    spinal c.
    Swan-Ganz c.
    Tracker c.
    Tracker infusion c.
    transducer-tipped c.
    transfemoral c.
cathode
catochus
cauda, pl. **caudae**
    c. equina
    c. equina avulsion
    c. equina syndrome
    c. fasciae dentatae
    c. nuclei caudati
    c. striati
caudal
    c. canal
    c. lamina resection
    c. neuropore
    c. regression syndrome
    c. transtentorial herniation
caudalis
    nucleus c.
    pars c.
    subnucleus c.
caudate
    c. nucleus
    c. volume
caudatolenticular
caudatum
caudolenticular
caumesthesia
causalgia
cava (*pl. of* cavum)
    inferior vena c.
cave
    Meckel's c.
cavernous
    c. aneurysm
    c. angioma
    c. hemangioma
    c. malformation
    c. plexus
    c. sinus
    c. sinus fistula

c. sinus syndrome
c. sinus thrombosis
c. sinus tumor
cavernous-carotid aneurysm
Cavitron
  C. laser
  C. ultrasonic aspirator
  C. ultrasonic surgical
    aspirator (CUSA)
cavity
  epidural c.
  oral c.
  c. of septum pellucidum
  subarachnoid c.
  subdural c.
cavum, pl. **cava**
  c. epidurale
  c. psalterii
  c. septi pellucidi (CSP)
  c. subarachnoidea
  c. subdurale
  c. veli interpositi (CVI)
  c. vergae
Cawthorne-Cooksey vestibular
  exercises
CBF
  cerebral blood flow
CBI
  convergent beam irradiation
CCA
  common carotid artery
    CCA clamp
CCF
  carotid-cavernous fistula
CCNU
  lomustine
CCT
  cranial computed tomography
    high-resolution CCT
C-D
  Cotrel-Dubousset

C-D device
C-D instrumentation
C-D instrumentation device
C-D instrumentation
  fixation strength
C-D instrumentation rigidity
C-D rod insertion
C-D screw modification
CeeNU
cefaclor
cefalothin sodium
cefamandole
  c. nafate
cefazedone
cefazolin
cefotaxime
cefoxitin
  c. sodium
ceftazidime
ceftizoxime
ceftriaxone
cefuroxime
celiac
  c. ganglia
  c. plexus
cell
  amacrine c.
  ameboid c.
  apolar c.
  astroglia c.
  auditory receptor c.'s
  basket c.
  Betz c.'s
  Bevan-Lewis c.'s
  bipolar c.
  border c.'s
  Böttcher's c.'s
  Cajal's c.
  chief c. of corpus pineale
  cochlear hair c.'s
  column c.'s

NOTES

cell *(continued)*
    commissural c.
    compound granule c.
    cone c. of retina
    corticotroph c.
    Corti's c.'s
    Deiters' c.'s
    Dogiel's c.'s
    effector c.
    ependymal c.
    external pillar c.'s
    Fañanás c.
    foam c.
    fusiform c.'s of cerebral
      cortex
    ganglion c.
    ganglion c.'s of dorsal
      spinal root
    ganglion c.'s of retina
    gemästete c.
    gemistocytic c.
    giant c.
    gitter c.
    glia c.'s
    glial c.
    globoid c.
    Golgi epithelial c.
    Golgi's c.'s
    gonadotroph c.
    granule c.'s
    gustatory c.'s
    gyrochrome c.
    hair c.'s
    Hensen's c.
    heteromeric c.
    horizontal c. of Cajal
    horizontal c.'s of retina
    Hortega c.'s
    internal pillar c.'s
    karyochrome c.
    lactotroph c.
    Langerhans' c.'s
    lymphokine-activated
      killer c.'s
    macroglia c.
    Martinotti's c.
    Mauthner's c.
    Merkel's tactile c.
    mesoglial c.'s
    Meynert's c.'s
    microglia c.'s, microglial c.'s
    midget bipolar c.'s
    mitral c.'s

    mossy c.
    motor c.
    Müller's radial c.'s
    multipolar c.
    Nageotte c.'s
    nerve c.
    neurilemma c.'s
    neuroendocrine c.
    neuroendocrine transducer c.
    neuroepithelial c.'s
    neuroglia c.'s
    neurolemma c.'s
    neurosecretory c.'s
    olfactory receptor c.'s
    oligodendroglia c.'s
    Opalski c.
    parenchymatous c. of
      corpus pineale
    phalangeal c.'s
    physaliphorous c.
    pillar c.'s
    pillar c.'s of Corti
    pineal c.'s
    c. proliferation
    pseudounipolar c.
    Purkinje's c.'s
    pyramidal c.'s
    reactive c.
    Renshaw c.'s
    rod c. of retina
    Rolando's c.'s
    satellite c.'s
    Schultze's c.'s
    Schwann c.'s
    somatotroph c.
    spider c.
    spindle c.
    stellate c.'s of cerebral
      cortex
    taste c.'s
    thyrotroph c.
    transducer c.
    tufted c.
    tunnel c.'s
    unipolar c.
    vestibular hair c.'s
    visual receptor c.'s
    wandering c.

cella, gen. and pl. **cellae**
    c. media
cellular kinetics
cellulose
    c. acetate polymer

oxidized c.
oxidized regenerated c.
CEM
CUSA electrosurgical module
cement
cenesthesia
cenesthesic, cenesthetic
center
anospinal c.
Broca's c.
Budge's c.
ciliospinal c.
expiratory c.
feeding c.
inspiratory c.
medullary c.
motor speech c.
respiratory c.
satiety c.
semioval c.
sensory speech c.
speech c.'s
vital c.
Wernicke's c.
centigray (cGy)
centra (*pl. of* centrum)
central
c. apnea
c. bradycardia
c. canal
c. chromatolysis
c. cord syndrome
c. dazzle
c. deafness
c. direct current bright spot
c. excitatory state
c. ganglioneuroma
c. gray substance
c. gyri
c. lobule
c. nervous system (CNS)

c. neuritis
c. paralysis
c. pit
c. pontine myelinolysis
c. somatosensory conduction
time (CSCT)
c. sulcus
c. tegmental fasciculus
c. tegmental tract
c. transactional core
c. venous pressure
Central European tick-borne fever
centre médian de Luys
centrencephalic
c. epilepsy
centrifugal
c. nerve
centripetal
c. nerve
centrokinesia
centrokinetic
centromedian nucleus
centrum, pl. **centra**
c. medianum
c. medullare
c. ovale
c. semiovale
Vicq d'Azyr's c. semiovale
Vieussens' c.
Willis' c. nervosum
cephalalgia
histaminic c.
Horton's c.
cephalea
c. agitata
c. attonita
cephaledema
cephalemia
cephalexin
cephalgia
cephalhematocele

NOTES

cephalhematoma
cephalhydrocele
cephalic
    c. flexure
    c. reflexes
    c. tetanus
cephalitis
cephalocele
cephalocentesis
cephalodynia
cephalogyric
cephalohematocele
cephalohematoma
cephalohemometer
cephalomedullary angle
cephalomeningitis
cephalometrography
cephalomotor
cephalo-oculocutaneous
  telangiectasia
cephalopalpebral reflex
cephalopathy
cephalorrhachidian index
cephalosporin
    third-generation c.
cephalothin
cephalotrigeminal angiomatosis
cephapirin
cepharadine
ceptor
    chemical c.
    contact c.
    distance c.
ceramic vertebral spacer
ceramidase
ceramide
    c. dihexoside
    c. trihexoside
    trihexosyl c.
cerebella (*pl. of* cerebellum)
cerebellar
    c. arachnoid cyst
    c. arteries
    c. ataxia
    c. atrophy
    c. cortex
    c. cortical degeneration
    c. cyst
    c. ectopia
    c. fissures
    c. fits
    c. gait
    c. gliosarcoma

    c. hematoma
    c. hemisphere
    c. hemisphere syndrome
    c. hemorrhage
    c. peduncle
    c. pyramid
    c. retraction
    c. rigidity
    c. speech
    c. sulci
    c. syndrome
    c. tonsil
    c. tremor
    c. veins
    c. vermian atrophy
    c. vermis dysgenesis
    c. volume
cerebelli
    pons c.
    tentorium c.
cerebellitis
cerebellolental
cerebellomedullary
    c. cistern
    c. fissure
    c. malformation syndrome
cerebello-olivary
    c.-o. degeneration
cerebellopontine
    c. angle
    c. angle approach
    c. angle cistern
    c. angle schwannoma
    c. angle syndrome
    c. angle tumor
    c. cisternography
    c. recess
cerebellorubral
    c. tract
cerebellothalamic tract
cerebellum, pl. cerebella
cerebra (*pl. of* cerebrum)
cerebral
    c. abscess
    c. agraphia
    c. amyloid angiopathy
    c. angiography
    c. anthrax
    c. aqueduct compression
    c. arterial gas tension of
      carbon dioxide (PaCO2)
    c. arteries
    c. arteriography

c. blindness
c. blood flow (CBF)
c. blood vessel
c. calculus
c. circulation
c. cladosporiosis
c. claudication
c. compression
c. contusion
c. convexity
c. cortex
c. death
c. decompression
c. decortication
c. diataxia
c. digital angiogram
c. dyschromatopsia
c. dysplasia
c. edema
c. embolism
c. embolus
c. fissures
c. flexure
c. foreign body embolization
c. gigantism
c. glioblastoma
c. gumma
c. hemicorticectomy
c. hemisphere
c. hemorrhage
c. hemosiderosis
c. hernia
c. hyperesthesia
c. hypoperfusion
c. infarction
c. ischemia
c. ischemia steal
c. layer of retina
c. lipidosis
c. localization

c. lymphoma
c. malaria
c. metabolism
c. metastasis
c. neuroblastoma
c. palsy
c. peduncle
c. perfusion pressure (CPP)
c. porosis
c. protection
c. ptosis
c. sclerosis
c. sensory input
c. sphingolipidosis
c. sulci
c. sulcus
c. tetanus
c. thrombosis
c. tuberculosis
c. vasodilating agent
c. vasoreactivity
c. vasospasm
c. veins
c. venous gas tension of oxygen (PvO2)
c. ventricles
c. ventriculography
c. vesicle

cerebralgia
cerebration
cerebri
    falx c.
    gliomatosis c.
    pseudotumor c.
cerebritis
    lupus c.
    suppurative c.
cerebroatrophic hyperammonemia
cerebrohepatorenal syndrome
cerebroma
cerebromalacia

NOTES

cerebromeningitis
cerebropathia
cerebropathy
cerebrosclerosis
cerebroside lipidosis
cerebrosidosis
cerebrosis
cerebrospinal
    c. axis
    c. fever
    c. fluid (CSF)
    c. fluid fistula
    c. fluid leakage
    c. fluid otorrhea
    c. fluid protein
    c. fluid rhinorrhea
    c. fluid volume
    c. index
    c. meningitis
    c. pressure
    c. system
cerebrospinant
cerebrotendinous
    c. cholesterinosis
    c. xanthomatosis
cerebrotomy
cerebrovascular
    c. accident (CVA)
    c. disease
    c. malformation
cerebrum, pl. **cerebra, cerebrums**
Ceretec ^{99m}**Tc HMPAO**
ceroid-lipofuscinosis
ceroid lipofuscinosis
ceruloplasmin deficiency
cerveau isolé
cervical
    c. aortic knuckle
    c. arthrodesis
    c. collar
    c. compression syndrome
    c. corpectomy
    c. decompression surgery
    c. discectomy
    c. disk excision
    c. disk herniation
    c. disk syndrome
    c. enlargement of spinal cord
    c. fibrositis
    c. flexure
    c. fusion
    c. fusion syndrome

    c. intersegmental vein
    c. interspace
    c. laminectomy
    c. medullary junction
    c. myositis
    c. myospasm
    c. nerve
    c. nerve root injury
    c. neural foramina
    c. perivascular sympathectomy
    c. plate
    c. radiculopathy
    c. rib syndrome
    c. screw insertion technique
    c. spinal stenosis
    c. spine
    c. spine arthritis
    c. spine decompression
    c. spine fixation
    c. spine fusion
    c. spine injury
    c. spine internal fixation
    c. spine kyphotic deformity
    c. spine laminectomy
    c. spine posterior fusion
    c. spine posterior ligament disruption
    c. spine rheumatoid disease
    c. spine screw-plate fixation
    c. spine stabilization
    c. spine stabilization procedure
    c. spine trauma
    c. spondylosis
    c. spondylosis without myelopathy
    c. spondylotic myelopathy
    c. spondylotic myelopathy fusion technique
    c. spondylotic myelopathy vertebrectomy
    c. stabilization
    c. steroid epidural nerve block
    c. sympathetic chain location
    c. tension syndrome
    c. trauma
    c. vertebra
    c. vertebrectomy
    c. vessel compression
cervices (*pl. of* cervix)

cervicis (*gen. of* cervix)
cervicocollic reflex
cervicodynia
cervicogenic
cervicolumbar phenomenon
cervicomedullary
    c. deformity
    c. junction compression
    c. kink
cervicothoracic
    c. ganglion
    c. junction
    c. junction stabilization
    c. junction surgery
    c. orthosis
    c. pedicle anatomy
    c. pedicle angle
cervix, gen. cervicis, pl. cervices
    c. of the axon
    c. columnae posterioris
cesarean resection
Cestan-Chenais syndrome
cesticidal
CFE
    colony-forming efficiency
C fibers
cGy
    centigray
Chaddock
    C. reflex
    C. sign
chain reflex
chair
    Combisit surgeon's c.
chamber
    drip c.
    flush c.
    Sechrist monoplace
      hyperbaric c.

Chamberlain's
    C. line
    C. palato-occipital line
Chance fracture
change
    degenerative discogenic
      vertebral c.
    personality c.
    trophic c.
    visual c.
Charcot-Bouchard aneurysm
Charcot-Marie-Tooth disease
Charcot's
    C. artery
    C. arthropathy
    C. disease
    C. gait
    C. joint
    C. triad
    C. vertigo
Charcot-Weiss-Baker syndrome
charring
Chaussier's line
checkerboard fields
cheirobrachialgia, chirobrachialgia
cheirocinesthesia, chirocinesthesia
cheirognostic, chirognostic
cheirokinesthesia, chirokinesthesia
cheirokinesthetic
cheirospasm, chirospasm
chemical
    c. ceptor
    c. hemostasis
    c. injury
    c. shift
    c. shift anisotrophy
    c. shift artifact
    c. sympathectomy
chemical-shift imaging
chemoceptor
chemodectoma

NOTES

chemoneurolysis
  glycerol c.
  percutaneous retrogasserian
    glycerol c.
chemonucleolysis
chemopallidectomy
chemopallidothalamectomy
chemopallidotomy
chemoreceptor
  medullary c.
  peripheral c.
  c. tumor
chemoreflex
chemosis
  orbital c.
chemothalamectomy
chemothalamotomy
chemotherapy
  blood-brain barrier
    disruption c.
  combination c.
  PCV c.
chemotransmitter
cherry-red
  c.-r. spot
  c.-r. spot myoclonus
    syndrome
chest
  flail c.
Cheyne-Stokes
  C.-S. breathing
  C.-S. respiration
CHI
  closed head injury
Chiari
  C. I malformation
  C. II malformation
  C. II syndrome
  C. III malformation
  C. malformation
chiasm
  optic c.
  prefixed c.
chiasma, pl. chiasmata
  c. opticum
  c. syndrome
chiasmal
  c. arachnoiditis
  c. compression
  c. epidermoid
  c. lesion

chiasmatic
chiasmatic-hypothalamic pilocytic
  astrocytoma
chief cell of corpus pineale
childhood muscular dystrophy
chin
  c. jerk
  c. reflex
chirobrachialgia (*var. of*
  cheirobrachialgia)
chirocinesthesia (*var. of*
  cheirocinesthesia)
chirognostic (*var. of* cheirognostic)
chirokinesthesia (*var. of*
  cheirokinesthesia)
chirospasm (*var. of* cheirospasm)
chitoneure
chitosan
chlorambucil
chloramphenicol
  c. sodium succinate
chlordiazepoxide
  amitriptyline hydrochloride
    and c.
  c. hydrochloride
chlorhexidine shampoo
chloride
  ammonium c.
  edrophonium c.
  ^{201}Tl c.
chloroma
Chloromycetin
chlorothiazide
chlorpheniramine maleate
chlorpromazine
  c. hydrochloride
chlorpropamide
chlorthalidone
Chlorthiazide
Chlor-Trimeton
chlorzoxazone and acetaminophen
Cho
  choline
Chodzko's reflex
cholecystokinin
cholesteatoma
cholesterinosis
  cerebrotendinous c.
cholesterol
  c. crystal
  c. cyst

c. embolism
c. granuloma
choline (Cho)
c. acetyltransferase
cholinergic
c. fibers
Cho:NAA ratio
chondritis
nasal c.
chondroblastoma
chondrocalcinosis
chondrohypoplasia
chondroma
chondromatous tumor
chondro-osteodystrophy
chondrosarcoma
Chopper-Dixon hybrid imaging
chord length
chordoma
chordotomy
chorea
automatic c.
chronic progressive c.
c. cordis
dancing c.
degenerative c.
c. dimidiata
electric c.
c. festinans
fibrillary c.
c. gravidarum
habit c.
hemilateral c.
Henoch's c.
hereditary c.
Huntington's c.
hysterical c.
juvenile c.
laryngeal c.
c. major
methodical c.

mimetic c.
c. minor
Morvan's c.
c. nutans
paralytic c.
posthemiplegic c.
procursive c.
rheumatic c.
rhythmic c.
c. rotatoria
saltatory c.
senile c.
Sydenham's c.
tetanoid c.
chorea-acanthocytosis
choreal
choreathetosis
choreic
c. abasia
c. movement
choreiform
c. disorder
choreoathetoid
choreoathetosis
dystonic c.
kinesogenic c.
choreoathetotic
choreoid
choreophrasia
choriocarcinoma
choriomeningitis
lymphocytic c.
chorionic gonadotropin
choristoma
c. nest
choroid
c. detachment
c. fissure
c. glomus
c. plexus
c. plexus adenoma

NOTES

choroid *(continued)*
- c. plexus of fourth ventricle
- c. plexus of lateral ventricle
- c. plexus of third ventricle
- c. skein
- c. tela of fourth ventricle
- c. tela of third ventricle
- c. vein

choroidal
- c. artery
- c. blush
- c. metastasis

choroidal-hippocampal fissure complex
choroidopathy
Christensen-Krabbe disease
Christmas disease
Christoferson's disk bony implant
chromaffinoma
chromaffinopathy
chromaffin tumor
chromatic
- c. audition
- c. granule

chromatinolysis
chromatolysis
- central c.
- retrograde c.
- transsynaptic c.

chromatolytic
chromesthesia
chromolysis
chromophil
- c. adenoma
- c. granule
- c. substance

chromophobe adenoma
chromosome
- c. study
- c. walking
- X c.

chronic
- c. acquired hepatic failure
- c. African sleeping sickness
- c. anterior poliomyelitis
- c. communicating hydrocephalus
- c. familial polyneuritis
- c. intractable pain
- c. migrainous neuralgia
- c. partial epilepsy
- c. progressive chorea

- c. trypanosomiasis
- c. vertigo

chronometry
- mental c.

chuck
- T-handled Jacob's c.

chunking
Churg-Strauss syndrome
Chvostek's sign
chylous leakage
chymopapain
cicatrix, pl. cicatrices
- brain c.
- meningocerebral c.

ciliary ganglion
ciliochoroid detachment
ciliospinal
- c. center
- c. reflex

ciliotomy
cimetidine
cinanesthesia
cinclisis
cincture sensation
cinerea
cinereal
cinereum
- tuber c.

cineritious
cineseismography
cingula (*pl. of* cingulum)
cingulate
- c. convolution
- c. gyrus
- c. gyrus dysgenesis
- c. gyrus eversion
- c. herniation

cingulectomy
cingulotomy
- rostral c.

cingulum, gen. cinguli, pl. cingula
- c. bundle

cinoxacin
ciprofloxacin
circle
- arterial c. of cerebrum
- Haller's c.
- Ridley's c.
- vascular c. of optic nerve
- c. of Willis
- Zinn's vascular c.

circuit
    Papez c.
    reverberating c.
circular
    c. fibers
    c. laminar hook with offset
      top
    c. sinus
    c. sulcus of Reil
circulation
    cerebral c.
    collateral c.
    thalamic c.
circulus, gen. and pl. **circuli**
    c. arteriosus cerebri
    c. arteriosus halleri
    c. vasculosus nervi optici
    c. venosus halleri
    c. venosus ridleyi
circumgemmal
circumscribed
    c. cerebral atrophy
    c. craniomalacia
    c. edema
    c. pyocephalus
circumscripta
    osteoporosis c.
circumventricular
    c. organs
cisplatin
cis-**platinum**
cistern
    cerebellomedullary c.
    cerebellopontine angle c.
    c. of chiasm
    c. of great vein of
      cerebrum
    interpeduncular c.
    c. of lateral fossa of
      cerebrum
    mesencephalic c.

    c. of nuclear envelope
    pontine c.
    quadrigeminal c.
    subarachnoidal c.'s
    suprasellar c.
cisterna, gen. and pl. **cisternae**
    c. ambiens, ambient c.
    c. basalis
    c. caryothecae
    c. cerebellomedullaris
    c. chiasmatis
    c. cruralis
    c. fossae lateralis cerebri
    c. interpeduncularis
    c. magna
    c. magna catheter
    c. pontis
    cisternae subarachnoideales
    c. superioris
    c. venae magnae
    c. venae magnae cerebri
cisternal
    c. puncture
cisternography
    cerebellopontine c.
    computed tomographic c.
    radionuclide c.
Citelli's angle
cladosporiosis
    cerebral c.
clamp
    CCA c.
    Crutchfield c.
    Dandy c.
    Duvol lung c.
    Halifax c.
    interlaminar c.
    Kocher c.
    Mayfield head c.
    Olivecrona aneurysm c.
    Selverstone c.

NOTES

clamp *(continued)*
 Selverstone type c.
 suture c.
clamping mechanism
Clarke's
 C. column
 C. nucleus
clasp-knife
 c.-k. effect
 c.-k. phenomenon
 c.-k. rigidity
 c.-k. spasticity
classic migraine
classification
 Hunt and Kosnik c.
 Kerohan system of
  glioma c.
 LeFort c.
 Spetzler-Martin c.
Claude's syndrome
claudication
 cerebral c.
 visual c.
claustral
 c. layer
claustrum, pl. claustra
clava
claval
clavulanic acid
clawhand deformity
clay-shoveler fracture
cleft
 pharyngeal c.
 Schmidt-Lanterman c.'s
 c. spine
 synaptic c.
Cleocin
Clevenger's fissure
climbing fibers
clindamycin
clinical
 c. electromagnetic flowmeter
 c. presentation
clinoidal
 c. aneurysm
 c. meningioma
 c. segment (ClinSeg)
clinoidectomy
 anterior extradural c.
 extradural c.
clinoid process
Clinoril

ClinSeg
 clinoidal segment
clip
 Adson scalp c.
 aneurysm c.
 c. application
 bayonet c.
 booster c.
 cross-legged c.
 Delrin plastic scalp c.
 Delrin scalp c.
 Drake c.
 Drake-Kees c.
 Drake's fenestrated c.
 Elgiloy c.
 fenestrated c.
 c. graft
 heavy-duty straight c.
 Heifetz c.
 Heifetz-Weck c.
 Iwabuchi c.
 Kerr c.
 Leroy-Raney scalp c.
 Mayfield c.
 Mayfield aneurysm c.
 McFadden c.
 McFadden cross-legged c.
 McFadden-Kees c.
 Michel scalp c.
 microvascular c.
 mini-Sugita c.
 Olivecrona c.
 c. placement
 plastic scalp c.
 primary c.
 Raney c.
 Raney scalp c.
 right-angle booster c.
 scalp c.
 Scoville c.
 Slimline c.
 straight c.
 Sugita c.
 Sugita aneurysm c.
 Sugita cross-legged c.
 Sugita-Ikakogyo c.
 Sundt c.
 Sundt booster c.
 Sundt cross-legged c.
 Sundt-Kees c.
 Sundt-Kees encircling
  patch c.
 Sundt-Kees graft c.

Sundt-Kees Slimline c.
Sundt straddling c.
temporary c.
towel c.
Weck c.
Yasargil c.
Yasargil-Aesculap spring c.
Yasargil cross-legged c.
Zimmer c.
clipping
aneurysm c.
proximal c.
clip-reinforced cotton sling
clival
clivus, pl. clivi
Blumenbach's c.
c. canal line
clonazepam
clonic
c. convulsion
c. spasm
clonicity
clonicotonic
clonidine
c. hydrochloride
topical c.
clonism
clonospasm
clonus
ankle c.
toe c.
wrist c.
clorazepate dipotassium
clorhexidine gluconate
Clorpactin
closed
c. angiography
c. Cotrel-Dubousset hook
c. head injury (CHI)
c. skull fracture

c. transverse process TSRH
hook
Clostridium
C. botulinum
C. difficile
closure
premature c.
c. pressure
scalp c.
watertight c.
clotting disorder
cloverleaf
c. skull
c. skull syndrome
Cloward
C. blade retractor
C. dural hook
C. elevator
C. operation
C. procedure
C. rongeur
C. technique
Cloward-Harper rongeur
Cloward-Hoen retractor
Cloward's PUKA
cloxacillin
CLQ
cognitive laterality quotient
cluster headache
CNR
contrast-to-noise ratio
CNS
central nervous system
Congress of Neurological
Surgeons
coagulation
bipolar c.
c. cascade
c. disorder
disseminated intravascular c.
(DIC)

NOTES

coagulation *(continued)*
>low current monopolar c.
>monopolar c.

coagulative necrosis

coagulator
>Fukushima's monopolar malleable c.
>Malis solid state c.
>solid state c.

coagulopathy
>consumptive c.

coagulum
>cryoprecipitate c.

coarctation
>aortic c.

coarse tremor

Coats' disease

coaxial cable

cobalt
>samarium c.
>c. samarium magnet

Cobb
>C. elevator
>C. periosteal elevator
>C. technique

Cobb's syndrome

cocaine abuse

Coccidiodes

coccidioidal meningitis

Coccidioides
>*C immitis*
>*C infection*

coccidioidomycosis

coccygeal
>c. ganglion
>c. part of spinal cord

coccygodynia

coccyx
>posterior surgical exposure of sacrum and c.

cochlea, pl. **cochleae**
>membranous c.

cochlear
>c. aqueduct
>c. duct
>c. hair cells
>c. implant
>c. microphonic potential
>c. nerve
>c. nuclei
>c. part of vestibulocochlear nerve
>c. recess

>c. root of vestibulocochlear nerve

cochleogram

cochleo-orbicular reflex

cochleopalpebral reflex

cochleopupillary reflex

cochleosacculotomy

cochleostapedial reflex

Cockayne's syndrome

coconut sound

codeine

Codman
>C. drill
>C. neurological headrest system
>C. scissors
>C. ventricular silicon catheter

coenesthesia

Cogan's
>C. lid twitch
>C. syndrome

Cogentin

cognition

cognitive
>c. disturbance
>c. laterality quotient (CLQ)

cogwheel
>c. phenomenon
>c. rigidity

coherence
>phase c.

coil
>body c.
>detachable c.
>Dixon's radiofrequency c.
>electrodetachable platinum c.
>c. embolization
>Golay gradient c.
>gradient c.
>Guglielmi detachable c. (GDC)
>head c.
>Hilal c.
>Ivalon wire c.
>occlusion c.
>platinum c.
>c. precision
>radiofrequency c.
>saddle c.
>shim c.
>surface c.

thrombogenic c.'s
transverse gradient c.
z-gradient c.

coiled spring
coin-counting
Colace
colchicine
coli
    Escherichia c.
colitis
    granulomatous c.
    pseudomembranous c.
    ulcerative c.
colla (*pl. of* collum)
collagen
    microfibrillar c.
collapse
    bone graft c.
    c. delirium
    hemispheric c.
    vertebral c.
collar
    cervical c.
    Philadelphia c.
    plastic c.
collateral
    c. blood flow
    c. circulation
    c. eminence
    c. fissure
    c. sulcus
    c. trigone
    c. vessel
Collet-Sicard syndrome
colliculus, pl. **colliculi**
    facial c.
    c. facialis
    c. inferior
    inferior c.
    c. superior
    superior c.

Collier's tract
collimation
collimator
    external c.
    c. helmet
    stereoguide c.
colloid cyst
collum, pl. **colla**
    c. distortum
coloboma
colon
colony-forming efficiency (CFE)
color
    c. anomia
    c. hearing
    c. taste
    c. vision
    c. vision disorder
    c. vision loss
color-flow
    c.-f. Doppler
    c.-f. Doppler sonography
    c.-f. imaging
colpocephaly
column
    anterior c. of medulla
      oblongata
    anterior c. of spinal cord
    anterolateral c. of spinal
      cord
    branchial efferent c.
    Burdach's c.
    c. cells
    Clarke's c.
    dorsal c. of spinal cord
    c. of fornix
    general somatic afferent c.
    general somatic efferent c.
    general visceral c.,
      splanchnic afferent c.,
      splanchnic efferent c.

NOTES

column *(continued)*
    Goll's c.
    Gowers' c.
    gray c.'s
    intermediolateral cell c. of
      spinal cord
    lateral c. of spinal cord
    posterior c. of spinal cord
    Rolando's c.
    special somatic afferent c.
    special visceral c.
    spinal c.
    splanchnic afferent c. (*var.
      of* general visceral c.)
    splanchnic efferent c. (*var.
      of* general visceral c.)
    Stilling's c.
    Türck's c.
    ventral c. of spinal cord
    vertebral c.
columna, gen. and pl. **columnae**
    c. anterior
    c. fornicis
    columnae griseae
    c. lateralis
    c. posterior
    c. vertebralis
coma
    barbiturate c.
    c. carcinomatosum
    diabetic c.
    hepatic c.
    hyperosmolar hyperglycemic
      nonketonic c.
    Kussmaul's c.
    metabolic c.
    c. scale
    thyrotoxic c.
    c. vigil
comatose
combination
    c. chemotherapy
    Isola spinal implant system
      plate-rod c.
    c. needle electrode
combined
    c. anterior and posterior
      approach
    c. flexion-distraction injury
      and burst fracture
    c. low cervical and
      transthoracic approach

    c. presigmoid-
      transtransversarium
      intradural approach
    c. sclerosis
    c. system disease
    c. transsylvian and middle
      fossa approach
Combisit surgeon's chair
Combitrans transducer
comma
    c. bundle of Schultze
    c. tract of Schultze
comminuted skull fracture
commissura,
  gen. and pl. **commissurae**
    c. alba
    c. anterior
    c. anterior grisea
    c. cinerea
    c. fornicis
    c. grisea
    c. habenularum
    c. hippocampi
    c. posterior cerebri
    c. posterior grisea
    commissurae supraopticae
    c. ventralis alba
commissural
    c. cell
    c. fibers
    c. myelotomy
    c. plate
commissure
    anterior c.
    anterior commissure-
      posterior c. (AC-PC)
    anterior white c.
    c. of cerebral hemispheres
    c. of fornix
    Ganser's c.'s
    Gudden's c.'s
    c. of habenulae
    habenular c.
    hippocampal c.
    Meynert's c.'s
    posterior cerebral c.
    supraoptic c.'s
    Wernekinck's c.
    white c.
commissurotomy
    percutaneous balloon c.
common
    c. carotid artery (CCA)

c. iliac artery injury
c. limb of membranous
  semicircular ducts
c. migraine
c. peroneal nerve
commotio
  c. cerebri
  c. spinalis
communicating hydrocephalus
communication
compartment syndrome
COMPASS
  C. arc-quadrant stereotactic
    system
  C. stereotactic system
compatibility
  ABO antigen c.
  MRI c.
Compazine
compensation
  gradient c.
compensatory scoliosis
competition
  hemisphere c.
complete
  c. iridoplegia
  c. lateral hemilaminectomy
complex
  c. absence
  ALD-AMN c.
  amygdaloid c.
  antigen-antibody c.
  brain wave c.
  choroidal-hippocampal
    fissure c.
  Dandy-Walker c.
  immune c.
  K c.
  mastoid c.
  occipito-atlanto-axial c.
  c. partial seizure (CPS)

c. precipitated epilepsy
spike and wave c.
ventrolateral nuclear c.
complicated fracture
complication
  Isola spinal implant
    system c.
  neurologic c.
component
  Isola spinal implant
    system c.
composite addition technique
composition
  device c.
compound
  c. fracture
  c. granule cell
  c. skull fracture
compressed spectral array
compression
  c. anesthesia
  axial c.
  c. of brain
  brainstem c.
  cerebral c.
  cerebral aqueduct c.
  cervical vessel c.
  cervicomedullary junction c.
  chiasmal c.
  c. fracture
  Harrington rod
    instrumentation c.
  c. instrumentation
  c. instrumentation posterior
    construct
  c. ophthalmodynamometer
  c. ophthalmodynamometry
  optic chiasm c.
  optic tract c.
  c. paralysis
  c. rod

NOTES

63

compression *(continued)*
  c. rod treatment
  spinal cord c.
  c. spring
  c. syndrome
  thecal sac c.
  c. U-rod instrumentation
compressive
  c. myelopathy
  c. rod
compromise
  adenohypophyseal c.
  adrenocorticotropic c.
  endocrinological c.
Compton scattering
computed
  c. tomographic
    cisternography
  c. tomographic metrizamide
    myelography (CTMM)
  c. tomographic myelography
    (CTM)
  c. tomography (CT)
computer
  Brown-Roberts-Wells c.
**computer-assisted stereotactic
  surgery (CASS)**
**computer-controlled neurological
  stimulation system**
**computerized infrared
  telethermographic imaging**
conarium
concentration
  hydrogen ion c.
  motion c.
concept
  three-column c.
concussion
  brain c.
  c. myelitis
  spinal c.
condition
  degenerative spine c.
conditioned
  c. reflex (CR)
  c. stimulus
conduction
  c. anesthesia
  c. aphasia
  bone c.
  c. disorder
  c. testing
condylar hypoplasia

condyle
  c. dissection
  c. resection
condylectomy
  mandibular c.
cone
  c. cell of retina
  c. fiber
  implantation c.
  medullary c.
  retinal c.'s
configuration
  Cotrel-Dubousset hook
    claw c.
  triangular base transverse
    bar c.
conflict
  intermanual c.
confluence of sinuses
confluens sinuum
confrontation testing
confusional migraine
congenita
  aplasia cutis c.
congenital
  c. aneurysm
  c. anomaly
  c. atonic pseudoparalysis
  c. cerebral aneurysm
  c. dilatation
  c. dysplastic angiomatosis
  c. dysplastic angiopathy
  c. facial diplegia
  c. hydrocephalus
  c. hypothesis
  c. kyphosis
  c. malformation
  c. muscular dystrophy
  c. nasal mass
  c. paramyotonia
  c. scoliosis
  c. spastic paraplegia
congestion
  brain c.
congestive heart failure
congophilic angiopathy
**Congress of Neurological Surgeons
  (CNS)**
coni (*pl. of* conus)
conjoined nerve root
conjugate paralysis
conjunctivitis
connective tissue disease

connector
    adjustable c.
    adjustable pedicle c.
    dual bypass c.'s
    intrinsic transverse c.
    longitudinal member to
      anchor c.
    stepdown c.
    straight c.
    tandem c.'s
    transverse c.
Conray
conscious
consciousness
constant current stimulator
construct
    anterior c.
    AO dynamic compression
      plate c.
    compression instrumentation
      posterior c.
    double-rod c.
    Edwards modular system
      bridging sleeve c.
    Edwards modular system
      compression c.
    Edwards modular system
      distraction-lordosis c.
    Edwards modular system
      kyphoreduction c.
    Edwards modular system
      neutralization c.
    Edwards modular system
      rod-sleeve c.
    Edwards modular system
      scoliosis c.
    Edwards modular system
      spondylo c.
    Edwards modular system
      standard sleeve c.
    hook-to-screw L4-S1
      compression c.
    iliosacral and iliac
      fixation c.
    pedicle screw c.
    posterior c.
    c. research
    rod-hook c.
    screw-to-screw
      compression c.
    segmental compression c.
    single-rod c.
    spondylo c.
    TSRH double-rod c.
    TSRH pedicle screw-laminar
      claw c.
    upper cervical spine
      anterior c.
    upper cervical spine
      posterior c.
    Wiltse system double-rod c.
    Wiltse system H c.
    Wiltse system single-rod c.
consumptive coagulopathy
contact
    c. ceptor
    c. compressive forceps
contents
    carotid c.
**contiguous nonoverlapping axial
CT**
continuous
    c. on-line recording
    c. positive airway pressure
    c. tremor
    c. venous oximetry
continuous-wave
    c.-w. Doppler
    c.-w. Doppler imaging
    c.-w. technique

NOTES

contour
field c.
contoured
c. anterior spinal plate
c. anterior spinal plate drill
guide
c. anterior spinal plate
technique
contouring
Isola spinal implant system
longitudinal member c.
contraceptive
oral c.
contraction
carpopedal c.
maximal voluntary c.
(MVC)
tetanic c.
contracture
functional c.
organic c.
Volkmann's c.
contrafissura
contralateral
c. hemiplegia
c. reflex
c. routing of sound (CROS)
c. sign
contrapulsion of saccades
contrast
c. agent
c. angiography
c. density
c. enhancement
inherent c.
c. media
paramagnetic c.
c. sensitivity reduction
contrast-enhanced
c.-e. CT
c.-e. CT scan
c.-e. MR image
c.-e. MR imaging
contrast-to-noise ratio (CNR)
Contraves stand
contrecoup
c. injury
c. injury of brain
control
airway c.
3-D positional c.
idiodynamic c.
motor c.

reflex c.
synergic c.
televised radiofluoroscopic c.
tonic c.
vestibulo-equilibratory c.
contusion
brain c.
cerebral c.
facial c.
scalp c.
wind c.
conus, pl. **coni**
c. avulsion
c. medullaris
c. medullaris root avulsion
convergence
c. abnormality
c. nucleus of Perlia
c. spasm
convergence-retraction nystagmus
convergent beam irradiation (CBI)
converse ocular dipping
conversion disorder
converter
digital-to-analog c.
convexity
cerebral c.
cortical c.
c. meningioma
c. metastatic tumor
convexobasia
convolution
angular c.
anterior central c.
ascending frontal c.
ascending parietal c.
callosal c.
cingulate c.
first temporal c.
hippocampal c.
inferior frontal c.
inferior temporal c.
middle frontal c.
middle temporal c.
posterior central c.
second temporal c.
superior frontal c.
superior temporal c.
supramarginal c.
third temporal c.
transitional c.
transverse temporal c.'s
Zuckerkandl's c.

convulsant
 c. threshold
convulsion
 clonic c.
 coordinate c.
 ether c.
 febrile c.
 hysterical c., hysteroid c.
 immediate posttraumatic c.
 infantile c.
 mimic c.
 puerperal c.'s
 salaam c.'s
 static c.
 tetanic c.
 tonic c.
convulsive
 c. reflex
 c. state
 c. tic
Cook stereotaxic guide
Cooley's anemia
cooling
 autocerebral c.
 brain c.
 c. helmet
 nasopharyngeal c.
 whole-body c.
coordinate convulsion
coordinated reflex
copper-constantan thermocouple
copper deposition
coprolalia
cord
 Bergmann's c.'s
 c. bladder
 spinal c.
 tethered spinal c.
 vocal c.'s
 Wilde's c.'s
cordectomy

Cordis Secor implantable pump
cordopexy
cordotomy
 anterolateral c.
 open c.
 percutaneous c.
 posterior column c.
 spinothalamic c.
 stereotactic c.
core
 central transactional c.
corectopia
Corgard
cornea
corneal
 c. anesthesia
 c. reflex
cornu, gen. cornus, pl. cornua
 c. ammonis
 c. anterius
 c. inferius
 c. inferius cartilaginis
  thyroideae
 c. inferius hiatus saphenus
 c. inferius ventriculi
  lateralis
 c. laterale
 cornua of lateral ventricle
 c. posterius, c. p. ventriculi
  lateralis
 cornua of spinal cord
corona, pl. coronae
 c. radiata
 Zinn's c.
coronal
 c. cleft vertebra
 c. plane
 c. plane deformity
 c. plane deformity sagittal
  translation

NOTES

67

coronal *(continued)*
    c. section
    c. synostosis
coronary
    c. artery disease
    c. bypass surgery
corpectomy
    anterior c.
    cervical c.
    median c.
    c. model
    vertebral c.
    vertebral body c.
corpus, gen. corporis, pl. corpora
    c. amygdaloideum
    c. aorticum
    corpora arenacea
    corpora bigemina
    c. callosotomy
    c. callosum
    c. callosum agenesis
    c. callosum dysgenesis
    c. dentatum
    c. fimbriatum
    c. fornicis
    c. geniculatum externum
    c. geniculatum internum
    c. geniculatum laterale
    c. geniculatum mediale
    c. luysii
    c. mamillare
    c. medullare cerebelli
    c. nuclei caudati
    c. olivare
    c. paraterminale
    c. pineale
    c. pontobulbare
    corpora quadrigemina
    c. quadrigeminum anterius
    c. quadrigeminum posterius
    c. restiforme
    c. striatum
    c. trapezoideum
corpuscle
    articular c.'s
    axis c., axile c.
    bulboid c.'s
    Dogiel's c.
    genital c.'s
    Golgi-Mazzoni c.
    lamellated c.'s
    Mazzoni's c.
    Meissner's c.

    Merkel's c.
    oval c.
    pacchionian c.'s
    pacinian c.'s
    Purkinje's c.'s
    Ruffini's c.'s
    tactile c.
    terminal nerve c.'s
    touch c.
    Valentin's c.'s
    Vater-Pacini c.'s
    Vater's c.'s
corpuscula
corpusculum, pl. corpuscula
    corpuscula articularia
    corpuscula bulboidea
    corpuscula genitalia
    corpuscula lamellosa
    corpuscula nervosa
    terminalia
    c. tactus, pl. corpuscula
    tactus
correction
    anterior c.
    King type IV curve
    posterior c.
    kyphosis c.
    mechanism of c.
    rotational c.
    surgical c.
correlation time
corsette
    lumbosacral c.
cortex, gen. corticis, pl. cortices
    agranular c.
    association c.
    auditory c.
    cerebellar c.
    c. cerebelli
    cerebral c.
    c. cerebri
    dysgranular c.
    frontal c.
    granular c.
    heterotypic c.
    homotypic c.
    insular c.
    laminated c.
    motor c.
    olfactory c.
    opercular c.
    orbitofrontal c.
    parastriate c.

peristriate c.
piriform c.
prefrontal c.
premotor c.
primary visual c.
secondary sensory c.
secondary visual c.
sensory c.
somatic sensory c.,
  somatosensory c.
striate c.
supplementary motor c.
temporal c.
vertebral body anterior c.
visual c.
Corti
  organ of C.
cortical
  c. apraxia
  c. atrophy
  c. blindness
  c. convexity
  c. deafness
  c. epilepsy
  c. hamartoma
  c. mapping
  c. mapping of memory
    function
  c. plate
  c. screw
  c. sensibility
  c. sulcus
  c. vein
corticalization
corticectomy
cortices (*pl. of* cortex)
corticifugal
corticipetal
corticis (*gen. of* cortex)
corticoafferent

corticobulbar
  c. fibers
  c. tract
corticocerebellum
corticoefferent
corticofugal
corticography
corticomedial
corticonuclear fibers
corticopontine
  c. fibers
  c. tract
corticoreticular fibers
corticospinal
  c. fibers
  c. tract
corticosteroid
  postoperative c.'s
corticothalamic
corticotomy
corticotroph cell
corticotropin
**corticotropin-releasing hormone
  (CRH)**
Corti's
  C. cells
  C. ganglion
  C. organ
  C. pillars
  C. rods
cortisol
  c. and sodium succinate
cortisone acetate
Cortone acetate
Cortrosyn
Corynebacterium diphtheriae
Cosman-Roberts-Wells (CRW)
  C.-R.-W. stereotactic frame
  C.-R.-W. stereotactic system
Cosman TeleSensor
costal arch reflex

NOTES

Costellano
costoclavicular syndrome
costopectoral reflex
cosyntropin
Cotrel
    C. pedicle screw
    C. pedicle screw fixation
      strength
    C. pedicle screw rigidity
Cotrel-Dubousset (C-D)
    C.-D. distraction system
    C.-D. dynamic transverse
      traction device
    C.-D. fixation
    C.-D. hook claw
      configuration
    C.-D. instrumentation
    C.-D. pedicle screw
      instrumentation
    C.-D. pedicular
      instrumentation
    C.-D. rod flexibility
    C.-D. screw-rod system
    C.-D. spinal instrumentation
Cotte presacral neurectomy
Cotte's operation
Cottle knife
Cottle-Neivert retractor
cotton
    oxidized c.
    c. paddies
    c. wool spot
    c. wrap
cottonoid
    c. pledget
Cotunnius'
    C. aqueduct
    C. canal
Cotunnius disease
couch
    Siemens c.
couch-mounted head frame
cough reflex
Coumadin
coup
    c. injury
    c. injury of brain
coupling
    spin-spin c.
covering
    titanium mini burr hole c.
CO$_2$-withdrawal seizure test
Coxsackie encephalitis

CPP
    cerebral perfusion pressure
CPS
    complex partial seizure
CR
    conditioned reflex
    crown-rump
craft palsy
cramp
    accessory c.
    intermittent c.
    miner's c.'s
    musician's c.
    pianist's c., piano-player's c.
    seamstress's c.
    shaving c.
    stoker's c.'s
    tailor's c.
    typist's c.
    violinist's c.
    waiter's c.
    watchmaker's c.
    writer's c.
crania (pl. of cranium)
cranial
    c. arteritis
    c. capacity
    c. computed tomography
      (CCT)
    c. dermal sinus
    c. dysmorphia
    c. epidural abscess
    c. extension
    c. flexure
    c. fracture
    c. Jacobs hook
    c. nerve dissection
    c. nerve manipulation
    c. nerve monitoring
    c. nerve neoplasm
    c. nerve palsy
    c. nerves
    c. neuropathy
    c. osteomyelitis
    c. osteopetrosis
    c. osteosynthesis
    c. osteosynthesis system
    c. perforator
    c. roots
    c. settling
    c. suture
    c. trauma
    c. vault

cranialis
cranialization
craniamphitomy
craniectomy
>linear c.
>partial-thickness c.
>retromastoid suboccipital c.
craniocardiac reflex
craniocele
craniocervical
>c. junction
>c. plate
>c. region
craniofacial
>c. disjunction
>c. dysostosis
>c. dysraphism
>c. malformation
>c. osteotomy
>c. reconstruction
>c. remodeling
>c. surgery
craniofrontonasal dysplasia
craniognomy
craniolacunia
craniology
>Gall's c.
craniomalacia
>circumscribed c.
craniomeningocele
craniometry
craniopathy
craniopharyngioma
>cystic papillomatous c.
cranioplasty
>aluminum c.
>metallic c.
>c. plate
>Tantalum c.
craniopuncture

craniorrhachischisis
craniosacral
>c. system
cranioschisis
craniosclerosis
cranioscopy
craniosinus fistula
craniospinal
>c. meningioma
>c. space
craniostenosis
craniosynostosis
craniotabes
craniotome
>Midas Rex c.
craniotomy
>attached c.
>bifrontal c.
>detached c.
>frontotemporal c.
>open stereotactic c.
>osteoplastic c.
>pterional c.
>right frontotemporal c.
>right temporoparietal c.
>stereotactic c.
>Yasargil c.
craniotonoscopy
craniotrypesis
craniovertebral junction
cranium, pl. crania
>c. bifidum, bifid c.
C-reactive
>C-r. protein
>C-r. protein test
>C-r. protein value
crease
>simian c.
creatine
creatinine

NOTES

creation
kyphosis c.
lordosis c.
creeping palsy
cremasteric reflex
crepitance
crepuscular
crescendo
c. sleep
c. transient ischemic attack
crescent
crescentic
c. lobules of the cerebellum
CREST
calcinosis, Raynaud's
phenomenon, esophageal
dysmotility, sclerodactyly, and
telangiectasia
CREST syndrome
crest
acoustic c.
acousticofacial c.
ampullary c.
basilar c. of cochlear duct
falciform c.
ganglionic c.
neural c.
transverse c.
trigeminal c.
vestibular c., c. of vestibule
Creutzfeldt-Jakob disease
CRH
corticotropin-releasing hormone
cribriform plate
Crichton-Browne's sign
cricoid ring
cricothyrotomy
Crigler-Najjar
C.-N. disease
C.-N. syndrome
Crile
C. hemostat
C. retractor
crisis, pl. **crises**
adrenal c.
gastric c.
laryngeal c.
oculogyric crises
tabetic c.
crispation
crista, pl. **cristae**
c. ampullaris

c. basilaris ductus cochlearis
c. quarta
c. transversa
c. vestibuli
criteria
Bartel c.
Nyquist sampling c.
Criticare
Crockard retractor
crocodile tears syndrome
Crohn's disease
Crooke's granules
CROS
contralateral routing of sound
cross
Ranvier's c.'s
cross-bracing
spinal rod c.-b.
Wiltse system c.-b.
crossed
c. adductor jerk
c. adductor reflex
c. adductor sign
c. anesthesia
c. extension reflex
c. hemianesthesia
c. hemiplegia
c. jerk
c. knee jerk
c. knee reflex
c. laterality
c. paralysis
c. phrenic phenomenon
c. pyramidal tract
c. reflex
c. reflex of pelvis
c. spino-adductor reflex
cross-facial nerve graft anastomosis
cross-legged clip
crosslink
Edwards modular system
rod c.
Galveston fixation with
TSRH c.
Texas Scottish Rite
Hospital c.
cross-sectional
c.-s. area (CSA)
c.-s. image
crossway
sensory c.
Crouzon's disease

crown
    Bremer halo c.
    radiate c.
crown-rump (CR)
    c.-r. length
cruciate ligament
crus, gen. cruris, pl. crura
    c. anterius capsulae internae
    c. cerebri
    c. fornicis
    c. of fornix
    crura membranacea
      ampullaria
    c. membranaceum commune
      ductus semicircularis
    c. membranaceum simplex
      ductus semicircularis
    crura ossea canales
      semicirculares
    c. posterius capsulae
      internae
crush injury
crus I
crus II
crusotomy
crutch
    c. palsy
    c. paralysis
Crutchfield clamp
Cruveilhier's disease
CRW
    Cosman-Roberts-Wells
    CRW arc system
    CRW base frame
    CRW head frame
    CRW system
cryalgesia
cryanesthesia
cryesthesia
crymodynia
cryoanalgesia

cryoglobulinemia
cryohypophysectomy
cryopallidectomy
cryoprecipitate
    c. coagulum
cryoprobe
cryopulvinectomy
cryospasm
cryostat
cryosurgery
cryothalamectomy
cryptococcal spondylitis
cryptococcoma
cryptococcosis
    intracranial c.
Cryptococcus
    C. infection
    C. neoformans
cryptotia
cry reflex
crystal
    cholesterol c.
CSA
    cross-sectional area
CSCT
    central somatosensory
    conduction time
CSF
    cerebrospinal fluid
    CSF shunt
C-shaped scalp flap
CSP
    cavum septi pellucidi
CT
    computed tomography
    CT bone windows
    contiguous nonoverlapping
    axial CT
    contrast-enhanced CT
    metrizamide-enhanced CT
    CT scan

NOTES

CT *(continued)*
    serial CT
    stable xenon CT
    xenon-enhanced CT
CT-guided
    CT-g. biopsy
    CT-g. stereotactic evacuation
CTI/Siemens 933 tomograph
CTM
    computed tomographic
    myelography
CTMM
    computed tomographic
    metrizamide myelography
cubital
    c. tunnel
    c. tunnel syndrome
cuboidodigital reflex
cuirass
    analgesic c.
    tabetic c.
culmen, pl. culmina
cuneate
    c. fasciculus
    c. funiculus
    c. nucleus
cunei (*pl. of* cuneus)
cuneiform
    c. lobe
cuneocerebellar tract
cuneus, pl. cunei
cup
    c. catheter
    c. forceps
    ocular c.
    optic c.
cupula, pl. cupulae
    c. cochleae
    c. cristae ampullaris
cupular part
cupulate part
cupulolithiasis
curare
curette
    blunt-ring c.
    bone c.
    disk c.
    downbiting Epstein c.
    Epstein c.
    flat back c.
    Hardy c.
    Rhoton blunt-ring c.
    secret c.

    Semmes c.
    straight ring c.
    uterine c.
current
    audiofrequency eddy c.
    demarcation c.
    direct c. (DC)
    eddy c.
    c. of injury
    radiofrequency eddy c.
curse
    Ondine's c.
curve
    accommodation c.
    double thoracic c.
    frequency dispersion c.
    King type I c.
    King type II c.
    King type III c.
    King type II thoracic and
    lumbar c.'s
    King type IV c.
    King type V c.
    low single thoracic c.
    lumbar c.
    right thoracic c.
    rigid c.
    severe rigid right
    thoracic c.
    signal intensity c.
    specific c.
    thoracolumbar c.
curved
    c. conventional microscissors
    c. electrode
    c. knot-tying forceps
    c. micro-needle holder
curved-tipped spatula
CUSA
    Cavitron ultrasonic surgical
    aspirator
    CUSA CEM system
    CUSA electrosurgical
    module (CEM)
Cushing
    C. bayonet forceps
    C. bivalve retractor
    C. brain forceps
    C. decompressive retractor
    C. effect
    C. phenomenon
    C. response

C. retractor
C. subtemporal retractor
Cushing-Landolt speculum
cushingoid
Cushing's
C. basophilism
C. disease
C. syndrome
C. ulcer
custom implant
cutaneomeningospinal angiomatosis
cutaneous
c. horn
c. meningioma
c. pupil reflex
c. reflex
cutaneous-pupillary reflex
cutter
dowel c.
CVA
cerebrovascular accident
CVI
cavum veli interpositi
cyanoacrylate
c. glue
cybernetics
cycle
brain wave c.
cyclic vomiting
cycling
phase c.
cyclobenzaprine hydrochloride
cyclooxygenase
c. inhibitor
cyclophosphamide
Cyclosporin A
cyclosporine
cylinder
axis c.
cylindraxis
cylindroma

cynic
c. spasm
Cyon's nerve
cyproheptadine
c. hydrochloride
cyst
aneurysmal bone c.
apoplectic c.
arachnoid c.
bilateral arachnoid c.
bilateral choroid plexus c.
brain c.
cerebellar c.
cerebellar arachnoid c.
cholesterol c.
colloid c.
Dandy-Walker c.
dermoid c.
enteric c.
ependymal c.
epidermoid c.
extradural c.
glial parenchymal c.
hydatid c.
interhemispheric c.
intraparenchymal c.
leptomeningeal c.
lumbar synovial c.
nasopharyngeal mucus
retention c.
neural c.
neuroenteric c.
neuroepithelial c.
paraphysial c.'s
perineurial c.
pineal c.
pontine hydatid c.
posttraumatic
leptomeningeal c.
quadrigeminal arachnoid c.
Rathke's cleft c.

NOTES

cyst *(continued)*
    Rathke's pouch c.
    recurrent enteric c.
    retinal c.
    sacral c.
    sacral nerve root c.
    sellar c.
    subperiosteal c.
    suprasellar c.
    synovial c.
    Tarlov's c.
cystadenoma
    apocrine c.
    eccrine c.
cystic
    c. encephalomalacia
    c. intraparenchymal
      meningioma
    c. lacunar infarct
    c. medial necrosis
    c. microadenoma
    c. myelomalacia
    c. necrosis
    c. papillomatous
      craniopharyngioma
cysticercal infection
cysticercosis
cytoarchitectonics
cytoarchitectural
cytoarchitecture
cytoid bodies
cytology
cytomegalic inclusion disease
cytomegalovirus
Cytomel
cytometry
    flow c.
cyton
cytopathy
    mitochondrial c.
cytoreductive surgery
cytoskeletal abnormality
cytotoxic edema

D

3-D
    three-dimensional
        3-D positional adjustability
        3-D positional control
        3-D titanium mini bone
        plates
DaCosta's syndrome
dacryoadenitis
dacryocystitis
dactinomycin
dactylospasm
DAG
    dianhydrogalactitol
damage
    anterior cervical surgery
    vocal cord d.
Dana posterior rhizotomy
Dana's operation
danazol
dance
    Saint Anthony's d., Saint
    John's d., Saint Vitus d.
dancing
    d. chorea
    d. disease
    d. spasm
Dandy
    D. clamp
    D. maneuver
    D. nerve hook
    D. operation
    D. suction tube
Dandy-Walker
    D.-W. complex
    D.-W. cyst
    D.-W. malformation
    D.-W. syndrome
Danielssen-Boeck disease
Danielssen's disease
Danocrine
Dantrium
dantrolene
    d. sodium
dapsone
Daraprim
Darvocet-N 100
Darvocet-N 50
Darvon
darwinian reflex

data
    d. acquisition bandwidth
    d. acquisition system
Davis guide
Dawson's encephalitis
dazoxidine
dazzle
    central d.
DBD
    Dibromodulcitol
DBS
    direct brain stimulation
DC
    direct current
DCS
    dorsal cord stimulation
DDAVP
    desmopressin acetate
dead space
deafferentation
    d. pain
    d. pain syndrome
deafness
    central d.
    cortical d.
    high frequency d.
    infantile X-linked d.
    midbrain d.
    nerve d., neural d.
    retrocochlear d.
    sensorineural d.
    word d.
death
    brain d.
    cerebral d.
    d. trance
Debakey forceps
debulk
debulking procedure
Decadron
decarboxylase
    glutamate d. (GAD)
decay
    free induction d. (FID)
decerebrate
    d. posturing
    d. rigidity
decerebration
    bloodless d.
decerebrize

decision theory
declive
declivis
decomposition of movement
decompression
    anterior d.
    bone graft d.
    cerebral d.
    cervical spine d.
    d. equipment
    extensive posterior d.
    foraminal d.
    interlaminar d.
    internal d.
    d. laminectomy
    laser disk d. (LDD)
    lumbar spine d.
    microvascular d. (MVD)
    nerve d.
    d. operations
    orbital d.
    posterior d.
    sacral d.
    sacral spine d.
    simple d.
    spinal d.
    suboccipital d.
    subtemporal d.
    surgical d.
    thoracic spine d.
    thoracolumbar spine d.
    timing of d.
    transantral ethmoidal
     orbital d.
    trigeminal d.
    vascular d.
    vertebral body d.
decompressive
    d. laminectomy
    d. surgery
decortication
    cerebral d.
    reversible d.
    d. technique
decortization
decubitus
    d. paralysis
    d. ulcer
decussate
decussatio, pl. decussationes
    d. brachii conjunctivi
    d. fontinalis
    d. lemniscorum

    d. motoria
    d. nervorum trochlearium
    d. pedunculorum
     cerebellarium superiorum
    d. pyramidum
    d. sensoria
    decussationes tegmenti
decussation
    d. of brachia conjunctiva
    dorsal tegmental d.
    d. of the fillet
    Forel's d.
    fountain d.
    Held's d.
    d. of medial lemniscus
    Meynert's d.
    motor d.
    optic d.
    pyramidal d.
    rubrospinal d.
    sensory d. of medulla
     oblongata
    d. of superior cerebellar
     peduncles
    tectospinal d.
    tegmental d.'s
    d. of trochlear nerves
    ventral tegmental d.
    Wernekinck's d.
decussationes
de-efferentation
deep
    d. abdominal reflexes
    d. cerebellar nuclei
    d. cerebral veins
    d. middle cerebral vein
    d. origin
    d. reflex
    d. retractors
    d. sensibility
    d. transitional gyrus
defect
    afferent pupillary d.
    developmental d.
    field d.
    galactosidase d.
    glycosphingolipid
     metabolic d.
    midline fusion d.
    neural tube d. (NTD)
    pursuit d.
    smooth pursuit d.
    visual field d.

defense reflex
deferent
deferoxamine
deferred shock
deficiency
    aldosterone d.
    antithrombin III d.
    aqueous humor d.
    bioenergetic d.
    ceruloplasmin d.
    idiopathic growth
     hormone d.
    protein C d.
    protein S d.
deficient spinous process
deficit
    attention d.
    auditory transfer d.
    bimanual coordination d.
    memory d.
    motor d.
    neurologic d.
    neuropsychological d.
    osteoporosis with vertebral
     collapse and neurologic d.
    perfusion d.
    proprioception d.
    reversible ischemic
     neurological d. (RIND)
    sensory d.
    d. syndrome
    tactile transfer d.
    transfer d.
    visual field d.
deflection force
deformans
    osteitis d.
deformation
    shear-strain d.
    trefoil tendon d.

deformity
    d. analysis
    Arnold-Chiari d.
    cervical spine kyphotic d.
    cervicomedullary d.
    clawhand d.
    coronal plane d.
    flat back d.
    hand d.
    hindbrain d.
    J-sella d.
    kyphotic d.
    lumbar spine kyphotic d.
    posttraumatic spinal d.
    saddle nose d.
    sagittal d.
    skeletal d.
    spinal d.
    spinal coronal plane d.
    swan neck d.
    thoracic spine kyphotic d.
    thoracic spine scoliotic d.
deformity/instability
    spinal d./i.
deganglionate
degeneracy
degenerate
degeneratio
degeneration
    acquired hepatocerebral d.
    adiposogenital d.
    ascending d.
    cerebellar cortical d.
    cerebello-olivary d.
    descending d.
    fascicular d.
    fibrinoid d.
    granulovacuolar d.
    gray d.
    hepatocerebral d.
    hepatolenticular d.

NOTES

degeneration *(continued)*
    hypertrophic olivary d.
    infantile neuronal d.
    lenticular progressive d.
    neurofibrillary d.
    Nissl d.
    olivary d.
    olivopontocerebellar d.
    orthograde d.
    primary neuronal d.
    primary progressive
      cerebellar d.
    retrograde d.
    secondary d.
    spinopontine d.
    spongy d.
    striatonigral d.
    subacute combined d. of
      the spinal cord
    transsynaptic d.
    Türck's d.
    wallerian d.
degenerative
    d. arthritis
    d. brain disease
    d. cervical disk disease
    d. chorea
    d. dementia
    d. discogenic end-plate
      disease
    d. discogenic vertebral
      change
    d. disease
    d. disk disease
    d. disorder
    d. hypothesis
    d. lumbar scoliosis
    d. lumbar spine fusion
    d. narrowing
    d. spine condition
    d. spondylolisthesis
    d. spondylosis
    d. spondylosis
      decompression and fusion
    d. subluxation
degloving
    midface d.
deglutition reflex
Degos disease
degustation
deiterospinal tract
Deiters'
    D. cells

    D. nucleus
    D. process
Dejerine-Lichtheim phenomenon
Dejerine-Roussy syndrome
Dejerine's
    D. anterior bulb syndrome
    D. disease
    D. hand phenomenon
    D. peripheral neurotabes
    D. reflex
    D. sign
Dejerine-Sottas disease
Delatestryl
delayed
    d. computed tomographic
      myelography
    d. hypersensitivity reaction
    d. postischemic
      hypoperfusion
    d. reflex
    d. sensation
    d. shock
deliriant
delirious
    d. shock
delirium
    acute d.
    anxious d.
    collapse d.
    low d.
    d. mussitans, muttering d.
    posttraumatic d.
    senile d.
    toxic d.
    d. tremens (DT)
delivery
    d. catheter
    d. guidewire
    intra-arterial drug d.
Delrin
    D. plastic scalp clip
    D. scalp clip
delta
    d. fornicis
    d. rhythm
    d. wave
Delta valve
demarcation
    d. current
    d. potential
demeclocycline
demented

dementia
  Alzheimer's d.
  degenerative d.
  dialysis d.
  epileptic d.
  hydrocephalic d.
  multi-infarct d.
  paralytic d., d. paralytica
  paretic d.
  posttraumatic d.
  presenile d., d. presenilis
  primary senile d.
  senile d.
  toxic d.
  vascular d.
Demerol
de Morsier's
  d. M. syndrome
demyelinating
  d. disease
  d. encephalopathy
  d. lesion
demyelination, demyelinization
demyelinative spinal fluid profile
dendraxon
dendriform
dendrite
  apical d.
dendritic
  d. process
  d. spines
  d. thorns
dendroid
dendron
denervate
denervation
  Krause d.
dens, pl. **dentes**
  d. anterior screw fixation
Densitometric analysis

density
  bone mineral d.
  contrast d.
  lumbosacral junction
   bone d.
  proton d.
  spectral d.
dental
  d. infection
  d. nerve
dentate
  d. fascia
  d. fissure
  d. gyrus
  d. ligament
  d. nucleus
  d. nucleus of cerebellum
dentatectomy
dentated serrations
dentatothalamic tract
dentatum
dentes (*pl. of* dens)
denticulate ligament
dentoliva
Denver valve
deoxygenation
deoxyhemoglobin
  intracellular d.
deoxyribonucleic acid (DNA)
Depakene
depersonalization
Depo-Medrol
deposit
  amyloid d.
deposition
  copper d.
depressed
  d. fracture
  d. skull fracture
depression
  spreading d.

NOTES

depressive stupor
depressomotor
depressor
    d. fibers
    d. nerve of Ludwig
depth
    d. guard
    d. recording
    wire penetration d.
derby hat fracture
derivative
    hematoporphyrin d.
dermatofibrosarcoma protuberans
dermatogenic torticollis
dermatome
dermatomyositis
dermatomyotome
dermatoneurosis
dermatosensory evoked potential
dermoid
    d. cyst
    nasal d.
    d. tumor
dermoneurosis
Derome
D'Errico retractor
De Sanctis-Cacchione syndrome
descendens
    d. cervicalis
    d. hypoglossi
descending
    d. degeneration
    d. neuritis
    d. nucleus of the trigeminus
    d. tract of trigeminal nerve
desiccated thyroid
design
    hook hollow-ground
        connection d.
    hook V-groove
        connection d.
    Isola spinal implant
        system d.
    mechanical plate d.
    pedicle screw linkage d.
    spinal implant d.
    transpedicular fixation
        system d.
    V-groove hollow-ground
        connection d.
desipramine
desmodynia

desmoplastic infantile ganglioglioma
desmopressin acetate (DDAVP)
desoxycorticosterone acetate
destruction
    bony element d.
destructive interference technique
desynchronous
detachable
    d. balloon
    d. coil
    d. silicone balloon
detached
    d. cranial section
    d. craniotomy
detachment
    choroid d.
    ciliochoroid d.
    retinal d.
detector
    phase-sensitive d.
deterioration
    alcoholic d.
determination
    fusion limit d.
detrusor
    d. areflexia
    d. reflex
deutencephalon
devascularized
developmental defect
deviation
    alternating skew d.
    ocular d.
    skew d.
    wrong-way d.
device
    anterior fixation d.
    anterior internal fixation d.
    antisiphon d. (ASD)
    Camino intraparenchymal
        fiberoptic d.
    C-D d.
    C-D instrumentation d.
    d. composition
    Cotrel-Dubousset dynamic
        transverse traction d.
    Dunn d.
    Dwyer d.
    dynamic transverse
        traction d.
    Edwards modular system
        sacral fixation d.
    Edwards sacral fixation d.

Egemen keyhole suction-
control d.
ferromagnetic monitoring d.
fixation d.
fracture fixation d.
Galtac d.
Harrington rod
instrumentation distraction
outrigger d.
head fixation d.
intravascular d.
Kostuik-Harrington d.
newer-generation d.
noise reduction d.
Novo-10a CBF
measuring d.
optical d.
Portnoy DPV d.
Silastic d.
Texas Scottish Rite Hospital
corkscrew d.
Texas Scottish Rite Hospital
mini-corkscrew d.
d. for transverse traction
(DTT)
ultrasonic aspirating d.
Viking II nerve
monitoring d.
Devic's disease
**Dewar posterior cervical fixation
procedure**
dexamethasone
d. suppression test
dextral
dextrality
dextran
dextroamphetamine
dextrocerebral
dextromanual
dextropedal
dextrorotoscoliosis

dextroscoliosis
Dextrostix Uristix
DFMO
dl-alpha-difluoromethylornithine
2DFT
two-dimensional Fourier
transform
2DFT gradient-echo imaging
2DFT GRASS
2DFT time-of-flight MR
angiography
3DFT
three-dimensional Fourier
transform
anisotropic 3DFT
3DFT gradient-echo imaging
3DFT gradient-echo MR
imaging
3DFT GRASS
isotropic 3DFT
diabetes
d. insipidus
d. mellitus
diabetic
d. amyotrophy
d. arthropathy
d. coma
d. myelopathy
d. neuropathy
d. puncture
Diabinese
diacele
diagastric line
diagnosis
intrauterine sonographic d.
noninvasive d.
diagnostic
d. anesthesia
d. apraxia
d. block

NOTES

diagram
    pulse timing d.
dialysis
    d. dementia
    d. encephalopathy syndrome
diamagnetism
diameter
    effective pedicle d.
    effective thread d.
    horizontal pedicle d.
    lumbar spine pedicle d.
    pedicle d.
    sagittal pedicle d.
    thoracic spine pedicle d.
    transpedicular fixation
      effective pedicle d.
    transverse pedicle d.
    vertical pedicle d.
diamond
    d. burr
    d. high-speed air drill
    d. knife
Diamox challenge testing
dianhydrogalactitol (DAG)
diaphemetric
diaphoresis
diaphragm
    d. of sella
diaphragma, pl. diaphragmata
    d. sella
    d. sellae
Diapid
diaplexus
diarrhea
    nocturnal d.
diaschisis
Diasonics magnetic resonance imaging
diastatic skull fracture
diastematocrania
diastematomyelia
diastole-phased pulsatile infusion
diataxia
    cerebral d.
diatela
diathesis
    spasmodic d.
    spasmophilic d.
diazepam
diazoxide
Dibenzyline
Dibromodulcitol (DBD)

DIC
    disseminated intravascular coagulation
Dick AO fixateur interne
dicloxacillin
dicoumarol
diencephala (*pl. of* diencephalon)
diencephalic
    d. astrocytoma
    d. epilepsy
    d. syndrome
    d. syndrome of infancy
    d. vein
diencephalohypophysial
diencephalon, pl. diencephala
diethylene triamine penta-acetic acid (DTPA)
Diferrante's disease
differential
    threshold d.
    d. threshold
differentiation
    retrogressive d.
difficile
    Clostridium d.
diffuse
    d. atrophy
    d. axonal injury
    d. brain injury
    d. cerebral atrophy
    d. cerebral histiocytosis
    d. cerebral sclerosis
    d. disseminated atheroembolism
    d. idiopathic skeletal hyperostosis
    d. infantile familial sclerosis
    d. intrinsic brainstem tumor
    d. necrotizing leukoencephalopathy
diffused reflex
diffusion
    d. imaging
    d. respiration
diffusion-weighted scanning
diffusum
    angiokeratoma corporis d.
difluoromethylornithin
digastric muscle
digital
    d. angiography
    d. intravenous angiography
    d. nerve

d. reflex
d. subtraction angiogram
d. subtraction angiography (DSA)
d. subtraction venography
d. temple massage
d. vascular imaging (DVI)
digitalgia paresthetica
digital-to-analog converter
digitationes hippocampi
digitoxin
digoxin
dihydromorphinone hydrochloride
Dilantin
dilatation
congenital d.
dilated intercavernous sinus
dilation
episcleral vascular d.
junctional d.
Dilaudid
diltiazem
dimeglumine
gadopentetate d.
dimenhydrinate
dimension
Isola spinal implant system d.'s
pedicle d.'s
dimethyl sulfoxide (DMSO)
Dingman oral retraction system
dinitrate
isosorbide d.
dioctyl sodium sulfosuccinate
dioxide
cerebral arterial gas tension of carbon d. (PaCO2)
diphasic milk fever
diphenhydramine
d. hydrochloride
diphenylhydantoin

diphtheriae
Corynebacterium d.
diphtheria, tetanus toxoids, and pertussis vaccine (DTP)
diphtheritic
d. neuropathy
d. paralysis
diphtheroid
diplegia
congenital facial d.
facial d.
infantile d.
masticatory d.
spastic d.
diploë
diploic vein
diplomyelia
diplopia
dipole
d. field
dipole-dipole
d.-d. interaction
d.-d. relaxation
dipotassium
clorazepate d.
dipping
converse ocular d.
ocular d.
dipyridamole
direct
d. auditory compound actional potential
d. brain stimulation (DBS)
d. current (DC)
d. embolectomy
d. fracture
d. multiplanar imaging
d. pyramidal tract
direction
flow d.
phase-encoding d.

NOTES

dirigation
dirigomotor
disability
    reversible ischemic
      neurologic d. (RIND)
disc (*var. of* disk)
Discase
discectomy
    anterior d.
    automated percutaneous
      lumbar d. (APLD)
    cervical d.
    lumbar d.
    thoracic d.
    transthoracic d.
discharge
    waning d.
disci (*pl. of* discus)
discitis
    intervertebral d.
    pyogenic d.
discogenic
    d. sclerosis
discogram
discography
discoid skin lesion
discomfort
    abdominal d.
disconnection syndrome
discontinuity
    Bruch's membrane d.
discopathy
    traumatic cervical d.
discotomy
discrimination
    pure tone d.
discus, pl. disci
    d. lentiformis
disease
    Adams-Stokes d.
    adaptation d.'s
    Addison's d.
    Akureyri d.
    Alexander's d.
    Alpers' d.
    Alzheimer's d.
    aortocranial d.
    Aran-Duchenne d.
    arterial occlusive d.
    atheromatous d.
    atherosclerotic d.
    Australian X d.
    Ayala's d.

    Azorean d.
    Ballet's d.
    Baló's d.
    Bamberger's d.
    Bannister's d.
    Batten-Mayou d.
    Batten's d.
    Baxter's d.
    Bayle's d.
    Bechterew's d.
    Begbie's d.
    Behçet's d.
    Bernard-Soulier d.
    Bernhardt's d.
    Bielschowsky's d.
    Biemond's d.
    Binswanger's d.
    Blocq's d.
    Bourneville-Pringle d.
    Bourneville's d.
    bowel d.
    brain d.
    Brissaud's d.
    Brodie's d.
    Brushfield-Wyatt d.
    Buschke's d.
    Busse-Buschke d.
    Camurati-Engelmann d.
    Canavan's d.
    cardiac d.
    cerebrovascular d.
    cervical spine rheumatoid d.
    Charcot-Marie-Tooth d.
    Charcot's d.
    Christensen-Krabbe d.
    Christmas d.
    Coats' d.
    combined system d.
    connective tissue d.
    coronary artery d.
    Cotunnius d.
    Creutzfeldt-Jakob d.
    Crigler-Najjar d.
    Crohn's d.
    Crouzon's d.
    Cruveilhier's d.
    Cushing's d.
    cytomegalic inclusion d.
    dancing d.
    Danielssen-Boeck d.
    Danielssen's d.
    degenerative d.
    degenerative brain d.

degenerative cervical disk d.
degenerative discogenic end-
  plate d.
degenerative disk d.
Degos d.
Dejerine's d.
Dejerine-Sottas d.
demyelinating d.
Devic's d.
Diferrante's d.
Dubini's d.
Duchenne-Aran d.
Duchenne's d.
Eales' d.
Engelmann's d.
enterococcal d.
Erb-Charcot d.
Erb's d.
Eulenburg's d.
exophytic joint d.
extracranial carotid
  occlusive d.
extracranial occlusive
  vascular d.
extrapyramidal d.
Fabry's d.
Fahr's d.
Feer's d.
Flatau-Schilder d.
Folling's d.
Forestier's d.
Fothergill's d.
Friedmann's d.
Friedreich's d.
Fuerstner's d.
Gaucher's d.
Gerhardt's d.
Gerlier's d.
Gerstmann-Straussler-
  Sheinker d.
Gilles de la Tourette's d.

Glanzmann's d.
Goldflam d.
Gowers d.
Graefe's d.
Graves' d.
Greenfield's d.
Guinon's d.
Hallervorden-Spatz d.
Hammond's d.
Hand-Schüller-Christian d.
Hartnup d.
hepatocerebral d.
hepatolenticular d.
Hippel-Lindau d.
Hippel's d.
Hodgkin's d.
Hoppe-Goldflam d.
Horton's d.
Hunter's d.
Huntington's d.
Hurler's d.
Hurler-Scheie d.
hydatid d.
iatrogenic d.
Iceland d.
infantile Refsum d.
inflammation bowel d.
intradural inflammatory d.
intrinsic d.
ischemic d.
Jakob-Creutzfeldt d.
Jansky-Bielschowsky d.
jumper d., jumper d. of
  Maine
kidney d.
kinky-hair d.
Klippel's d.
Krabbe's d.
Kufs d.
Kugelberg-Welander d.
labyrinthine d.

NOTES

disease *(continued)*
    Lafora body d., Lafora's d.
    L4-5 disk d.
    Leigh's d.
    Letterer-Siwe d.
    Lhermitte-Duclos d.
    Lindau's d.
    Little's d.
    liver d.
    L5-S1 disk d.
    Luft's d.
    lumbar disk d.
    lumbar facet d.
    Lyme d.
    Machado-Joseph d.
    Marchiafava-Bignami d.
    Marie-Strümpell d.
    Maroteaux-Lamy d.
    Ménière's d.
    Merzbacher-Pelizaeus d.
    metastatic d.
    Milton's d.
    Minamata d.
    Mitchell's d.
    Möbius d.
    Morgagni's d.
    Morquio's d.
    Morvan's d.
    motor neuron d.
    moyamoya d.
    multicore d.
    myelinoclastic d.
    Neftel's d.
    neuro-Behçet's d.
    neurodegenerative d.
    Niemann-Pick d.
    nonneoplastic d.
    occlusive d.
    occlusive cerebrovascular d.
    Ollier's d.
    Oppenheim's d.
    Paget's d.
    Parkinson's d.
    Pelizaeus-Merzbacher d.
    periatrial d.
    periventricular d.
    Pette-Döring d.
    Pick's d.
    Portuguese-Azorean d.
    Pott's d.
    pulseless d.
    Quincke's d.
    Recklinghausen's d.

    Refsum's d.
    Rendu-Osler-Weber d.
    rheumatic d.
    rheumatic heart d.
    rheumatoid d.
    Romberg's d.
    Roth-Bernhardt's d.
    Roth's d.
    Roussy-Lévy d.
    Rust's d.
    Sandhoff's d.
    Sanfilippo d.
    Schaumberg's d.
    Scheie's d.
    Scheuermann's d.
    Schilder's d.
    Scholz' d.
    Seitelberger's d.
    Selter's d.
    severe degenerative disk d.
    sickle cell d.
    Siemerling-Creutzfeldt d.
    Sly's d.
    Spielmeyer-Sjögren d.
    Spielmeyer-Vogt d.
    spinal metastatic d.
    Steele-Richardson-
      Olszewski d.
    Steinert's d.
    Stokes-Adams d.
    Strümpell-Marie d.
    Strümpell's d.
    Strümpell-Westphal d.
    Sturge's d.
    Sturge-Weber d.
    Sydenham's d.
    Takayasu's d.
    Talma's d.
    Tay-Sachs d.
    Thomsen's d.
    thoracolumbar
      degenerative d.
    Tourette's d.
    Unverricht's d.
    van Bogaert-Canavan d.
    van Bogaert's d.
    venous occlusive d.
    Virchow's d.
    vitreous d.
    Vogt-Spielmeyer d.
    von Economo's d.
    von Hippel-Lindau d.
    von Recklinghausen's d.

Werdnig-Hoffmann d.
Wernicke's d.
Westphal's d.
white matter d.
Wilson's d.
Winkelman's d.
Wohlfart-Kugelberg-
  Welander d.
Wolman's d.
Ziehen-Oppenheim d.
disengagement mechanism
disequilibrium
dishpan fracture
disjunction
craniofacial d.
disk, disc
d. curette
embryonic d.
free fragment d.
herniated d.
herniated cervical d.
d. herniation
intervertebral d.
intraspinal herniated d.
magnetic d.
Merkel's tactile d.
optic d.
protruded d.
Ranvier's d.'s
d. rongeur
ruptured d.
d. space
d. syndrome
tactile d.
vacuum d.
dislocation
C6-C7 d.
fracture d.
temporomandibular joint d.
dislodgement
hook d.

disodium
carbenicillin d.
d. etidronate
moxalactam d.
disorder
accommodation d.
affect d.
affective d.
attention deficit d.
autoimmune d.
autonomic d.
balance d.
behavioral d.
bleeding d.
breathing d.
choreiform d.
clotting d.
coagulation d.
color vision d.
conduction d.
conversion d.
degenerative d.
eye movement d.
gastrointestinal d.
genetic d.
glycoprotein storage d.
hyperkinetic d.
joint d.
language d.
lipid metabolism d.
lung d.
mastication d.
mitral valve d.
motor d.
mouth d.
movement d.
neoplastic d.
neurogenic d.
neuropsychologic d.
obsessive-compulsive d.
optokinetic d.

NOTES

disorder *(continued)*
    organic brain d.
    organic mental d.
    psychiatric d.
    psychophysiologic d.
    psychosomatic d.
    reading d.
    reflex d.
    respiratory d.
    rheumatoid d.
    sleep d.
    smell d.
    speech d.
    substance abuse d.'s
    substantia nigra d.
    swallowing d.
    taste d.
    traumatic d.
    vestibular d.
    visceral d.
    visual image movement d.
    wakefulness d.
    writing d.
disorganization
    segmental arterial d.
disorientation
    visuospatial d.
dispersion
    intravoxel phase d.
    nuclear magnetic
      relaxation d.
displacement
    significant d.
    spondylolisthesis with
      significant d.
    traumatic d.
disruption
    anterior column d.
    cervical spine posterior
      ligament d.
    pedicle cortex d.
dissecting
    d. aneurysm
    d. basilar artery aneurysm
    d. forceps
dissection
    bone d.
    bone/ligament d.
    bony d.
    carotid artery d.
    condyle d.
    cranial nerve d.
    flank d.

    hard palate d.
    incisural d.
    intradural d.
    jugular vein d.
    middle fossa
      floor/petrous d.
    muscle d.
    nasal d.
    neck d.
    parotid d.
    soft tissue d.
    subperiosteal d.
    subtemporal d.
    suction d.
    sylvian d.
    vertebral d.
dissector
    Freier d.
    Hardy d.
    needle d.
    neural d.
    Olivecrona d.
    Penfield d.
    spatula d.
    teardrop d.
    tissue plane d.
    ultrasonic d.
disseminated
    d. CNS histoplasmosis
    d. encephalomyelitis
    d. intravascular coagulation
    (DIC)
    d. sclerosis
dissociated anesthesia
dissociation
    albuminocytologic d.
    d. sensibility
    sleep d.
    syringomyelic d.
    tabetic d.
dissociative anesthesia
distal
    d. anterior cerebral artery
      aneurysm
    d. carotid
    d. catheter
    d. catheter lengthening
    d. occlusion
    d. part of anterior lobe of
      hypophysis
    d. tingling on percussion
    (DTP)

distance
  d. ceptor
  internodal d. (IND)
  interpedicular d.
  interuncal d.
distant metastasis
distortion
  local field d.
distraction
  apical d.
  d. bar
  d. force
  Harrington d.
  d. instrumentation
  d. instrumentation
    biomechanics
  d. rod
distraction/compression scoliosis
  treatment
distribution
  butterfly d.
  nervous d.
  sensory d.
disturbance
  cognitive d.
  gait d.
  metabolic d.
  psychiatric d.
  speech d.
disulfiram
Ditropan
Diuril
divergence
divergent
diving reflex
Dix-Hallpike test
Dixon method opposed imaging
Dixon's radiofrequency coil
dl-alpha-difluoromethylornithine
DMSO
  dimethyl sulfoxide

DNA
  deoxyribonucleic acid
dobutamine
Dobutrex
docosahexanoic acid
documented pseudarthrosis
Dogiel's
  D. cells
  D. corpuscle
dol
Dolenc technique
dolichoectasia
dolichoectatic artery
doll's
  d. eye maneuver
  d. eye sign
Dolophine
dolor
  d. capitis
dolorific
dolorimetry
dolorogenic zone
dolorology
dolorosa
  analgesia d.
  anesthesia d.
  hypalgesia d.
domain
  analog d.
  particle d.
dominant
  d. frequency
  d. hemisphere
domperidone
Doose syndrome
dopamine hydrochloride
dopaminergic
Doppler
  color-flow D.
  continuous-wave D.
  D. effect

NOTES

Doppler *(continued)*
    D. frequency spectrum
    D. imaging
    D. monitoring
    D. precordial end-tidal
      carbon dioxide monitoring
    D. probe
    pulsed D.
    pulse wave D.
    D. sonography
    transcranial D.
    D. ultrasound monitor
Dorello's canal
dorsal
    d. accessory olivary nucleus
    d. column of spinal cord
    d. column stimulation
    d. cord stimulation (DCS)
    d. enteric fistula
    d. funiculus
    d. horn
    d. longitudinal fasciculus
    d. mesencephalic syndrome
    d. midbrain syndrome
    d. motor nucleus of vagus
    d. nucleus
    d. nucleus of vagus
    d. part of pons
    d. plate of neural tube
    d. rami
    d. reflex
    d. rhizotomy
    d. root
    d. root entry zone (DREZ)
    d. root entry zone lesion
    d. root entry zone lesioning
    d. root ganglion
    d. scapular nerve
    d. spine
    d. spinocerebellar tract
    d. tegmental decussation
dorsum of foot reflex
Dorsey dural separator
dorsolateral
    d. fasciculus
    d. tract
dorsomedial
    d. hypothalamic nucleus
    d. mesencephalic syndrome
    d. nucleus
dorsum pedis reflex
dose
    equivalent d. (ED)

dosimetry
dot
    line frequency noise d.
dotage
dotardness
double
    d. athetosis
    d. compartment
      hydrocephalus
    d. congenital athetosis
    d. curve scoliosis
    d. fishhook retractor
    d. fragment sign
    d. hemiplegia
    d. major curve pattern
    d. major curve scoliosis
    d. thoracic curve
    d. thoracic curve scoliosis
    d. vision
    d. Zielke instrumentation
double-L
    d.-L rod
    d.-L spinal rod
double-lumen Swan-Ganz catheter
double-point threshold
double-pore vent system
double-rod
    d.-r. construct
    d.-r. technique
double-vector
    d.-v. blade
    d.-v. brain spatula
douloureux
    tic d.
dowel cutter
downbeat nystagmus
downbiting Epstein curette
downsized circular laminar hook
Down's syndrome
downward gaze paresis
doxepin hydrochloride
doxorubicin
    d. hydrochloride
doxycycline
Doyen rib spreader
Doyère's eminence
DR
    reaction of degeneration
dracunculiasis
drain
    Hemovac d.
    Jackson-Pratt d.

Penrose d.
subgaleal d.
drainage
burr hole d.
external ventricular d.
lumbar d.
serial percutaneous
    needle d.
spinal d.
stereotactic catheter d.
ventricular d.
draining vein
Drake
D. clip
D. tourniquet
Drake-Kees clip
Drake's
D. fenestrated clip
D. tandem clipping
    technique
Dramamine
draping
drawing
pain d.
dream pain
dreamy state
Dressing
DuoDerm D.
dressing
d. forceps
OpSite d.
surgical d.
DREZ
dorsal root entry zone
DREZ lesioning
DREZ procedure
DREZ surgery
Dridol
drill
air d.
air-powered d.

Anspach d.
Anspach 65K d.
Caspar d.
Codman d.
diamond high-speed air d.
electric d.
Fisch d.
d. guide
Hall Surgairtome II d.
Hudson d.
Midas Rex d.
power d.
right-angle d.
twist d.
drilling technique
drip chamber
drive
kinetic d.
driver's thigh
driving
photic d.
dromic
drop
d. attack
d. foot
d. hand
d. metastasis
drop-entry (closed body) hook
droperidol
drowsiness
drug
d. abuse
d. fever
d. infusion pump
nonsteroidal anti-
    inflammatory d. (NSAID)
d. reaction
d. tetanus
d. toxicity
drug-induced anemia

NOTES

Drummond's spinous wiring technique
drusen
dry

    d. beriberi
    d. eye syndrome
    d. leprosy
    d. mouth

DSA

    digital subtraction angiography

DT

    delirium tremens
    duration tetany

DTP

    diphtheria, tetanus toxoids, and pertussis vaccine
    distal tingling on percussion

DTPA

    diethylene triamine penta-acetic acid
        gadolinium DTPA

DTT

    device for transverse traction
        DTT implant

dual

    d. bypass connectors
    d. compression scoliosis treatment

dual-isotope SPECT
Duane's retraction syndrome
Dubini's disease
Duchenne-Aran disease
Duchenne-Erb paralysis
Duchenne's

    D. disease
    D. dystrophy
    D. muscular dystrophy
    D. paralysis
    D. sign
    D. syndrome

duck-billed anodized spatula
Duckworth's phenomenon
duct

    cochlear d.
    endolymphatic d.
    Hensen's d.
    lacrimal d.
    parotid d.
    perilymphatic d.
    semicircular d.'s
    Stensen's d.

    uniting d.
    utriculosaccular d.

ductus, gen. and pl. ductus

    d. cochlearis
    d. endolymphaticus
    d. perilymphaticus
    d. reuniens
    d. semicirculares
    d. semicircularis anterior
    d. semicircularis lateralis
    d. semicircularis posterior
    d. utriculosaccularis

dumbbell ganglioneuroma
dumbell-shaped spinal cavernous hemangioma
Duncan's

    D. syndrome
    D. ventricle

Dunn device
duodenal ulcer
DuoDerm Dressing
duplex

    d. scanning
    d. transmission

duplication anomaly
Dura

    Tutoplast D.

dura

    lyophilized d.
    d. mater

dural

    d. arteriovenous fistula
    d. arteriovenous malformation
    d. ectasia
    d. incision
    d. margins
    d. ring
    d. sheath
    d. sinus
    d. sinus occlusion
    d. tail
    d. venous sinus

dura mater

    d. m. of the brain
    d. m. encephali
    d. m. of the spinal cord
    d. m. spinalis

duramatral
duraplasty
duration tetany (DT)
Dürck's nodes
Duret hemorrhage

Duret's lesion
dust
    angel d.
    bone d.
Duvol lung clamp
DVI
    digital vascular imaging
dwarfism
    pituitary d.
Dwyer
    D. device
    D. instrument
    D. instrumentation
      biomechanics
Dymelor
dynamic
    d. bed
    d. compression plate
      instrumentation
    flow d.'s
    d. single photon emission
      computed tomography
    d. transverse traction device
dynamometer
Dynapen
dynorphin
dysacusis
dysantigraphia
dysaphia
dysaphic
dysarthria
    d. literalis
    d. syllabaris spasmodica
dysarthria-clumsy hand syndrome
dysarthric
dysarthrosis
dysautonomia
    familial d.
dysbasia
    d. lordotica progressiva
dyscalculia

dyscheiral, dyschiral
dyscheiria, dyschiria
dyschiria
dyschromatopsia
    cerebral d.
dyscinesia
dyscoimesis
dysconjugate movement
dyscontrol
dysdiadochokinesia,
    dysdiadochocinesia
dyserethism
dysergia
dysesthesia
dysfunction
    autonomic d.
    hypothalamic-pituitary d.
    lacrimal gland d.
    mental d.
    minimal brain d.
    oculosympathetic d.
    pituitary d.
    salivary gland d.
dysgenesis
    cerebellar vermis d.
    cingulate gyrus d.
    corpus callosum d.
dysgeusia
dysgnosia
dysgranular cortex
dysgraphia
dyskinesia
    d. algera
    biliary d.
    extrapyramidal d.'s
    tardive d.
    tardive oral d.
dyskinetic
dyslexia
dyslexic
dyslogia

NOTES

dysmegalopsia
dysmetria
    ocular d.
dysmnesic
    d. psychosis
    d. syndrome
dysmorphia
    cranial d.
dysmyelination
dysmyotonia
dysnystaxis
dysostosis
    craniofacial d.
dyspallia
dysphagia
dysphasia
    Broca's d.
dysphonia
    d. spastica
dysphrasia
dysplasia
    bony d.
    cerebral d.
    craniofrontonasal d.
    fibromuscular d.
    fibrous d.
    odontoid d.
    septo-optic d.
dysplastic gangliocytoma
dyspraxia
dysprosium-DTPA
dysraphism
    craniofacial d.
    occult spinal d.
    spinal d.
dysrhythmia
    electroencephalographic d.
    paroxysmal cerebral d.
dyssomnia
dysspondylism
dyssynergia
    d. cerebellaris myoclonica
    d. cerebellaris progressiva
dystaxia

dystonia
    d. lenticularis
    d. musculorum deformans
    torsion d.
dystonic
    d. choreoathetosis
    d. reaction
    d. torticollis
dystopia
    orbital d.
dystrophia
    d. adiposogenitalis
    d. myotonica
dystrophoneurosis
dystrophy
    adiposogenital d.
    adult pseudohypertrophic
      muscular d.
    Barnes' d.
    Becker's muscular d.
    Becker-type tardive
      muscular d.
    childhood muscular d.
    congenital muscular d.
    Duchenne's d.
    Duchenne's muscular d.
    facioscapulohumeral
      muscular d.
    Fukuyama-type congenital
      muscular d.
    infantile neuroaxonal d.
    Landouzy-Dejerine d.
    Leyden-Möbius muscular d.
    limb-girdle muscular d.
    muscular d.
    myotonic d.
    myotonic muscular d.
    neuroaxonal d.
    pelvofemoral muscular d.
    progressive muscular d.
    pseudohypertrophic
      muscular d.
    reflex sympathetic d.
    sympathetic reflex d.

EAE
  experimental allergic
    encephalitis
Eagle's minimum essential medium
Eagle syndrome
Eales' disease
ear cartilage inflammation
Earle's salts
early posttraumatic epilepsy
East
  E. African sleeping sickness
  E. African trypanosomiasis
**eastern equine encephalomyelitis
  (EEE)**
eating epilepsy
ECA
  external carotid artery
ECA-PCA bypass surgery
ecchondrosis
  e. physaliformis, e.
    physaliphora
ecchymosis
  periorbital e.
eccrine
  e. cystadenoma
  e. gland
echinococcosis
echo
  gradient e.
  Hahn e.
  radiofrequency-induced e.
  e. reaction
  e. speech
  e. time (TE)
  T1-weighted spin e.
  T2-weighted spin e.
echocardiogram
  bubble e.
echocardiography
  transesophageal e.
echoencephalography
echographia
echokinesis, echokinesia
echolalia
echomatism
echomimia
echomotism
echopathy
echophrasia
echoplanar imaging

echopraxia
eclampsia
  puerperal e.
eclamptic
eclamptogenic, eclamptogenous
ECoG
  electrocorticogram
  electrocorticography
  ECoG monitoring
ECS
  electrocerebral silence
E2CS
  Edinburgh 2 Coma Scale
ecstasy
ecstatic
ectal origin
ectasia
  dural e.
ectoderm
  neural e.
ectopia
  cerebellar e.
  posterior pituitary gland e.
ectopic
  e. ACTH syndrome
  e. pinealoma
ectoretina
ectropion
ED
  equivalent dose
EDAS
  encephaloduroarteriosynangiosis
eddy
  e. current
  e. current heating
edema
  airway e.
  angioneurotic e.
  blue e.
  brain e.
  brainstem e.
  cerebral e.
  circumscribed e.
  cytotoxic e.
  hereditary angioneurotic e.
    (HANE)
  periodic e.
  Quincke's e.
  retroauricular e.

edge enhancement
Edinburgh 2 Coma Scale (E2CS)
Edinger-Westphal nucleus
EDRF
    endothelium-derived relaxing
    factor
edrophonium
    e. chloride
    e. chloride test
Edwards
    E. instrumentation
    E. modular system
    E. modular system bridging
    sleeve construct
    E. modular system
    compression construct
    E. modular system construct
    selection
    E. modular system
    distraction-lordosis
    construct
    E. modular system dynamic
    loading
    E. modular system
    kyphoreduction construct
    E. modular system load
    sharing
    E. modular system
    neutralization construct
    E. modular system rod
    crosslink
    E. modular system rod-
    sleeve construct
    E. modular system sacral
    fixation device
    E. modular system scoliosis
    construct
    E. modular system spinal
    rod-sleeve
    E. modular system
    spinal/sacral screw
    E. modular system spondylo
    construct
    E. modular system standard
    sleeve construct
    E. modular system universal
    rod
    E. sacral fixation device
    E. sacral screw
    E. spinal/sacral screw
EEE
    eastern equine encephalomyelitis

EEG
    electroencephalogram
    electroencephalography
    EEG activation
effect
    adverse side e.
    blast e.
    Bohr e.
    clasp-knife e.
    Cushing e.
    Doppler e.
    flow e.
    inflow e.
    magnetohydrodynamic e.
    missile e.
    muscarinic e.
    Orbeli e.
    phase e.
    phase-shift e.
    radiation e.'s
    side e.
    susceptibility e.
    sympathectomy e.
    time-of-flight e.
    Vulpian's e.
effected pain
effective
    e. pedicle diameter
    e. thread diameter
effectiveness
    relative biological e. (RBE)
effector
    e. cell
efferent
    gamma e.
    e. nerve
efficacy study
efficiency
    colony-forming e. (CFE)
effort syndrome
Egemen keyhole suction-control
   device
egersis
eggcrate mattress
Ehlers-Danlos syndrome
Ehrenritter's ganglion
Eichhorst's neuritis
eicosapentaenoic acid
eighth
    e. cranial nerve
    e. nerve herpetic neuritis
    e. nerve neuritis
    e. nerve tumor

Eisenhardt
Eisenlohr's syndrome
eisodic
ejection fraction
Ekbom syndrome
elasticity
elasticum
     pseudoxanthoma e.
Elavil
elbow
     e. jerk
     e. reflex
elective mutism
electric
     e. chorea
     e. drill
     e. knife
     e. shock
     e. sleep
electrical stimulation
electroanalgesia
electroaxonography
electrocautery
electrocerebral silence (ECS)
electrocoagulation
     RF e.
electrocoagulator
electrocochleogram
electrocontractility
electroconvulsive
electrocorticogram (ECoG)
electrocorticography (ECoG)
electrode
     active surface e.
     combination needle e.
     curved e.
     El-Naggar-Nashold right-
       angled nucleus caudalis
       DREZ e.
     e. migration
     monopolar e.

     needle e.
     straight needle e.
     subdural grid e.
     subdural strip e.
     wolfram needle e.
electrodetachable
     e. balloon
     e. platinum coil
electrodiagnostic testing
electroencephalogram (EEG)
     flat e., isoelectric e.
electroencephalograph
electroencephalographic
     e. burst-suppression
     e. dysrhythmia
electroencephalography (EEG)
electromagnetic
     e. flow meter
     e. flow probe
electromicturation
electromuscular sensibility
electromyelography
electromyogram (EMG)
electromyographic (EMG)
     e. response
electromyography
     facial e.
     needle e.
electron
     e. micrograph
     e. microscopy
electron-coupled nuclear spin-spin
   interaction
electroneurogram (ENoG)
electroneurography
     facial e.
electroneurolysis
electroneuromyography
electronystagmography (ENG)
electropathology

NOTES

electrophoresis
    agarose gel e.
    thin-layer agarose gel e.
electrophrenic
    e. respiration
electrophysiological
    e. guidance
    e. mapping
    e. stimulation
electroretinography
electroshock
electrospectrography
electrospinogram
electrospinography
electrostimulation
electrotherapeutic
    e. sleep
    e. sleep therapy
electrothrombosis
electrotonic
    e. junction
    e. synapse
electrotonus
elephantiasis
    e. neuromatosa
elevation
    flap e.
    e. paresis
elevator
    Cloward e.
    Cobb e.
    Cobb periosteal e.
    Jarit periosteal e.
    Langenbach e.
    periosteal e.
    round-tipped periosteal e.
eleventh cranial nerve
elfin facies
Elgiloy
    E. clip
    E. clip material
ELISA
    enzyme-linked immunosorbent
    assay
El-Naggar-Nashold right-angled
   nucleus caudalis DREZ electrode
emarginate
emargination
embolalia
embolectomy
    direct e.
emboli (pl. of embolus)
embolic apoplexy

emboliform
    e. nucleus
embolism
    air e.
    artery-to-artery e.
    cardiac e.
    cerebral e.
    cholesterol e.
    fat e.
    paradoxic e.
    paradoxical air e. (PAE)
    paradoxical cerebral e.
    pulmonary e.
    retinal e.
    therapeutic e.
    venous e.
embolization
    cerebral foreign body e.
    coil e.
    flow-directed e.
    particulate e.
    percutaneous intra-arterial e.
    selective e.
    staged e.
    therapeutic e.
    transarterial platinum coil e.
    transtorcular e.
embolalia
embolophasia
embolophrasia
embolotherapy
embolus, pl. emboli
    air e.
    calcium e.
    cerebral e.
    fat e.
    fibrin-platelet-fibrin e.
    Gelfoam powder emboli
    organism e.
    platelet-fibrin e.
    septic e.
embryogenesis
embryology
embryonic
    e. cervical somite
    e. disk
emergence
emerogene
EMG
    electromyogram
    electromyographic
    EMG biofeedback
    EMG stimulator

eminence
    collateral e.
    Doyère's e.
    facial e.
    hypoglossal e.
    malar e.
    medial e.
    median e.
    olivary e.
    restiform e.
    round e.
    thenar e.
eminentia, pl. **eminentiae**
    e. abducentis
    e. collateralis
    e. facialis
    e. hypoglossi
    e. medialis
    e. mediana
    e. restiformis
    e. teres
emissary vein
emission computed tomography
emphysema
    subgaleal e.
emprosthotonos
empty
    e. delta sign
    e. sella
    e. sella sign
    e. sella syndrome
    e. triangle sign
empyema
EMV
    eyes, motor, voice/verbal
enanthate
    testosterone e.
encephala (*pl. of* encephalon)
encephalalgia
encephalatrophic
encephalatrophy

encephalauxe
encéphale isolé
encephalemia
encephalic
    e. angioma
    e. vesicle
encephalitic
encephalitides
encephalitis, pl. **encephalitides**
    acute hemorrhagic e.
    acute necrotizing e.
    Australian X e.
    bunyavirus e.
    California e.
    Coxsackie e.
    Dawson's e.
    epidemic e.
    experimental allergic e.
    (EAE)
    Far East Russian e.
    fulminant necrotizing e.
    e. hemorrhagica
    herpes e.
    herpes simplex e.
    hyperergic e.
    Ilhéus e.
    inclusion body e.
    Japanese B e.
    e. japonica
    lead e.
    e. lethargica
    Mengo e.
    Murray Valley e.
    necrotizing e.
    e. neonatorum
    e. periaxialis concentrica
    e. periaxialis diffusa
    postvaccinal e.
    Powassan e.
    purulent e.
    e. pyogenica

NOTES

encephalitis *(continued)*
Russian autumn e.
Russian spring-summer e.
(Eastern subtype)
Russian spring-summer e.
(Western subtype)
Russian tick-borne e.
secondary e.
subacute inclusion body e.
e. subcorticalis chronica
suppurative e.
tick-borne e. (Central
European subtype)
tick-borne e. (Eastern
subtype)
varicella e.
vernal e.
von Economo's e.
woodcutter's e.
encephalitogen
encephalitogenic
encephalization
encephalocele
anterior basal e.
frontoethmoidal e.
frontosphenoidal e.
nasoethmoidal e.
nasofrontal e.
naso-orbital e.
occipital e.
orbital e.
parietal e.
sphenoid e.
transsphenoidal e.
encephaloclastic microcephaly
**encephaloduroarteriosynangiosis
(EDAS)**
encephalodynia
encephalodysplasia
encephalogram
encephalography
encephaloid
encephalolith
encephalology
encephaloma
encephalomalacia
cystic e.
encephalomeningitis
encephalomeningocele
encephalomeningopathy
encephalometer
encephalomyelitis
acute disseminated e.

benign myalgic e.
disseminated e.
eastern equine e. (EEE)
epidemic myalgic e.
experimental allergic e.
granulomatous e.
Venezuelan equine e. (VEE)
virus e.
western equine e. (WEE)
zoster e.
encephalomyelocele
encephalomyeloneuropathy
nonspecific e.
encephalomyelonic axis
encephalomyelopathy
carcinomatous e.
epidemic myalgic e.
mitochondrial e.
necrotizing e.
paracarcinomatous e.
encephalomyeloradiculitis
encephalomyeloradiculopathy
encephalomyocarditis
encephalomyopathy
mitochondrial e.
encephalomyosynangiosis
encephalon, pl. encephala
encephalonarcosis
encephalopathia
e. addisonia
encephalopathy
bilirubin e.
Binswanger's e.
demyelinating e.
familial e.
hepatic e.
hypernatremic e.
hypertensive e.
lead e.
metabolic e.
mitochondrial e.
palindromic e.
pancreatic e.
portal-systemic e.
progressive subcortical e.
recurrent e.
saturnine e.
spongiform e.
spongiform virus e.
subacute spongiform e.
subcortical arteriosclerotic e.
thyrotoxic e.
traumatic e.

traumatic progressive e.
Wernicke-Korsakoff e.
Wernicke's e.
encephalopsy
encephalopyosis
encephalorrhachidian
encephalorrhagia
encephaloschisis
encephalosclerosis
encephaloscope
encephaloscopy
encephalosis
encephalospinal
encephalothlipsis
encephalotome
encephalotomy
encephalotrigeminal
    e. angiomatosis
    e. vascular syndrome
encoding
    frequency e.
    phase e.
end
    e. bulb
    e. organ
    e. plate
endarterectomy
    carotid e.
endbrain
end-brush
endemic
    e. neuritis
    e. paralytic vertigo
end-feet
ending
    annulospiral e.
    calyciform e., caliciform e.
    epilemmal e.
    flower-spray e.
    free nerve e.'s

    grape e.'s
    hederiform e.
    nerve e.
    sole-plate e.
    synaptic e.'s
endoaneurysmoplasty
endoaneurysmorrhaphy
endocarditis
    bacterial e.
    infective e.
    marantic e.
endoceliac
endocrine-inactive pituitary adenoma
endocrine system
endocrinological compromise
endocrinopathy
endodermal sinus
endogenous fibers
endolymphatic
    e. duct
    e. sac
endomeninx
endoneuritis
endoneurium
endonuclease
    restriction e.
endoperineuritis
end organ
endorphin
endorphinergic
endorrhachis
endoscopic
    e. sinus surgery
    e. sphenoidal biopsy
endoscopy
    intraventricular e.
endothelial injury
endothelin

NOTES

endothelin-1 platinum-Dacron
microcoil
endothelium-derived relaxing factor
(EDRF)
endotracheal tube
endovascular
e. balloon occlusion
e. technique
e. therapy
e. treatment
endplate, end-plate
motor e.
end-tidal nitrogen monitoring
end-to-end anastomosis
endyma
energy requirement
enervation
enflurane
ENG
electronystagmography
Engelmann's disease
engram
engraphia
enhancement
contrast e.
edge e.
gadolinium e.
MR imaging with
gadolinium e.
nodular e.
paramagnetic contrast e.
relaxation rate e.
selective relaxation e.
vertebral end-plate e.
enhancing ring
enkephalin
enkephalinergic
enlargement
cervical e. of spinal cord
lumbar e. of spinal cord
moyamoya collateral e.
sulcal e.
ENoG
electroneurogram
enophthalmos
en plaque meningioma
Ensure Plus
ental origin
Entamoeba histolytica
entasia, entasis
entatic
enteral alimentation
enteric cyst

entering roots
enteritis
regional e.
enterococcal disease
enterogastric reflex
enteropathic arthritis
enthlasis
entoderm
entoretina
entorhinal area
entrapment
median nerve e.
nerve e.
e. neuropathy
entropion
entry
e. point
e. zone
e. zone lesion
enucleation
eye e.
enucleator
Hardy microsurgical e.
enuresis
nocturnal e.
enuretic absence
environmental factor
enzyme
Hind III e.
enzyme-linked immunosorbent
assay (ELISA)
eosinophil adenoma
eosinophilic
e. granuloma
e. granulomastosis
e. meningoencephalitis
ependyma
ventricular e.
ependymal
e. cell
e. cyst
e. layer
e. zone
ependymitis
e. granularis
ependymoblastoma
ependymocyte
ependymoma
exophytic e.
myxopapillary e.
sacrococcygeal
myxopapillary e.
spinal e.

subcutaneous sacrococcygeal
   myxopapillary e.
ephapse
ephaptic
ephedrine sulfate
epicondylectomy
   medial e.
epicranium
epicritic
   e. sensibility
epidemic
   e. cerebrospinal meningitis
   e. encephalitis
   e. myalgic encephalomyelitis
   e. myalgic
    encephalomyelopathy
   e. neuromyasthenia
   e. tetany
   e. vertigo
epidermal
   e. growth factor
   e. necrolysis
epidermoid
   chiasmal e.
   e. cyst
   e. lipoma
   e. tumor
epidural
   e. abscess
   e. abscess evacuation
   e. angiolipoma
   e. block
   e. cavernous hemangioma
   e. cavity
   e. hematoma
   e. infection
   e. injection
   e. meningitis
   e. pneumatosis
   e. pneumocephalus
   e. space

   e. steroid injection
   e. tumor
   e. tumor evacuation
   e. venous plexus
epidurography
epigastric reflex
epilemma
epilemmal ending
epilepsia
   e. nutans
   e. partialis continua
epilepsy
   activated e.
   akinetic e.
   anosognosic e.
   atonic e.
   audiogenic e.
   automatic e.
   autonomic e.
   centrencephalic e.
   chronic partial e.
   complex precipitated e.
   cortical e.
   diencephalic e.
   early posttraumatic e.
   eating e.
   focal e.
   generalized tonic-clonic e.
   grand mal e.
   idiopathic e.
   e. implant
   intractable e.
   jacksonian e.
   juvenile myoclonic e.
   Kojewnikoff's e.
   Lafora's familial
    myoclonic e.
   laryngeal e.
   late e.
   local e.
   major e.

NOTES

epilepsy *(continued)*
    masked e.
    matutinal e.
    myoclonic astatic e.
    myoclonus e.
    nocturnal e.
    partial e.
    pattern sensitive e.
    petit mal e.
    photogenic e.
    posttraumatic e.
    primary generalized e.
    procursive e.
    psychomotor e.
    reflex e.
    rolandic e.
    secondary generalized e.
    sensory e.
    sensory precipitated e.
    sleep e.
    somnambulic e.
    startle e.
    e. surgery
    symptomatic e.
    tardy e.
    temporal lobe e.
    tonic e.
    tornado e.
    uncinate e.
    vasomotor e.
    vasovagal e.
    visceral e.
epileptic
    e. absence
    e. dementia
    e. focus
epilepticus
    status e.
epileptiform
    e. neuralgia
epileptogenic, epileptogenous
    e. zone
epileptoid
epileptologist
epiloia
epinephrine
epinephrine-anesthetic mixture
epineural
epineurectomy
epineurial
epineurium
epineurolysis
epiphora

epiphysiopathy
epiphysis, pl. **epiphyses**
    e. cerebri
epipial
episcleral vascular dilation
episcleritis
episodic
    e. apnea
    e. paroxysmal hemicrania
    e. syndrome
epispinal
epistaxis
epithalamus
epithelial
    e. choroid layer
    e. lamina
epithelioma
epitheliopathy
    multifocal placoid
      pigment e.
    placoid pigment e.
    retinal pigment e.
epithelium
    retinal pigment e.
epsilon-aminocaproic acid
epsilon opiate receptor
Epstein curette
Epstein's
    E. staging system
    E. symptom
e-PTFE
    expanded
    polytetrafluoroethylene
    e-PTFE ventricular catheter
    e-PTFE ventricular shunt
      catheter
Equanil
equation
    Bloch e.
    Larmor e.
    Poiseuille e.
    Solomon-Bloembergen e.
equilibrium
equina
    cauda e.
equine gait
equipment
    decompression e.
    insertion e.
    stainless steel e.
    Vitallium e.
equivalent dose (ED)
Erb-Charcot disease

Erb's
    E. atrophy
    E. disease
    E. palsy
    E. paralysis
    E. point
    E. sign
    E. spinal paralysis
Erb-Westphal sign
Erdheim tumor
erector-spinal reflex
erethism
erethismic, erethistic, erethitic
Ergomar
ergonomic
ergonovine
Ergostat
ergotamine
    e. tartrate
    e. tartrate and caffeine
ergotropic
erosion
    vascular e.
error
    frequency e.
erythema multiforme
erythematosus
    lupus e.
    systemic lupus e. (SLE)
erythermalgia
erythralgia
erythredema polyneuritis
erythroblastosis fetalis
erythrocyte sedimentation rate
erythrocytosis
erythroderma
erythromelalgia
erythromycin
erythroprosopalgia
escape phenomenon
eschar

Escherichia coli
Escherich's sign
ESEP
    extreme somatosensory evoked
    potential
Esidrix
esmolol
esodic
    e. nerve
esoethmoiditis
esophageal
    e. achalasia
    e. airway
    e. perforation
esophagosalivary reflex
esotropia
essential
    e. anosmia
    e. tremor
ESSF
    external spinal skeletal fixator
Essick's cell bands
esthematology
esthesia
esthesic
esthesiodic
    e. system
esthesiogenesis
esthesiogenic
esthesiography
esthesiology
esthesiometer
esthesiometry
esthesioneuroblastoma
    olfactory e.
esthesioneurocytoma
esthesioneurosis
esthesionosus
esthesiophysiology
esthesioscopy
esthesodic

NOTES

esthetic
estradiol
    ethinyl e.
estrogen
état
    e. criblé
etat lacunaire
ethacrynic acid
ethanol
ether
    e. convulsion
    e. screen
Ethicon Ligaclip
ethinyl estradiol
ethmoidal osteotomy
ethmoidectomy
ethmoid sinus
ethopropazine
ethosuximide
ethylene vinyl alcohol copolymer
  liquid
etidocaine
etidronate
    disodium e.
etomidate
    e. injection
eugnosia
Eulenburg's disease
eumetria
euosmia
eupraxia
eurycephalic, eurycephalous
eutonic
evacuation
    CT-guided stereotactic e.
    epidural abscess e.
    epidural tumor e.
    hematoma e.
    transsphenoidal e.
evagination
evaluation
    neurologic e.
    pedicle e.
    preoperative e.
even-echo rephasing
eversion
    cingulate gyrus e.
evisceroneurotomy
EVM grading of Glasgow Coma
  Scale

evoked
    e. potential
    e. response
Ewald-Hudson forceps
Ewing's sarcoma
examination
    tangent screen e.
Excedrin
exchange
    blood gas e.
    e. force
excision
    C2-C3 cervical disk e.
    cervical disk e.
    extratemporal e.
    retropulsed bone e.
excitability test
excitable area
excitations
    number of e. (NEX)
excitomotor
excitoreflex nerve
excitor nerve
excyclotorsion
exencephalia
exencephalic
exencephalocele
exencephalous
exencephaly
exenteration
exercises
    Cawthorne-Cooksey
      vestibular e.
Exner's plexus
exodic nerve
exogenous fibers
exophthalmos
exophytic
    e. ependymoma
    e. joint disease
exorbitism
exostosis
exotropia
    paralytic pontine e.
expanded polytetrafluoroethylene (e-
  PTFE)
expansion
    field e.
    volume e.
expenditure
    caloric e.

experimental
  e. allergic encephalitis
    (EAE)
  e. allergic encephalomyelitis
expiratory center
explosive speech
exposure
  anterior surgical e.
  bone e.
  bony e.
  extradural e.
  half-and-half e.
  e. keratopathy
  middle fossa e.
  midline e.
  surgical e.
  thoracolumbar junction
    surgical e.
  thoracolumbar spine
    anterior e.
  upper cervical spine
    anterior e.
  vertebral e.
expressed skull fracture
expressive aphasia
extended
  e. sector ultrasonic probe
  e. subfrontal approach
extension
  cranial e.
  e. injury
  e. injury posterior
    atlantoaxial arthrodesis
  intrasellar e.
  radiolucent operating room
    table e.
  subependymal e.
extension-type cervical spine injury
extensive
  e. neoplasm
  e. posterior decompression

extensor tetanus
external
  e. arcuate fibers
  e. bracing
  e. capsule
  e. carotid artery (ECA)
  e. collimator
  e. cuneate nucleus
  e. hydrocephalus
  e. intercostal muscle
  e. malleolar sign
  e. meningitis
  e. oblique reflex
  e. pillar cells
  e. pyocephalus
  e. spinal fixation
  e. spinal skeletal fixator
    (ESSF)
  e. support
  e. ventricular drainage
exteroceptive
exteroceptor
exterofective
  e. system
extinction phenomenon
extraaxial cavernous hemangioma
extracerebral cavernous angioma
**extracorporeal membrane
  oxygenation**
extracranial
  e. carotid occlusive disease
  e. mass lesion
  e. occlusive vascular disease
  e. pneumatocele
  e. pneumocele
extracranial-intracranial
  e.-i. bypass
  e.-i. bypass surgery
extradural
  e. clinoidectomy
  e. cyst

NOTES

extradural *(continued)*
  e. exposure
  e. hematorrhachis
  e. hemorrhage
  e. phase
  e. space
  e. tumor
  e. vertebral artery
extraintracranial bypass
extraocular muscle involvement
extrapineal pinealoma
extrapyramidal
  e. disease
  e. dyskinesias
  e. motor system
  e. nucleus
  e. syndrome
extratemporal excision
extreme
  e. capsule
  e. lateral transcondylar
    approach

  e. narrowing limit
  e. somatosensory evoked
    potential (ESEP)
extremity
  anterior e. of caudate
    nucleus
extrusion
  bone graft e.
  wire e.
extubation
  postoperative e.
eye
  e. enucleation
  e. movement disorder
  e. muscle weakness
  raccoon e.'s
  redness of e.
eye-closure reflex
eyelash sign
eyes, motor, voice/verbal (EMV)

F

Fabry's disease
face
    masklike f.
facet, facette
    f. excision technique
    f. fracture stabilization
      wiring
    f. hypertrophy
    f. joint
    f. joint preparation
    locked f.'s
    f. replacement
    f. rhizotomy
    f. subluxation stabilization
      wiring
    f. syndrome
    f. wiring
facetectomy
    partial f.
facial
    f. artery
    f. colliculus
    f. contusion
    f. diplegia
    f. electromyography
    f. electroneurography
    f. eminence
    f. fracture
    f. habit spasm
    f. hematoma
    f. hemiatrophy
    f. hemiplegia
    f. hillock
    f. motor nucleus
    f. myokymia
    f. nerve
    f. neuralgia
    f. neuroma
    f. neuropathy
    f. osteosynthesis
    f. pain
    f. palsy
    f. paralysis
    f. reanimation
    f. reflex
    f. root
    f. spasm
    f. tattoo
    f. tic

    f. trophoneurosis
    f. vision
facialis phenomenon
facies, pl. facies
    elfin f.
    Hutchinson's f.
    f. inferior cerebri
    f. inferior hemispherii
      cerebelli
    mask f.
    f. medialis cerebri
    myasthenic f.
    myopathic f.
    Parkinson's f.
    f. superior hemispherii
      cerebelli
    f. superolateralis cerebri
facilitation
    Wedensky f.
faciocephalalgia
faciocephalic pain
faciolingual
facioplegia
facioscapulohumeral
    f. atrophy
    f. muscular dystrophy
factor-α
    recombinant human tumor
      necrosis f.
factor
    biomechanical f.
    endothelium-derived
      relaxing f. (EDRF)
    environmental f.
    epidermal growth f.
    fibroblast growth f.
    growth f.
    Hageman f.
    plasma f.
    platelet activating f.
    platelet-derived growth f.
    rheumatoid f.
    Stuart-Power f.
Fahr's
    F. disease
    F. syndrome
failed
    f. back surgery syndrome
    (FBSS)
    f. back syndrome

failed *(continued)*
    f. back syndrome with
      documented pseudarthrosis
failure
    chronic acquired hepatic f.
    congestive heart f.
    fatigue f.
    Harrington rod
      instrumentation f.
    hepatic f.
    instrumentation f.
    metal f.
    myoglobinuric renal f.
    renal f.
    spinal implant load to f.
faint
falcate
falces (*pl. of* falx)
falcial
falciform
    f. crest
    f. lobe
falcine
Falconer lobectomy
Falcon plastic flask
falcula
falcular
falling sickness
fallopian neuritis
false neuroma
falx, pl. **falces**
    f. cerebelli
    f. cerebri
familial
    f. aggregation
    f. amyloid neuropathy
    f. amyloidosis
    f. dysautonomia
    f. encephalopathy
    f. glioma
    f. hemiplegic migraine
    f. hypercholesterolemia
    f. periodic paralysis
    f. spinal muscular atrophy
    f. splenic anemia
    f. tremor
Fañanás cell
Fanconi's syndrome
fan sign
Faraday's law of induction
Farber's lipogranulomatosis
Far East Russian encephalitis

**far lateral inferior suboccipital
  approach**
fascia, pl. **fasciae**
    f. cinerea
    f. dentata hippocampi
    dentate f.
    infraspinous f.
    vertebral f.
fascia-muscle-fascia sandwich
fascicle
    nerve f.
fascicular
    f. degeneration
    f. graft
    f. ophthalmoplegia
fasciculation
    f. potential
fasciculus, gen. and pl. **fasciculi**
    f. anterior proprius
    arcuate f.
    Burdach's f.
    calcarine f.
    central tegmental f.
    f. circumolivaris pyramidis
    f. corticospinalis anterior
    f. corticospinalis lateralis
    cuneate f.
    f. cuneatus
    dorsal longitudinal f.
    dorsolateral f.
    f. dorsolateralis
    Flechsig's fasciculi
    Foville's f.
    fronto-occipital f.
    f. gracilis
    hooked f.
    inferior longitudinal f.
    interfascicular f.
    f. interfascicularis
    intersegmental fasciculi
    f. lateralis proprius
    f. lenticularis
    Lissauer's f.
    fasciculi longitudinales
      pontis
    f. longitudinalis dorsalis
    f. longitudinalis inferior
    f. longitudinalis medialis
    f. longitudinalis superior
    f. macularis
    mamillotegmental f.
    f. mamillotegmentalis
    mamillothalamic f.

f. mamillothalamicus
f. marginalis
medial longitudinal f.
Meynert's f.
f. obliquus pontis
occipitofrontal f.
f. occipitofrontalis
oval f.
f. pedunculomamillaris
perpendicular f.
proper fasciculi
fasciculi proprii
f. pyramidalis anterior
f. pyramidalis lateralis
retroflex f.
f. retroflexus
f. rotundus
fasciculi rubroreticulares
semilunar f.
f. semilunaris
septomarginal f.
f. septomarginalis
slender f.
f. solitarius
subcallosal f.
f. subcallosus
superior longitudinal f.
f. thalamicus
f. thalamomamillaris
unciform f., uncinate f.
uncinate f. of Russell
f. uncinatus
wedge-shaped f.
fasciola, pl. **fasciolae**
    f. cinerea
fasciolar
    f. gyrus
fast
    f. Fourier transformation
      spectrum analyzer
    f. imaging

    f. imaging with steady
      precession (FISP)
    f. low angle shot (FLASH)
    f. rhythm
fastigatum
fastigiobulbar tract
fastigium
fast-scan magnetic resonance
fat
    f. embolism
    f. embolus
fatigue
    f. failure
    implant f.
    metal f.
fat-patch graft
fat-suppression
    f.-s. MR imaging
    f.-s. technique
fatty streak
fat-water
    f.-w. chemical shift
    f.-w. signal cancellation
faucial
    f. paralysis
    f. reflex
FBSS
    failed back surgery syndrome
febrile convulsion
feedback
    negative f.
    positive f.
    f. system
feeding center
Feer's disease
felt
    shredded Teflon f.
    Teflon f.
feltwork
Felty's syndrome

NOTES

femoral
    f. cutaneous nerve
    f. introducer sheath
    f. nerve
    f. reflex
femoroabdominal reflex
fenestrated clip
fenestration
fenoprofen
    f. calcium
fentanyl
    f. citrate
Féréol-Graux palsy
Ferguson suction
Ferris
    F. Smith-Kerrison punch
    F. Smith-Kerrison rongeur
ferrite
    barium f.
ferromagnetic
    f. artifact
    f. implant
    f. monitoring device
ferromagnetism
ferrugination
festinant
festinating gait
festination
fetal
    f. adenoma
    f. substantia nigra
    f. transfusion
fetalis
    erythroblastosis f.
Feulgen-cytophotometry
fever
    Central European tick-
      borne f.
    cerebrospinal f.
    diphasic milk f.
    drug f.
    meningotyphoid f.
    South African tick-bite f.
    spotted f.
    trypanosome f.
    Zika f.
feverfew plant
[^{18}F] fluoride solution
FI
    fixateur interne
fiber, fibre
    A f.'s
    accelerator f.'s

adrenergic f.'s
afferent f.'s
alpha f.'s
anastomosing f.'s,
  anastomotic f.'s
arcuate f.'s
association f.'s
augmentor f.'s
B f.'s
Bergmann's f.'s
beta f.'s
C f.'s
cholinergic f.'s
circular f.'s
climbing f.'s
commissural f.'s
cone f., inner cone f., outer
  cone f.
corticobulbar f.'s
corticonuclear f.'s
corticopontine f.'s
corticoreticular f.'s
corticospinal f.'s
depressor f.'s
endogenous f.'s
exogenous f.'s
external arcuate f.'s
gamma f.'s
Gratiolet's f.'s
gray f.'s
inhibitory f.'s
inner cone f. (*var. of*
  cone f.)
internal arcuate f.'s
intrafusal f.'s
intrinsic f.'s
medullated nerve f.
mossy f.'s
motor f.'s
Müller's f.'s
myelinated nerve f.
Myer's loop f.'s
nerve f.
nonmedullated f.'s
outer cone f. (*var. of*
  cone f.)
periventricular f.'s
pilomotor f.'s
pressor f.'s
projection f.'s
pyramidal f.'s
Reissner's f.
Remak's f.'s

Retzius' f.'s
rod f.
Rosenthal f.
striatopetal f.
sudomotor f.'s
sustentacular f.'s of retina
tautomeric f.s
transverse f.'s of pons
unmyelinated f.'s
fiberoptics
fibra, pl. **fibrae**
    fibrae arcuatae cerebri
    fibrae arcuatae externae
    fibrae arcuatae internae
    fibrae circulares
    fibrae corticonucleares
    fibrae corticopontinae
    fibrae corticoreticulares
    fibrae corticospinales
    fibrae periventriculares
    fibrae pontis transversae
    fibrae pyramidales
fibre (*var. of* fiber)
fibrillary
    f. astrocyte
    f. astrocytoma
    f. chorea
    f. myoclonia
    f. neuroma
    f. tremor
fibrillation
    atrial f.
    paroxysmal atrial f.
    f. potential
    ventricular f.
fibrin
    f. film
    f. glue
fibrinogen
fibrinoid degeneration
fibrinolysin

fibrinolysis
fibrin-platelet-fibrin embolus
fibroblast growth factor
fibrogliosis
fibrolipoma
fibroma
    ossifying f.
    psammomatoid ossifying f.
    sinonasal psammomatoid
      ossifying f.
fibromatosis
    juvenile f.
fibromuscular
    f. dysplasia
    f. hyperplasia
fibroneuroma
fibropsammoma
fibrosarcoma
fibrosis
    leptomeningeal f.
    postradiation f.
fibrositic headache
fibrositis
    cervical f.
fibrosus
    annulus f.
fibrous
    f. astrocyte
    f. dysplasia
    f. plaque
fibroxanthoma
fibroxanthosarcoma
fibular
    f. allograft
    f. grafting
    f. peg
FID
    free induction decay
fiducial
    f. marker
    radiopaque f.

NOTES

field
>Broca's f.
>checkerboard f.'s
>f. contour
>f. defect
>dipole f.
>f. expansion
>f.'s of Forel
>fringing f.
>gradient f.
>gradient magnetic f.
>H f.'s
>harmonic f.
>harmonic error f.
>f. homogeneity
>f. inhomogeneity
>lattice f.
>f. magnet
>main f.
>nerve f.
>f. pattern
>prerubral f.
>radiofrequency f.
>radiofrequency
> electromagnetic f.
>radiofrequency magnetic f.
>f. shift
>static magnetic f.
>f. strength
>tegmental f.'s of Forel
>vector f.
>f. of view
>Wernicke's f.
>z-gradient f.

Fielding's membrane
fifth
>f. cranial nerve
>f. ventricle

Figueira's syndrome
figure
>fortification f.'s
>myelin f.

fila (*pl. of* filum)
filament
>root f.'s

fillet
>lateral f.
>f. layer
>medial f.

filling
>zero f.

film
>absorbable gelatin f.

>fibrin f.
>Instat fibrin f.

filovaricosis
filter
>analog f.
>low-pass f.
>shunt f.

filtering
>antialias f.
>signal f.

filum, pl. **fila**
>f. durae matris spinalis
>fila olfactoria
>fila radicularia
>terminal f.
>f. terminale

fimbria, pl. **fimbriae**
>f. hippocampi

fimbriodentate sulcus
fine-cup forceps
fine-tipped up-and-down-angled
  bipolar forceps
fine tremor
finger
>f. agnosia
>f. fracture technique
>f. indicator
>jerk f.
>lock f.
>f. phenomenon
>snap f.
>spring f.
>stuck f.
>trigger f.

finger-nose test
finger-thumb reflex
finger-to-finger test
Finochietto retractor
Fiorinal
first
>f. cranial nerve
>f. temporal convolution

Fisch drill
Fisher's
>F. exact test
>F. syndrome

Fishgold's line
FISP
>fast imaging with steady
> precession

fissura, pl. **fissurae**
>f. calcarina
>fissurae cerebelli

f. cerebri lateralis
f. choroidea
f. collateralis
f. dentata
f. hippocampi
f. horizontalis cerebelli
f. longitudinalis cerebri
f. mediana anterior
  medullae oblongatae
f. mediana anterior
  medullae spinalis
f. parietooccipitalis
f. posterolateralis
f. prima cerebelli
f. secunda cerebelli
f. transversa cerebelli
f. transversa cerebri

fissure

anterior median f. of
  medulla oblongata
anterior median f. of spinal
  cord
ape f.
Bichat's f.
Broca's f.
calcarine f.
callosomarginal f.
cerebellar f.'s
cerebellomedullary f.
cerebral f.'s
choroid f.
Clevenger's f.
collateral f.
dentate f.
great horizontal f.
great longitudinal f.
hippocampal f.
horizontal f. of cerebellum
interhemispheric f.
lateral cerebral f.
longitudinal f. of cerebrum

lunate f.
optic f.
Pansch's f.
paracentral f.
parieto-occipital f.
postcentral f.
posterior median f. of the
  medulla oblongata
posterior median f. of
  spinal cord
posterolateral f.
posthippocampal f.
postlingual f.
postlunate f.
postpyramidal f.
postrhinal f.
prenodular f.
primary f. of the
  cerebellum
rhinal f.
f. of Rolando
secondary f. of the
  cerebellum
simian f.
superior orbital f.
superior temporal f.
sylvian f., f. of Sylvius
transverse f. of cerebellum
transverse f. of cerebrum
vestibular f. of cochlea
zygal f.

fistula, pl. **fistulae, fistulas**

arteriovenous f.
carotid-cavernous f. (CCF)
carotid-cavernous sinus f.
carotid-dural f.
cavernous sinus f.
cerebrospinal fluid f.
craniosinus f.
dorsal enteric f.

NOTES

fistula *(continued)*
    dural arteriovenous f.
    radiculomedullary f.
fit
    cerebellar f.'s
    uncinate f.
fixateur interne (FI)
fixation
    adjunctive f.
    adjunctive screw f.
    anterior C1-C2 f.
    anterior C1-C2 screw f.
    anterior metallic f.
    anterior plate f.
    anterior screw f.
    anterior spinal f.
    Caspar anterior plate f.
    cervical spine f.
    cervical spine internal f.
    cervical spine screw-plate f.
    Cotrel-Dubousset f.
    dens anterior screw f.
    f. device
    external spinal f.
    Galveston f.
    Halifax clamp posterior
     cervical f.
    Harrington rod f.
    hook-plate f.
    iliac f.
    internal f.
    internal spinal f.
    lumbar pedicle f.
    lumbar spine f.
    lumbar spine segmental f.
    lumbar spine
     transpedicular f.
    Luque-Galveston f.
    Luque loop f.
    Magerl posterior C1-C2
     screw f.
    mandibular f.
    multiple-point sacral f.
    occipitocervical f.
    odontoid fracture internal f.
    pedicle f.
    pedicle screw-rod f.
    pedicular f.
    pelvic f.
    plate f.
    plate-screw f.
    posterior cervical f.
    posterior segmental f.

    ReFix non-invasive f.
    rigid internal f.
    Roy-Camille posterior screw
     plate f.
    sacral f.
    sacral pedicle screw f.
    sacral spine f.
    sacrum fusion screw f.
    scoliotic curve f.
    screw f.
    segmental f.
    SOF'WIRE spinal f.
    spinal f.
    sublaminar f.
    f. technique
    Texas Scottish Rite Hospital
     rod f.
    transpedicular f.
    transpedicular screw-rod f.
    transverse f.
    visual f.
fixator
    AO internal f.
    external spinal skeletal f.
    (ESSF)
    Vermont spinal f.
fixed
    f. pupil
    f. torticollis
[^{18}F]-labeled fluorodeoxyglucose
flail chest
Flamm's technique
flank dissection
flap
    axial pattern scalp f.
    bone f.
    C-shaped scalp f.
    f. elevation
    free bone f.
    I-shaped scalp f.
    island pedicle scalp f.
    liver f.
    myocutaneous f.
    neurovascular f.
    osteoplastic bone f.
    pericranial temporalis f.
    scalp f.
    sickle f.
    skin f.
    supraorbital pericranial f.
    U-shaped scalp f.
flapping tremor

FLASH
    fast low angle shot
flashing pain syndrome
flask
    Falcon plastic f.
    tissue culture f.
flat
    f. back curette
    f. back deformity
    f. back syndrome
    f. electroencephalogram
    f. top waves
Flatau-Schilder disease
Flatau's law
Flechsig's
    F. areas
    F. fasciculi
    F. ground bundles
    F. tract
Flexeril
flexibility
    Cotrel-Dubousset rod f.
flexible arm retractor
flexion
    flicker thumb f.
    f. injury posterior
    atlantoaxial arthrodesis
flexion-compression spine injury
  stabilization
flexion-distraction injury
flexion-extension injury
flexor
    f. reflex
    f. tetanus
flexura, pl. **flexurae**
flexure
    basicranial f.
    cephalic f.
    cerebral f.
    cervical f.
    cranial f.

    mesencephalic f.
    pontine f.
    telencephalic f.
    transverse
    rhombencephalic f.
F.L. Fischer modular stereotaxy
  system
flicker thumb flexion
flip angle
flittering scotoma
floating-forehead operation
floccular
floccule
flocculonodular
    f. arteriovenous
    malformation
    f. lobe
    f. node
flocculus, pl. **flocculi**
    accessory f.
flow
    blood f.
    cerebral blood f. (CBF)
    collateral blood f.
    f. cytometry
    f. detection technique
    f. direction
    f. dynamics
    f. effect
    hypothalamic blood f.
    f. imaging
    intraarterial f.
    f. misregistration
    regional cerebral blood f.
    (rCBF)
    f. regulated suction tube
    retrograde blood f.
    f. theory
    f. velocity
flow-directed embolization
flower basket of Bochdalek

NOTES

flower-spray
    f.-s. ending
    f.-s. organ of Ruffini
flowmeter
    clinical electromagnetic f.
flow-sensitive MR imaging
fludrocortisone
fluid
    f. balance
    cerebrospinal f. (CSF)
    f. retention
    ventricular f.
fluke infestation
flunarizine
fluorocytosine
fluorodeoxyglucose
    $[^{18}F]$-labeled f.
    positron emission
      tomography with $[^{18}F]$-
      labeled f. (PET-FDG)
fluorography
    pulsed f.
fluoroptic
    f. thermometry probe
    f. thermometry system
fluoroscopic imaging
fluoroscopy
    C-arm f.
fluorosis
5-fluorouracil
fluoxetine
fluoxymesterone
fluphenazine hydrochloride
flush chamber
flushing
flutter
    ocular f.
Flynn-Aird syndrome
foam
    f. cell
    gelatin f.
    polyvinyl alcohol f.
    PV f.
focal
    f. epilepsy
    f. sclerosis
focus, pl. foci
    epileptic f.
focused radiation therapy
Foix-Alajouanine
    F.-A. myelitis
    F.-A. syndrome
Foix's syndrome

fold
    neural f.'s
foldover
    image f.
Foley catheter
folium, pl. folia
    folia cerebelli
    f. vermis
follicle
    hair f.
Folling's disease
fontanel
fontanelle
fonticulus nasofrontalis
foot
    drop f.
    f. of hippocampus
foot-drop
foramen, pl. foramina
    arachnoid f.
    Bichat's f.
    f. cecum medullae
      oblongatae
    f. cecum posterius
    cervical neural foramina
    great f.
    interventricular f.
    f. interventriculare
    jugular f.
    f. of Key-Retzius
    f. lateralis ventriculi quarti
    f. of Luschka
    f. of Magendie
    Magendie's f.
    f. magnum
    f. magnum line
    f. of Monro
    Monro's f.
    foramina nervosa
    f. ovale
    parietal f.
    Retzius' f.
    f. rotundum
    f. of Vesalius
    Vicq d'Azyr's f.
foraminal
    f. approach
    f. decompression
    f. herniation
    f. stenosis
foraminotomy
foraminulum, pl. foraminula

force
 f. application
 deflection f.
 distraction f.
 exchange f.
 fraction maximal voluntary
  contraction f.
 f. nucleus
 f. transducer
forced grasping reflex
forceps
 Adson f.
 Adson-Brown f.
 alligator cup f.
 f. anterior
 bayonet f.
 bipolar f.
 bipolar bayonet f.
 bipolar coagulating f.
 bipolar electrocautery f.
 bipolar long-shaft f.
 Brown-Adson f.
 Castroviejo eye suture f.
 contact compressive f.
 cup f.
 curved knot-tying f.
 Cushing bayonet f.
 Cushing brain f.
 Debakey f.
 dissecting f.
 dressing f.
 Ewald-Hudson f.
 fine-cup f.
 fine-tipped up-and-down-
  angled bipolar f.
 Fox bipolar electrocautery f.
 Gerald f.
 Hardy bayonet dressing f.
 Hardy microsurgical bayonet
  bipolar f.
 Heifetz cup serrated ring f.

 Hunt angled serrated ring f.
 Hunt angled tip f.
 Hunt grasping f.
 Jannetta f.
 Jansen-Middleton f.
 Jerald f.
 jeweler's f.
 jeweler's bipolar f.
 Knight f.
 Luc ethmoid f.
 MacCarty f.
 f. major
 Malis angled bayonet f.
 McGill f.
 microcup f.
 Miles punch biopsy f.
 f. minor
 mosquito f.
 Moynihan f.
 Oldberg pituitary f.
 Péan f.
 plain f.
 f. posterior
 Rhoton f.
 ringed formed f.
 round-handled f.
 Spencer biopsy f.
 straight f.
 straight knot-tying f.
 straight line bayonet f.
 f. tip
 tissue f.
 tying f.
 Yasargil flat serrated ring f.
forebrain
 f. vesicle
forehead
 remodeled f.
foreign
 f. body
 f. body granuloma

NOTES

Forel's decussation
Forestier's disease
fork
    Hardy 3-prong f.
    Sugita f.
formatio, pl. formationes
    f. hippocampalis
    f. reticularis
formation
    hemostatic plug f.
    reticular f.
formed visual hallucination
formication
fornices
fornix, gen. fornicis, pl. fornices
    transverse f.
Forte
    Aristocort F.
    Parafon F.
fortification
    f. figures
    f. spectrum
fossa, gen. and pl. fossae
    infratemporal f.
    interpeduncular f.
    f. interpeduncularis
    lateral f. of brain
    lateral cerebral f.
    f. lateralis cerebri
    middle cranial f.
    posterior f.
    posterior pituitary f.
    rhomboid f.
    f. rhomboidea
    f. of Sylvius
    temporal f.
fossula, pl. fossulae
Foster Kennedy syndrome
Fothergill's
    F. disease
    F. neuralgia
foudroyant
fountain decussation
Fourier
    F. synthesis
    F. transform
    F. transform technique
four-poster frame
fourth
    f. cranial nerve
    f. nerve palsy
    f. ventricle
fovea, pl. foveae

    f. anterior
    f. centralis retinae
    f. inferior
    f. superior
Foville's
    F. fasciculus
    F. syndrome
Fox bipolar electrocautery forceps
fraction
    ejection f.
    f. maximal voluntary
    contraction force
    S-phase f.
fractionated StaRT
fractionation protocol
fracture
    acute f.
    articular mass separation f.
    atlantal f.
    atlas f.
    atlas-axis combination f.
    axial loading f.
    axis-atlas combination f.
    basal skull f.
    basilar skull f.
    blow-out f.
    burst f.
    capillary f.
    Chance f.
    clay-shoveler f.
    closed skull f.
    combined flexion-distraction
    injury and burst f.
    comminuted skull f.
    complicated f.
    compound f.
    compound skull f.
    compression f.
    f. by contrecoup
    cranial f.
    depressed f.
    depressed skull f.
    derby hat f.
    diastatic skull f.
    direct f.
    dishpan f.
    f. dislocation
    expressed skull f.
    facial f.
    f. fixation device
    growing f.
    gutter f.
    hairline f.

hangman's f.
indirect f.
Jefferson's f.
linear f.
linear skull f.
low lumbar f.
low lumbar spine f.
lumbar spine burst f.
lumbosacral junction f.
maxillofacial f.
neurogenic f.
odontoid f.
open skull f.
orbital f.
ping-pong f.
pond f.
f. reduction
rib f.
sagittal slice f.
seatbelt f.
sentinel spinous process f.
simple skull f.
skull f.
slice f.
slot f.
spinous process f.
f. stabilization
stellate skull f.
teardrop f.
thoracic spine f.
thoracolumbar f.
thoracolumbar burst f.
T8-L3 thoracolumbar
  burst f.
T11-L5 thoracolumbar
  burst f.
translational f.
vertebral f.
wedge-compression f.
f. with scoliosis
zygomatic f.

fracture-dislocation
  f.-d. reduction
  thoracolumbar spine f.-d.
  f.-d. with anterior ligament
fraise
frame
  Andrews f.
  Brown-Roberts-Wells head f.
  Cosman-Roberts-Wells
    stereotactic f.
  couch-mounted head f.
  CRW base f.
  CRW head f.
  f. fixation-scanner assisted
    target localization
  four-poster f.
  Greenberg retractor f.
  Leksell f.
  Leksell stereotactic f.
  Olivier-Bertrand-Tipal f.
  operative wedge f.
  Reichert-Mundinger
    stereotactic head f.
  Relton-Hall f.
  Riechert-Mundinger
    stereotactic f.
  self-retaining brain
    retractor f.
  stereotactic f.
  Sugita multipurpose head f.
  Talairach stereotactic f.
  ZD f.
Frankenhäuser's ganglion
Frazier
  F. dural guide
  F. stylet
  F. suction tip
  F. suction tube
Frazier's needle

NOTES

Frazier-Spiller
    F.-S. operation
    F.-S. rhizotomy
free
    f. bone flap
    f. fragment disk
    f. induction decay (FID)
    f. nerve endings
    f. radical
Freier dissector
French
    F. catheter
    F. polio
    F. rod bender
Frenkel's symptom
frenulum, pl. **frenula**
    f. cerebelli
    f. of Giacomini
    f. of superior medullary
      velum
    f. veli medullaris superius
frequency
    f. aliasing
    f. dispersion curve
    dominant f.
    f. encoding
    f. error
    Larmor f.
    Nyquist f.
    f. offset
    offset f.
    precessional f.
    f. range
    resonant f.
    f. shift
    spatial f.
frequency-encoding gradient
fressreflex
Frey's
    F. irritation hairs
    F. syndrome
Friedmann's disease
Friedreich's
    F. ataxia
    F. disease
fringing field
Fröhlich's syndrome
Frohse
    arcade of F.
Froin's syndrome
Froment's sign
frontal
    f. area

    f. artery
    f. cortex
    f. grooves
    f. gyrectomy
    f. gyrus
    f. horn
    f. lobe
    f. lobe syndrome
    f. pole
frontoethmoidal encephalocele
frontonasomaxillary osteotomy
fronto-occipital fasciculus
fronto-orbital
    f.-o. area
    f.-o. osteotomy
frontopontine tract
frontosphenoidal encephalocele
frontotemporal
    f. approach
    f. craniotomy
    f. tract
front-tap reflex
Froriep's ganglion
frozen section
fucosidosis
Fuerstner's disease
fugax
    amaurosis f.
Fukushima's
    F. cavernous bypass
    F. monopolar malleable
      coagulator
**Fukuyama-type congenital muscular
  dystrophy**
fulgurant
fulgurating
    f. migraine
fulminant
    f. necrotizing encephalitis
fumigatus
    Aspergillus f.
function
    allomeric f.
    arousal f.
    cortical mapping of
      memory f.
    harmonic f.
    isomeric f.
    Legendre f.
    psychosocial f.
    secretory f.
    spectral density f.
    vestibular f.

functional
- f. activation PET scanning
- f. anosmia
- f. aphasia
- f. apoplexy
- f. contracture
- f. neuroimaging
- f. neurosurgery
- f. spasm
- f. stereotaxy
- f. terminal innervation ratio

fungal infection
fungus, pl. fungi
- f. cerebri

funicular
- f. graft
- f. myelitis
- f. myelosis

funiculitis
funiculus, pl. funiculi
- anterior f.
- f. anterior
- cuneate f.
- dorsal f.
- f. dorsalis
- f. gracilis
- f. lateralis
- lateral f. of spinal cord
- funiculi medullae spinalis
- f. posterior
- posterior f.
- f. separans
- f. solitarius
- f. teres

funnel
- pial f.

furor epilepticus
furosemide
Fused Rhymed Dichotic Words Test

fusiform
- f. aneurysm
- f. cells of cerebral cortex
- f. gyrus
- f. layer

fusimotor
fusion
- anterior cervical discectomy and f.
- anterior interbody f.
- anterior lumbar spine interbody f.
- atlantoaxial f.
- Brooks type f.
- cervical f.
- cervical spine f.
- cervical spine posterior f.
- degenerative lumbar spine f.
- degenerative spondylosis decompression and f.
- Gallie spinal f.
- interbody f.
- interfacet wiring and f.
- f. limit determination
- long segment f.
- long segment spinal f.
- lower cervical spine f.
- lumbar f.
- lumbar interbody f.
- lumbar spinal f.
- lumbar spine f.
- lumbosacral f.
- f. nonunion rate
- occipitocervical f.
- posterior-interbody lumbar spinal f.
- posterior-lateral lumbar spinal f.
- posterior lumbar interbody f. (PLIF)
- posterior spinal f.

NOTES

fusion *(continued)*
    posterolateral f.
    posterolateral lumbosacral f.
    sacral spine f.
    selective thoracic f.
    selective thoracic spine f.
    short segment f.
    short segment spinal f.
    single-level spinal f.

    in situ spinal f.
    spinal f., spine f.
    f. stiffness
    f. technique
    thoracic spinal f.
    upper cervical spine f.
    vertebral f.
    Wiltberger's f.

G

GAD
glutamate decarboxylase
gadolinium
    g. diethylenetriamine pentaacetic acid (Gd-DTPA)
    g. DTPA
    g. enhancement
gadolinium-enhanced
    g.-e. MRI
    g.-e. MR imaging
gadopentetate dimeglumine
gag
    g. reflex
    g. reflex loss
Gagel's granuloma
gain
    weight g.
gait
    g. abnormality
    ataxic g.
    cerebellar g.
    Charcot's g.
    g. disturbance
    equine g.
    festinating g.
    helicopod g.
    hemiplegic g.
    high steppage g.
    scissor g.
    spastic g.
    steppage g.
galactose
galactosidase defect
Galant's reflex
Galassi's pupillary phenomenon
galea
    g. aponeurotica
galeatomy
Galen
    vein of G.
Galen's
    G. anastomosis
    G. nerve
gallamine triethiodide
Gallie
    G. spinal fusion
    G. technique
    G. wiring technique
gallium-67

Gall's craniology
Galtac device
galvanic
    g. skin reaction
    g. skin reflex
    g. skin response (GSR)
    g. vertigo
Galveston
    G. fixation
    G. fixation with TSRH crosslink
Gambian trypanosomiasis
gamma
    g. efferent
    g. efferent system
    g. fibers
    g. irradiation
    g. knife
    g. knife radiosurgery
    g. loop
    g. motor neuron
    g. motor system
    g. radiosurgery
    201-source cobalt-60 g. unit
    g. thalamotomy
gamma-acetylenic-GABA
Gamma Maxicamera
gamma-vinyl-GABA
gammopathy
    monoclonal g.
ganglia (*pl. of* ganglion)
gangliectomy
gangliitis
gangliocyte
gangliocytoma
    dysplastic g.
ganglioglioma
    desmoplastic infantile g.
    infantile g.
gangliolysis
    percutaneous radiofrequency g.
ganglioma
    intracerebral g.
ganglion, pl. ganglia, ganglions
    aberrant g.
    acousticofacial g.
    Andersch's g.
    aorticorenal ganglia
    ganglia aorticorenalia

ganglion *(continued)*
   Arnold's g.
   auditory g.
   Auerbach's ganglia
   auricular g.
   autonomic ganglia
   ganglia of autonomic
     plexuses
   basal ganglia
   Bezold's g.
   Bochdalek's g.
   Bock's g.
   Böttcher's g.
   cardiac ganglia
   ganglia cardiaca
   carotid g.
   celiac ganglia
   ganglia celiaca
   g. cell
   g. cells of dorsal spinal
     root
   g. cells of retina
   g. cervicale inferius
   g. cervicale medium
   g. cervicale superius
   cervicothoracic g.
   g. cervicothoracicum
   g. ciliare
   ciliary g.
   coccygeal g.
   Corti's g.
   dorsal root g.
   Ehrenritter's g.
   g. extracraniale
   g. of facial nerve
   Frankenhäuser's g.
   Froriep's g.
   gasserian g.
   geniculate g.
   g. geniculi
   Gudden's g.
   g. habenulae
   hypogastric ganglia
   g. impar
   inferior cervical g.
   inferior g. of
     glossopharyngeal nerve
   inferior mesenteric g.
   inferior g. of vagus
   g. inferius nervi
     glossopharyngei
   g. inferius nervi vagi
   intercrural g.

ganglia intermedia
intermediate ganglia
g. of intermediate nerve
interpeduncular g.
intervertebral g.
intracranial g.
g. isthmi
jugular g.
Laumonier's g.
Lee's g.
lenticular g.
Lobstein's g.
Ludwig's g.
ganglia lumbalia
lumbar ganglia
Meckel's g.
g. mesentericum inferius
g. mesentericum superius
middle cervical g.
nasal g.
nerve g., neural g.
nodose g.
otic g.
g. oticum
parasympathetic ganglia
paravertebral ganglia
pelvic ganglia
ganglia pelvina
petrosal g., petrous g.
phrenic ganglia
ganglia phrenica
ganglia plexuum
   autonomicorum
prevertebral ganglia
pterygopalatine g.
g. pterygopalatinum
Remak's ganglia
renal ganglia
ganglia renalia
Ribes' g.
sacral ganglia
ganglia sacralia
Scarpa's g.
Schacher's g.
semilunar g.
sensory g.
Soemmering's g.
solar ganglia
sphenopalatine g.
spinal g.
g. spinale
spiral g. of cochlea
g. spirale cochleae

splanchnic g.
g. splanchnicum
stellate g.
g. stellatum
sublingual g.
g. sublinguale
submandibular g.
g. submandibulare
submaxillary g.
superior cervical g.
superior g. of
  glossopharyngeal nerve
superior mesenteric g.
superior g. of the vagus
  nerve
g. superius nervi
  glossopharyngei
g. superius nervi vagi
sympathetic ganglia
ganglia of sympathetic trunk
terminal g.
g. terminale
thoracic ganglia
ganglia thoracica
trigeminal g.
g. trigeminale
ganglia trunci sympathici
g. of trunk of vagus
tympanic g.
g. tympanicum
Valentin's g.
vertebral g.
g. vertebrale
vestibular g.
g. vestibulare
Vieussens' g.
Walther's g.
Wrisberg's ganglia
ganglionectomy
  Meckel's sphenopalatine g.

sphenopalatine g.
superior cervical g.
ganglioneuroblastoma
ganglioneuroma
  central g.
  dumbbell g.
ganglioneuromatosis
ganglionic
  g. blocking agent
  g. crest
  g. layer of cerebellar cortex
  g. layer of cerebral cortex
  g. layer of optic nerve
  g. layer of retina
  g. motor neuron
ganglionitis
ganglionostomy
ganglions (*pl. of* ganglion)
ganglioplegic
ganglioside lipidosis
gangliosidosis
  G_{M1} g.
  G_{M2} g.
  generalized g.
gangrene
  trophic g.
GANS
  isolated granulomatous angiitis
    of the central nervous system
Ganser's commissures
gantry rotation
gap junction
Garamycin
Garcin's syndrome
Gardner
  G. headholder
  G. meningocele repair
Gardner-Wells tongs
Garrett
  G. line
  G. orientation line

NOTES

Gaskell's nerves
gasserian
  g. ganglion
Gasserian ganglion area
gastric
  g. crisis
  g. neurasthenia
  g. tetany
  g. vertigo
gastrocolic reflex
gastroileac reflex
gastrointestinal disorder
gastroparalysis
gastroparesis
gastrostomy
gate
gate-control
  g.-c. hypothesis
  g.-c. theory
gating
  cardiac g.
  g. mechanism
Gaucher's disease
gauge
  pressure g.
  strain g.
gauss
gaze
  horizontal g.
  g. palsy
  g. paralysis
  g. paresis
  ping-pong g.
  vertical g.
gaze-evoked visual loss
GCS
  Glasgow Coma Scale
GDC
  Guglielmi detachable coil
Gd-DTPA
  gadolinium diethylenetriamine
    pentaacetic acid
Gd-DTPA-enhanced cranial MR
  imaging
"gearshift" probe
GE 9800 CT system
gegenhalten
Geigel's reflex
gelatin
  g. foam
  g. phantom
  g. sponge

gelatinous substance
Gelfoam
  G. pad
  Papaverine-soaked G.
  G. powder emboli
Gélineau's syndrome
gelotripsy
Gelpi retractor
Gelusil
gemästete cell
gemistocyte
gemistocytic
  g. astrocyte
  g. astrocytoma
  g. cell
  g. reaction
gemistocytoma
gemmule
genera (pl. of genus)
general
  g. sensation
  g. somatic afferent column
  g. somatic efferent column
  g. visceral column
general-adaptation
  g.-a. reaction
  g.-a. syndrome
General Electric CT 9800 scanner
generalized
  g. gangliosidosis
  g. tetanus
  g. tonic-clonic epilepsy
  g. tonic-clonic seizure
generation
  lesion g.
generator
  high-frequency g.
  programmable pulse g.
  pulse g.
  radiofrequency g.
  Radionics RF lesion g.
gene therapy
genetic
  g. disorder
  g. screening
genicula (pl. of geniculum)
geniculate
  g. body
  g. ganglion
  g. neuralgia
  g. nucleus
  g. otalgia

geniculocalcarine
    g. radiation
    g. tract
geniculum, pl. **genicula**
    g. of facial nerve
    g. nervi facialis
genital
    g. corpuscles
    g. ulceration
genitofemoral nerve
genitourinary tract
Gennari
    stripe of G.
Gennari's
    G. band
    G. stria
gentamicin
    g. sulfate
genu, gen. **genus**, pl. **genua**
    g. capsulae internae
    g. corporis callosi
    g. of corpus callosum
    g. of facial nerve
    g. of internal capsule
    g. nervi faciallis
genus, pl. **genera**
Geopen
Gerald forceps
Gerhardt's disease
Gerhardt-Semon law
Gerlier's disease
germ cell tumor
germinal matrix
germinoma
geromorphism
Gerstmann's syndrome
Gerstmann-Straussler-Sheinker disease
Gerstmann-Sträussler syndrome
G_{MI} **gangliosidosis**

ghost
    g. image
    I/Q imbalance g.
giant
    g. aneurysm
    g. axonal neuropathy
    g. cavernous aneurysm
    g. cell
    g. cell arteritis
    g. cell astrocytoma
    g. cell glioblastoma
    g. cell tumor
    g. glomus tumor
    g. hives
    g. motor unit action potential
    g. urticaria
Gibbs
    G. artifact
    G. phenomenon
Gierke's respiratory bundle
Gifford's reflex
gigantism
    cerebral g.
gigantocellular glioma
Gigli
    G. guide
    G. saw
Gill
    G. laminectomy
    G. procedure
    G. Thomas locator
Gilles
    G. de la Tourette's disease
    G. de la Tourette's syndrome
"gimmick"
ginger paralysis
girdle
    Ace halo pelvic g.
    g. anesthesia

NOTES

girdle *(continued)*
    Hitzig's g.
    g. pain
    g. sensation
Girdlestone laminectomy
githagism
gitter cell
gitterzelle
glabella
glabellar exposure osteotomy
gland
    adrenal g.
    apocrine g.
    eccrine g.
    lacrimal g.
    master g.
    pacchionian g.'s
    pineal g.
    pituitary g.
    salivary g.
    thyroid g.
glandula, pl. **glandulae**
    g. basilaris
    g. pituitaria
Glanzmann's disease
Glasgow
    G. Coma Scale (GCS)
    G. Outcome Scale (GOS)
glass
    optical g.
Glasscock's triangle
glasses
    protective g.
glaucoma
    angle-closure g.
    low tension g.
glia
    g. cells
gliacyte
glial
    g. cell
    g. fibrillary acidic protein
    g. parenchymal cyst
glioblastoma
    cerebral g.
    giant cell g.
    g. multiforme
    occipital g.
glioblastosis cerebri
glioma
    familial g.
    gigantocellular g.
    malignant g.

    medullary g.
    mixed g.
    multifocal g.
    nasal g.
    optic g.
    g. of optic chiasm
    optic nerve g.
    g. of the spinal cord
    subependymal mixed g.
    supratentorial g.
    tectal g.
    telangiectatic g., g.
      telangiectodes
    thalamic g.
gliomatosis
    arachnoidal g.
    g. cerebri
gliomatous
gliomyxoma
glioneuroma
gliosarcoma
    cerebellar g.
gliosis
    isomorphous g.
    piloid g.
global
    g. amnesia
    g. aphasia
    g. paralysis
globe
    pale g.
globoid
    g. cell
    g. cell leukodystrophy
globus, pl. **globi**
    g. hystericus
    g. pallidus
glome
glomectomy
glomera (*pl. of* glomus)
glomerule
glomerulonephritis
    hypocomplementemic g.
glomerulus, pl. **glomeruli**
    olfactory g.
glomus, pl. **glomera**
    g. aorticum
    g. arteriovenous
    malformation
    g. body
    choroid g.
    g. choroideum
    g. intravagale

g. jugulare
g. jugulare tumor
g. jugulotympanicum
g. pulmonale
g. vagale
glossokinesthetic, glossocinesthetic
glossolabiolaryngeal paralysis
glossolabiopharyngeal paralysis
glossolysis
glossopharyngeal
g. nerve
g. neuralgia
g. neuropathy
g. tic
glossoplegia
glossospasm
glossotomy
labiomandibular g.
glossy skin
glottidospasm
glove anesthesia
glucagon
glucocorticoid
glucomineralocorticoid
gluconate
clorhexidine g.
glue
cyanoacrylate g.
fibrin g.
glue-sniffing
glutamate
g. decarboxylase (GAD)
monosodium g.
glutaraldehyde
glutaric
g. acid
g. aciduria type I
gluteal
g. nerve
g. reflex

glycerol
g. chemoneurolysis
g. rhizotomy
glyceryl trinitrate
glycogeusia
glycoprotein storage disorder
glycopyrrolate
glycorrhachia
glycosaminoglycan
glycoside
cardiac g.
glycosphingolipid metabolic defect
G_{M2} gangliosidosis
gnosia
GnRH
gonadotropin-releasing hormone
Golay gradient coil
Goldflam disease
Goldman perimetry
Goldscheider's test
Goldstein's toe sign
Golgi
G. epithelial cell
G. tendon organ
G. type II neuron
G. type I neuron
Golgi-Mazzoni corpuscle
Golgi's cells
Goll's column
Gombault's triangle
gonadotroph cell
gonadotropin
beta-human chorionic g.
chorionic g.
human chorionic g.
gonadotropin-producing adenoma
gonadotropin-releasing hormone (GnRH)
Gordon reflex

NOTES

Gordon's
- G. sign
- G. symptom

Gore-Tex

Gorlin's
- G. sign
- G. syndrome

GOS
- Glasgow Outcome Scale

Gosling pulsatility

gouge
- AO g.

gouty arthritis

Gowers'
- G. column
- G. syndrome
- G. tract

Gowers disease

gracile tubercle

grade
- g. I astrocytoma
- g. II astrocytoma
- g. III astrocytoma
- g. IV astrocytoma
- g. IV spondylolisthesis

Gradenigo's syndrome

gradient
- g. amplifier
- bipolar g.
- g. coil
- g. compensation
- g. echo
- g. field
- frequency-encoding g.
- g. magnetic field
- g. moment
- g. moment nulling
- phase-encoding g.
- readout g.
- rewinder g.
- slice-select encoding g.
- steep-dose g.
- x g.
- y g.

gradient-echo
- g.-e. MR image
- g.-e. MR imaging

gradient-recalled acquisition in the steady state (GRASS)

gradient-refocused
- g.-r. imaging
- g.-r. sequence

Graefe's
- G. disease
- G. sign
- G. spots

graft
- adipose g.
- autogenous bone g.
- autologous fat g.
- bone g.
- bypass g.
- cable g.
- carotid-vertebral vein bypass g.
- clip g.
- fascicular g.
- fat-patch g.
- funicular g.
- human dural substitute g.
- hydroxyapatite g.
- interbody g.
- intracranial-extracranial nerve g.
- intracranial-intratemporal nerve g.
- Keystone g.
- g. material alternative
- g. migration
- nerve g.
- petrous carotid-to-intradural carotid saphenous vein g.
- posterior bone g.
- posterolateral bone g.
- rib g.
- roof-patch g.
- saphenous vein g.
- saphenous vein bypass g.
- saphenous vein patch g.
- g. site
- in situ tricortical iliac-crest block bone g.
- sleeve g.
- sural nerve bridge g.
- sural nerve cable g.
- Teflon tube g.
- tricortical iliac crest bone g.
- vascular patch g.

grafting
- allograft bone g.
- g. anastomosis
- autograft bone g.
- bone g.
- fibular g.

posterolateral bone g.
strut g.
grand
g. mal
g. mal epilepsy
g. mal seizure
Granit's loop
granular
g. cell myoblastoma
g. cell tumor
g. cortex
g. layers of cerebral cortex
g. layers of retina
granularis
ependymitis g.
granulatio, pl. granulationes
granulationes arachnoideales
granulation
arachnoidal g.'s
pacchionian g.'s
granulationes
granule
Birbeck g.
g. cells
chromatic g.
chromophil g.
Crooke's g.'s
Nissl g.'s
granulocyte
granulocytic sarcoma
granuloma
cholesterol g.
eosinophilic g.
foreign body g.
Gagel's g.
lethal midline g.
parenchymal g.
petroclival cholesterol g.
granulomastosis
eosinophilic g.
Langerhans cell g.

granulomatosis
lymphomatoid g.
Wegener's g.
granulomatous
g. angiitis
g. arteritis
g. colitis
g. encephalomyelitis
g. ileocolitis
granulovacuolar degeneration
grape endings
graphanesthesia
graphesthesia
graphic
2D g. localization
graphic aphasia
graphomotor
g. aphasia
graphospasm
grasping reflex
grasp reflex
GRASS
gradient-recalled acquisition in
the steady state
2DFT GRASS
3DFT GRASS
interleaved GRASS
sequential GRASS
Grasset-Gaussel phenomenon
Grasset's
G. law
G. phenomenon
G. sign
grass seed
Gratiolet's
G. fibers
G. radiation
Graves'
G. disease
G. ophthalmopathy

NOTES

gravidarum
    chorea g.
gravireceptors
gravis
    myasthenia g.
Gravol
gray (Gy)
    g. columns
    g. degeneration
    g. fibers
    g. layer of superior
      colliculus
    g. matter
    periaqueductal g.
    periventricular g.
    g. substance
    g. tuber
    g. tubercle
    g. wing
great
    g. anterior medullary artery
    g. cerebral vein
    g. foramen
    g. horizontal fissure
    g. longitudinal fissure
    g. vein of Galen
greater
    g. occipital nerve
    g. rhomboid muscle
    g. superficial petrosal nerve
great-toe reflex
Greenberg
    G. retracting system
    G. retractor
    G. retractor frame
    G. retractor set
    G. and Sugita retractor
Greenberg-type bar
Greenfield's disease
grid
    subdural g.
Griesinger's sign
grip
    pencil g.
    pincer g.
    pistol g.
    syringe g.
groove
    anterior intermediate g.
    anterolateral g.
    anteromedian g.
    frontal g.'s
    neural g.

    olfactory g.
    pontomedullary g.
    posterior intermediate g.
    posterolateral g.
    vascular g.
ground bundles
group
    AO g.
    Pittsburgh Gamma Knife g.
    Swedish Gamma Knife g.
growing
    g. fracture
    g. pains
growth
    g. factor
    g. hormone
    g. hormone-producing
      adenoma
    g. hormone-secreting
      adenoma
Gruca-Weiss spring
gryochrome
GSR
    galvanic skin response
guanethidine sulfate
guard
    depth g.
Gubler's
    G. hemiplegia
    G. line
    G. paralysis
    G. syndrome
Gudden's
    G. commissures
    G. ganglion
    G. tegmental nuclei
Guglielmi detachable coil (GDC)
guidance
    electrophysiological g.
    stereotactic g.
    ultrasonographic g.
guide
    AO-stopped drill g.
    contoured anterior spinal
      plate drill g.
    Cook stereotaxic g.
    Davis g.
    drill g.
    Frazier dural g.
    Gigli g.
    nut alignment g.
    stereotaxic g.

guidepin
    AO g.
guidewire
    delivery g.
    J-tipped g.
Guillain-Barré
    G.-B. reflex
    G.-B. syndrome
guinea worm infestation
Guinon's disease
Guiot
gumma
    cerebral g.
gun
    Omni clip g.
Gunn phenomenon
Gunn's syndrome
gunshot wound
gustation
gustatory
    g. anesthesia
    g. audition
    g. cells
    g. hyperesthesia
    g. lemniscus
    g. nucleus
    g. organ
    g. sweating syndrome
gustatory-sudorific reflex
gutter fracture
gutters
gutturotetany
Guyon's canal
Gy
    gray
Gynergen
gyrate
gyration
gyrectomy
    frontal g.
gyrencephalic

gyri (*gen. and pl. of* gyrus)
gyriform calcification
gyrochrome
    g. cell
gyromagnetic ratio
gyrosa
gyrose
gyrospasm
gyrus, gen. and pl. **gyri**
    angular g.
    g. angularis
    annectent g.
    anterior central g.
    anterior piriform g.
    ascending frontal g.
    ascending parietal g.
    gyri breves insulae
    callosal g.
    central gyri
    gyri cerebri, gyri of cerebrum
    cingulate g.
    g. cinguli
    deep transitional g.
    dentate g.
    g. dentatus
    fasciolar g.
    g. fasciolaris
    g. fornicatus
    frontal g.
    g. frontalis inferior
    g. frontalis medius
    g. frontalis superior
    fusiform g.
    g. fusiformis
    Heschl's gyri
    hippocampal g.
    inferior frontal g.
    inferior occipital g.
    inferior parietal g.
    inferior temporal g.
    gyri insulae

NOTES

gyrus *(continued)*
 interlocking gyri
 lateral occipitotemporal g.
 lingual g.
 g. lingualis
 long g. of insula
 g. longus insulae
 marginal g.
 medial occipitotemporal g.
 middle frontal g.
 middle temporal g.
 occipital gyri
 g. occipitotemporalis
  lateralis
 g. occipitotemporalis
  medialis
 orbital gyri
 gyri orbitales
 parahippocampal g.
 g. parahippocampalis
 paraterminal g.
 g. paraterminalis
 postcentral g.
 g. postcentralis
 posterior central g.

 precentral g.
 g. precentralis
 prepiriform g.
 g. rectus
 Retzius' g.
 short gyri of the insula
 splenial g.
 straight g.
 subcallosal g.
 g. subcallosus
 superior frontal g.
 superior occipital g.
 superior parietal g.
 superior temporal g.
 supracallosal g.
 supramarginal g.
 g. supramarginalis
 gyri temporales transversi
 g. temporalis inferior
 g. temporalis medius
 g. temporalis superior
 transitional g.
 transverse temporal gyri
 uncinate g.

habena, pl. habenae
habenula, pl. habenulae
    habenulae perforata
    pineal h.
habenular
    h. commissure
    h. nucleus
habenulointerpeduncular tract
habit
    h. chorea
    h. spasm
    h. tic
habituation
Hachinski ischemic score
haemaccel
Haemophilus
    H. aerophilus
    H. influenzae
    H. influenzae meningitis
    H. parainfluenzae
Haenel's symptom
Hageman factor
Hagen-Poiseuille law
Hahn echo
Haid universal bone plate system
hair
    h. cells
    h. follicle
    Frey's irritation h.'s
    h. loss
hairline fracture
Håkanson's technique
Hakim's syndrome
Hakim valve
Hakuba
    medial triangle of H.
Haldol
half-and-half exposure
half-Fourier imaging
half-NEX imaging
Halifax
    H. clamp
    H. clamp posterior cervical
      fixation
Haller's
    H. ansa
    H. circle
    H. unguis

Hallervorden-Spatz
    H.-S. disease
    H.-S. syndrome
Hallervorden syndrome
Hallpike test
Hall Surgairtome II drill
hallucination
    formed visual h.
    hypnagogic h.
    lilliputian h.
    palinoptic h.
    stump h.
    unformed visual h.
hallucinatory neuralgia
hallucinogen
hallucinogenic
halo
    Ace low profile MR h.
    Ace Mark III h.
    h. apparatus
    h. brace
    hypoechogenic
      peritumoral h.
    h. phenomenon
    h. retractor system
    h. ring
    h. vest
haloperidol
Halotestin
halothane
    h. anesthesia
hamartoma
    cortical h.
    hypothalamic h.
    subependymal h.
hamartomatous lipoma
hammock bandage
Hammond's disease
hand
    accoucheur's h.
    h. ataxia
    h. deformity
    drop h.
    Marinesco's succulent h.
    obstetrical h.
    writing h.
handedness
handle
    bayonet h.
    Hardy lateral knife h.

Hand-Schüller-Christian disease
HANE
    hereditary angioneurotic edema
hangman's fracture
haphalgesia
happy puppet syndrome
haptics
haptometer
hard palate dissection
Hardy
    H. attachment
    H. bayonet dressing forceps
    H. bivalve speculum
    H. curette
    H. dissector
    H. lateral knife handle
    H. lip retractor
    H. microsurgical bayonet
      bipolar forceps
    H. microsurgical enucleator
    H. 5 mm mirror
    H. pituitary spoon
    H. 3-prong fork
    H. sella punch
    H. speculum
    H. suction tube
Hardy-Rand-Rittler plate
harmonic
    h. error field
    h. field
    h. function
harmonics
Harm's posterior cervical plate
Harriluque
    H. sublaminar wiring
      modification
    H. technique
Harrington
    H. distraction
    H. instrumentation
    H. pedicle hook
    H. rod
    H. rod fixation
    H. rod and hook system
    H. rod instrumentation
    H. rod instrumentation
      compression
    H. rod instrumentation
      distraction outrigger device
    H. rod instrumentation
      failure
    H. rod instrumentation
      force application

    H. scissors
    H. spreader
Harris' migraine
Hartel technique
Hartnup disease
Hartshill
    H. Ransford loop
    H. rectangle
Haubenfelder
Haversian canals
head
    h. coil
    h. fixation device
    h. injury
    h. movement
    3-point h. rest
    h. ring
    swelled h.
    h. tetanus
    h. trauma
headache
    bilious h.
    blind h.
    cluster h.
    fibrositic h.
    histaminic h.
    Horton's h.
    migraine h.
    nodular h.
    organic h.
    reflex h.
    sick h.
    spinal h.
    symptomatic h.
    tension h.
    vacuum h.
    vascular h.
head-bobbing doll syndrome
head-dropping test
headholder
    Gardner h.
    Mayfield h.
    pin h.
    pinion h.
    Sugita h.
headlamp
    Keeler video h.
headrest
    horseshoe h.
Head's
    H. lines
    H. zones
head-tilt

hearing
    color h.
heart
    irritable h.
    h. reflex
    soldier's h.
heating
    eddy current h.
    radiofrequency h.
heat loss
heavy-duty straight clip
heavy particle radiotherapy
hecateromeric
hecatomeral, hecatomeric
hederiform ending
heel
    h. jar
    h. tap
heel-tap
    h.-t. reaction
    h.-t. test
Heifetz
    H. carotid occluder
    H. clip
    H. cup serrated ring forceps
    H. skull perforator
Heifetz-Weck clip
height vertigo
Heilbronner's thigh
Held's
    H. bundle
    H. decussation
helicopod gait
helicopodia
heliencephalitis
heliotrope rash
helmet
    collimator h.
    cooling h.
Helweg's bundle
Hemaclip

hemangioblastoma
    third ventricular h.
hemangioendothelioma
hemangioma
    calvarial h.
    cavernous h.
    dumbell-shaped spinal
        cavernous h.
    epidural cavernous h.
    extraaxial cavernous h.
    infantile hemangioblastic h.
    vertebral h.
hemangiopericytoma
hematencephalon
hematocephaly
hematocrit
hematoma
    acute subdural h.
    cerebellar h.
    epidural h.
    h. evacuation
    facial h.
    intracerebral h.
    intracranial h.
    intraparenchymal h.
    isodense subdural h.
    retropharyngeal h.
    subdural h.
    subgaleal h.
    subperiosteal h.
    sylvian h.
    traumatic h.
Hematome system
hematomyelia
hematomyelopore
hematoporphyrin derivative
hematorrhachis
    h. externa
    extradural h.
    h. interna
    subdural h.

NOTES

hematuria
hemiacrosomia
hemialgia
hemiamyosthenia
hemianalgesia
hemianesthesia
    alternate h.
    crossed h.
hemianopia
    homonymous h.
hemianopic scotoma
hemianopsia
    homonymous h.
hemiapraxia
hemiasynergia
hemiataxia
hemiathetosis
hemiatrophy
    facial h.
    progressive lingual h.
hemiballism
hemiballismus
hemicephalalgia
hemicerebrum
hemichorea
hemicord
hemicorticectomy
    cerebral h.
hemicrania
    episodic paroxysmal h.
hemicranial pain
hemicraniectomy
hemicraniosis
hemicraniotomy
hemidysesthesia
hemiepilepsy
hemifacial spasm
hemihydranencephaly
hemihypalgesia
hemihyperesthesia
hemihyperkinesis
hemihypertonia
hemihypertrophy
hemihypesthesia
hemihypoesthesia
hemihypotonia
hemilaminectomy
    complete lateral h.
    lumbar h.
    partial h.
    unilateral h.
hemilateral chorea
hemimegalencephaly

hemimyelomeningocele
hemineglect
hemiopalgia
hemiparanesthesia
hemiparaplegia
hemiparesis
    ataxic h.
    herald h.
    hypesthetic ataxic h.
hemiparkinsonian stiffness
hemiplegia
    alternating h.
    alternating hypoglossal h.
    contralateral h.
    crossed h.
    double h.
    facial h.
    Gubler's h.
    infantile h.
    pure motor h.
    spastic h.
    superior alternating h.
hemiplegic
    h. amyotrophy
    h. gait
    h. migraine
hemisensory
hemispasm
hemisphere
    cerebellar h.
    cerebral h.
    h. competition
    dominant h.
hemispherectomy
hemispheric
    h. collapse
    h. disconnection syndrome
hemispherium
    h. cerebelli
    h. cerebri
hemithermoanesthesia
hemitonia
hemitremor
hemivertebra
hemochromatosis
Hemoclip
    Samuels-Weck H.
hemoclip
hemodialysis
hemodilution
    isovolemic h.
hemoglobinopathy
hemolysis

hemolytic anemia
hemophilia
hemorrhachis
hemorrhage
    aneurysmal h.
    arterial h.
    brainstem h.
    cerebellar h.
    cerebral h.
    Duret h.
    extradural h.
    Icelandic form of
     intracranial h.
    intracapsular h.
    intracerebral h.
    intracranial h.
    intraocular h.
    intraventricular h.
    lobar h.
    mesencephalic h.
    neonatal intraventricular h.
    nonaneurysmal
     perimesencephalic
     subarachnoid h.
    perianeurysmal h.
    petechial h.
    pontine h.
    slit h.
    subarachnoid h. (SAH)
    subconjunctival h.
    subcortical h.
    subdural h.
    subgaleal h.
    subhyaloid h.
    subintimal h.
    syringomyelic h.
    thalamic-subthalamic h.
    vitreous h.
hemorrhagic
    h. metastasis
    h. necrosis

    h. pachymeningitis
    h. shearing injury
hemosiderin
    h. scar
hemosiderosis
    cerebral h.
hemostasis
    chemical h.
    immaculate h.
hemostat
    Avitene microfibrillar
     collagen h.
    Crile h.
hemostatic plug formation
hemotympanum
Hemovac drain
Hendler test
Henle's
    H. fiber layer
    H. nervous layer
    H. sheath
Henoch-Schönlein purpura
Henoch's chorea
Hensen's
    H. canal
    H. cell
    H. duct
    H. node
heparin
hepatic
    h. coma
    h. encephalopathy
    h. failure
    h. porphyria
hepatitis B virus infection
hepatocerebral
    h. degeneration
    h. disease
hepatolenticular
    h. degeneration
    h. disease

NOTES

herald hemiparesis
hereditary
  h. angioneurotic edema
    (HANE)
  h. ataxia
  h. branchial myoclonus
  h. cerebellar ataxia
  h. chorea
  h. hemorrhagic telangiectasia
  h. hypertrophic neuropathy
  h. myokymia
  h. neuropathy
  h. photomyoclonus
  h. posterior column ataxia
  h. sensory radicular
    neuropathy
  h. spastic paraplegia
  h. spinal ataxia
heredoataxia
heredofamilial tremor
heredopathia atactica
  polyneuritiformis
Hering-Breuer reflex
Hering's sinus nerve
Hering-Traube waves
Hermetian symmetry
hernia
  cerebral h.
  meningeal h.
herniated
  h. cervical disk
  h. disk
  h. nucleus pulposus
herniation
  brain h.
  caudal transtentorial h.
  cervical disk h.
  cingulate h.
  disk h.
  foraminal h.
  lumbar disk h.
  rostral transtentorial h.
  sphenoidal h.
  subfalcial h.
  tentorial h.
  thoracic disk h.
  tonsillar h.
  transtentorial h.
  traumatic cervical disk h.
  uncal h.
heroin
herophili
  torcular h.

herpes
  h. encephalitis
  h. simplex
  h. simplex encephalitis
  h. zoster
  h. zoster ophthalmicus
  h. zoster oticus
herpetic
  h. meningoencephalitis
  h. neuritis
Herring bodies
Herrmann's syndrome
hersage
Heschl's gyri
Hess
  Hunt and H.
hetacillin
heteresthesia
heterokinesia
heterokinesis
heterolalia
heterologous stimulus
heteromeral
heteromeric
  h. cell
heteromerous
heteropathy
heterophasia
heterophemia, heterophemy
heterotopia
  band h.
  incomplete band h.
heterotopic
  h. ossification
  h. pain
heterotypic cortex
Heubner
  recurrent artery of H.
Hexabrix
hexamethylpropyleneamineoxime
hexamethyl-propyleneamine oxime
  (HMPAO)
hexose
Heyer-Pudenz valve
H fields
HFPV
  high-frequency percussive
    ventilation
hiccups
Hickman catheter
hidradenoma
hidrocystoma

h. frequency deafness
h. steppage gait
higher order motion
high-force Sundt clip system
high-frequency
    h.-f. generator
    h.-f. percussive ventilation
    (HFPV)
high-grade spondylolisthesis
high-intensity
    h.-i. lesion
    h.-i. signal
high-resolution
    h.-r. brain SPECT system
    h.-r. CCT
    h.-r. 3DFT MR imaging
high-speed microdrill
hila (*pl. of* hilum)
Hilal
    H. coil
    H. microcoil
hilar
hillock
    axon h.
    facial h.
Hilton's
    H. law
    H. method
hilum, pl. **hila**
    h. of dentate nucleus
    h. nuclei dentati
    h. nuclei olivaris
    h. of olivary nucleus
    h. ovarii
    h. of ovary
hilus
hindbrain
    h. deformity
    h. vesicle
Hind III enzyme

hinged cast
hip-flexion phenomenon
Hippel-Lindau disease
Hippel's disease
hip phenomenon
hippocampal
    h. atrophy
    h. commissure
    h. convolution
    h. fissure
    h. gyrus
    h. sclerosis
hippocampectomy
hippocampus
    h. major
    h. minor
Hirano body
Hirschberg test
His' perivascular space
histamine
histaminic
    h. cephalalgia
    h. headache
histiocytoma
histiocytosis
    diffuse cerebral h.
    kerasin h.
histiocytosis X
histogram
histolytica
    Entamoeba h.
histonectomy
histoneurology
histopathology
Histoplasma
    H. capsulatum
    H. infection
histoplasmosis
    disseminated CNS h.
histotoxic hypoxia

NOTES

145

histrionic spasm
Hitachi scanning electron microscope
Hitzig's girdle
HIV
    human immunodeficiency virus
hives
    giant h.
HMPAO
    hexamethyl-propyleneamine
    oxime
      Ceretec ^{99m}Tc HMPAO
Hoche's
    H. bundle
    H. tract
Hodgkin's disease
Hoen
    H. intervertebral disk
      rongeur
    H. pituitary rongeur
Hoffmann's
    H. muscular atrophy
    H. phenomenon
    H. reflex
    H. sign
holder
    curved micro-needle h.
    needle h.
    Texas Scottish Rite Hospital
      hook h.
    vari-angled clip h.
    Webster needle h.
hole
    burr h.
    h. preparation method
Hollander test
Hollenhorst plaque
Holmes-Adie
    H.-A. pupil
    H.-A. syndrome
holocord
    h. hydromyelia
holoprosencephaly
holorachischisis
holotelencephaly
Holter-Hausner valve
Holter valve
Homans' sign
homeostasis
homocystinuria
homogeneity
    field h.
    spatial h.
homolateral

homologous stimulus
homonymous
    h. hemianopia
    h. hemianopsia
homotopic pain
homotypic cortex
homunculus
hook
    anatomic h.
    André h.
    André anatomical h.
    ball tip nerve h.
    blunt nerve h.
    Bobechko's sliding barrel h.
    calvarial h.
    circular laminar h. with
      offset top
    closed Cotrel-Dubousset h.
    closed transverse process
      TSRH h.
    Cloward dural h.
    cranial Jacobs h.
    Dandy nerve h.
    h. dislodgement
    downsized circular
      laminar h.
    drop-entry (closed body) h.
    Harrington pedicle h.
    h. hollow-ground connection
      design
    intermediate C-D h.
    Isola spinal implant
      system h.
    laminar h.
    laminar C-D h.
    large ball nerve h.
    Leatherman h.
    microball h.
    Moe h.
    Moe alar h.
    multispan fracture h.
    Murphy ball h.
    nerve h.
    open h.
    open C-D h.
    pear-shaped nerve h.
    pediatric h.
    pediatric C-D h.
    pediatric TSRH h.
    pedicle h.
    pedicle C-D h.
    ribbed h.
    side-opening laminar h.
    h. site

Smithwick h.
Smithwick ganglion h.
square-ended h.
straight nerve h.
Texas Scottish Rite
  Hospital h.
Texas Scottish Rite Hospital
  trial h.
top-entry (open body) h.
TSRH buttressed laminar h.
TSRH circular laminar h.
TSRH pedicle h.
h. V-groove connection
  design
von Graefe strabismus h.
Zielke bifid h.
Hookean body
hooked
  h. bundle of Russell
  h. fasciculus
hook-plate fixation
**hook-to-screw L4-S1 compression
  construct**
Hoover's signs
Hoppe-Goldflam disease
horizontal
  h. cell of Cajal
  h. cells of retina
  h. fissure of cerebellum
  h. gaze
  h. gaze paresis
  h. pedicle diameter
  h. vertigo
hormone
  adrenocorticotropic h.
    (ACTH)
  antidiuretic h. (ADH)
  corticotropin-releasing h.
    (CRH)
  gonadotropin-releasing h.
    (GnRH)

growth h.
luteinizing hormone-
  releasing h.
thyroid-stimulating h. (TSH)
thyrotropin-releasing h.
horn
  Ammon's h.
  anterior h.
  cutaneous h.
  dorsal h.
  frontal h.
  inferior h.
  inferior h. of lateral
    ventricle
  lateral h.
  occipital h.
  posterior h.
  temporal h.
  ventral h.
Horner's syndrome
Horrax
horseshoe
  h. headrest
  h. incision
Horsley rongeur
Horsley's bone wax
Hortega cells
Horton's
  H. arteritis
  H. cephalalgia
  H. disease
  H. headache
hot-cell
hotfoot
hot knife
hot-spot phantom
Hounsfield unit (HU)
House-Brackmann Score
Housepian
H reflex
HTLV-1-associated myelopathy

NOTES

HU
   Hounsfield unit
Hudson
   H. brace
   H. brace burr
   H. drill
human
   h. chorionic gonadotropin
   h. dural substitute
   h. dural substitute graft
   h. immunodeficiency virus
      (HIV)
Hunt
   H. angled serrated ring
      forceps
   H. angled tip forceps
   H. grasping forceps
   H. and Hess
   H. and Kosnik classification
Hunt-Early technique
hunterian ligation
Hunter's
   H. disease
   H. operation
Huntington's
   H. chorea
   H. disease
Hunt's
   H. atrophy
   H. neuralgia
   H. paradoxical phenomenon
   H. syndrome
Hurler-Scheie disease
Hurler's disease
Hutchinson's
   H. facies
   H. mask
   H. pupil
hyaline
   h. arteriosclerosis
   h. bodies of pituitary
   h. thickening
hybridoma
hydatid
   h. cyst
   h. disease
hydralazine
   h. hydrochloride
hydranencephaly
hydrencephalocele
hydrencephalomeningocele
hydrencephalus
hydrobulbia

hydrocele
   h. spinalis
hydrocephalic
   h. dementia
hydrocephalocele
hydrocephaloid
hydrocephalus
   chronic communicating h.
   communicating h.
   congenital h.
   double compartment h.
   external h.
   h. ex vacuo
   internal h.
   noncommunicating h.
   normal-pressure h.
   obstructive h.
   occult h.
   otitic h.
   postmeningitic h.
   posttraumatic h.
   primary h.
   secondary h.
   thrombotic h.
   toxic h.
hydrocephaly
hydrochloride
   amantadine h.
   amitriptyline h.
   chlordiazepoxide h.
   chlorpromazine h.
   clonidine h.
   cyclobenzaprine h.
   cyproheptadine h.
   dihydromorphinone h.
   diphenhydramine h.
   dopamine h.
   doxepin h.
   doxorubicin h.
   fluphenazine h.
   hydralazine h.
   hydromorphone h.
   hydroxyzine h.
   imipramine h.
   isoetharine h.
   meperidine h.
   methadone h.
   nalbuphine h.
   naloxone h.
   perphenazine and
      amitriptyline h.
   procarbazine h.
   promethazine h.

proparacaine h.
propoxyphene h.
propranolol h.
ticlopidine h.
trifluoperazine h.
trihexyphenidyl h.
trimethobenzamide h.
hydrochlorothiazide
hydrodipsomania
HydroDIURIL
hydroencephalocele
hydroflumethiazide
hydrogen ion concentration
hydroma
hydromeningocele
hydromeningoencephalocele
hydromicrocephaly
hydromorphone hydrochloride
hydromyelia
holocord h.
hydromyelocele
hydrophobia
hydrophobic
h. tetanus
hydrophorograph
hydrops
hydrosyringomyelia
hydroxide
aluminum hydroxide and
magnesium h.
magnesium aluminum h.
hydroxyapatite graft
6-hydroxydopamine (OHDA)
2-hydroxyethylmethacrylate
hydroxyethyl methacrylate
polymerizing solution
5-hydroxytryptophan
hydroxyurea
hydroxyzine
h. hydrochloride
h. pamoate

hygroma
subdural h.
hyla
hyoid bone
hypalgesia
h. dolorosa
hypalgesic, hypalgetic
hypalgia
Hypaque
hypaxial
hyperabduction
h. syndrome
hyperactivity
spontaneous neuronal h.
hyperacusis, hyperacusia
hyperadrenergic response
hyperalgesia
auditory h.
hyperalgesic, hyperalgetic
hyperalgia
hyperammonemia
cerebroatrophic h.
hyperaphia
hyperaphic
hyperbaric oxygen
hypercalcemia
hypercapnia
hypercarbia
hypercatabolism
hypercholesterolemia
familial h.
hypercinesis, hypercinesia
hypercoagulability
hypercoagulable state
hypercoagulation
hypercortisolism
hypercryalgesia
hypercryesthesia
hyperdynamia
hyperdynamic
hyperemia

NOTES

hyperergasia
hyperergic encephalitis
hyperesthesia
    auditory h.
    cerebral h.
    gustatory h.
    muscular h.
    olfactory h., h. olfactoria
    h. optica
    tactile h.
hyperesthetic
hyperextension
    intraoperative neck h.
hyperextension-hyperflexion injury
hyperflexion
hyperfractionated
    h. irradiation
    h. radiotherapy
hyperfractionation
hypergammaglobulinemia
hypergasia
hypergeusia
hyperglycemia
    nonketotic h.
hyperglycorrhachia
hyperintensity
    incidental punctate white
      matter h.
    punctate white matter h.
hyperkalemia
hyperkalemic periodic paralysis
hyperkinesis, hyperkinesia
hyperkinetic
    h. disorder
    h. syndrome
hyperkyphoscoliosis
    neuropathic h.
hyperlexia
hyperlipidemia
hyperlysinemia
hypermetamorphosis
hypermetria
hypermimia
hypermyesthesia
hypermyotonia
hypernatremic encephalopathy
hyperosmia
hyperosmolar hyperglycemic
  nonketonic coma
hyperosmolarity
hyperosphresia, hyperosphresis

hyperostosis
    diffuse idiopathic skeletal h.
    h. frontalis interna
hyperostotic spondylosis
hyperparathyroidism
hyperpathia
hyperperfusion syndrome
hyperphagia
hyperpipecolatemia
hyperpituitarism
hyperplasia
    arachnoidal h.
    fibromuscular h.
hyperpolarization
hyperponesis
hyperpraxia
hyperprolactinemia
hyperpyrexia
hyperreflexia
hypersecretion
hypersecretory adenoma
hypersensitivity
    h. vasculitis
hypersomnia
Hyperstat I.V.
hyperstimulation
    adrenergic h.
hypertarachia
hypertelorism
    orbital h.
hypertension
    venous h.
hypertensive encephalopathy
hypertensor
hyperthermalgesia
hyperthermia
    malignant h.
hyperthermoesthesia
hyperthyroidism
hypertonia
    sympathetic h.
hypertonic absence
hypertrichosis
hypertrophic
    h. arthritis
    h. cervical pachymeningitis
    h. interstitial neuropathy
    h. olivary degeneration
hypertrophied frenula syndrome
hypertrophy
    facet h.
    pseudomuscular h.
    uncovertebral joint h.

hypertropia
  over-right h.
hyperuricemia
hypervascularity
  intratumoral h.
hyperventilation
  h. test
  h. tetany
hypervolemia
hypervolemic treatment
hypesthesia
  brachiofacial cortical h.
  olfactory h.
hypesthetic ataxic hemiparesis
hyphema
hypnagogic hallucination
hypnalgia
hypnesthesia
hypnocinematograph
hypnogenic spot
hypnolepsy
hypnosis
hypnotic
hypoadrenalism
hypoalgesia
hypocalcemia
hypocapnia
hypochondria
hypochondrial reflex
hypochondroplasia
hypocomplementemic
  glomerulonephritis
hypocortisolemia
hypoechogenic peritumoral halo
hypoergia, hypoergy
hypoesthesia
hypofibrinogenemia
hypofunction
hypoganglionosis

hypogastric
  h. ganglia
  h. reflex
hypogenetic corpus callosum
hypogeusia
hypoglossal
  h. eminence
  h. nerve
  h. neuropathy
  h. nucleus
hypoglossal-facial nerve
  anastomosis
hypoglycorrhachia
hypogonadism
  h. with anosmia
hypohypnotic
hypointensity
hypokalemia
hypokalemic
  h. metabolic acidosis
  h. periodic paralysis
hypokinesia
hypokinetic syndrome
hypokyphosis
  right thoracic curve with h.
  thoracic h.
hypologia
hypometria
hypomyelination,
  hypomyelinogenesis
hypoparathyroidism
hypoparathyroid tetany
hypoperfusion
  cerebral h.
  delayed postischemic h.
hypophyseal
  h. aneurysm
hypophysectomize
hypophysectomy
  partial central h.
  total h.

NOTES

hypophysectomy *(continued)*
    transsphenoidal h.
    unilateral h.
hypophysial
    h. cachexia
    h. syndrome
hypophysio-sphenoidal syndrome
hypophysis
    h. cerebri
    pharyngeal h.
hypophysitis
    lymphocytic h.
    lymphoid h.
hypopituitarism
hypoplasia
    condylar h.
    optic nerve h.
hypopraxia
hyporeflexia
hyposensitivity
hyposmia
hyposomnia
hyposomniac
hyposphresia
hyposthenia
hypostheniant
hyposthenic
hypotaxia
hypotelorism
hypotension
    intracranial h.
    orthostatic h.
hypotensive
    h. retinopathy
    h. surgery
hypothalamic
    h. astrocytoma
    h. blood flow
    h. hamartoma
    h. infundibulum
    h. obesity
    h. sulcus
hypothalamic-pituitary dysfunction

hypothalamohypophysial
    h. portal system
    h. tract
hypothalamus
Hypotherm Gel Kap
hypothermia
    regional h.
hypothermic metabolic index
hypothesis
    congenital h.
    degenerative h.
    gate-control h.
    lipid h.
    mnemic h.
hypothyroidism
hypotonia
hypotonicity
hypotonus, hypotony
hypotropia
hypoventilation
hypovolemia
hypovolemic shock
hypoxemia
hypoxia
    histotoxic h.
    stagnant h.
hypsarhythmia, hypsarrhythmia
hypsicephalic
hypsicephaly
hypsocephaly
hysteresis
hysteria
    major h.
hysterical
    h. anesthesia
    h. chorea
    h. convulsion
    h. syncope
hystericoneuralgic
hysteroepilepsy
hysterogenic, hysterogenous
hysteroid convulsion

IAP
    intermittent acute porphyria
iatrogenic
    i. disease
    i. lumbar kyphosis
ibuprofen
ICA
    internal carotid artery
ICA-occluded stable Xe/CT CBF study
Iceland disease
Icelandic form of intracranial hemorrhage
ICP
    intracranial pressure
ictal
ictus
    i. epilepticus
    i. paralyticus
ideal spinal implant
ideation
    suicidal i.
ideational
    i. agnosia
    i. apraxia
ideatory apraxia
ideokinetic
    i. apraxia
ideomotion
ideomotor
    i. apraxia
idiocy
    amaurotic familial i.
idiodynamic
    i. control
idiomuscular
idiopathic
    i. epilepsy
    i. growth hormone deficiency
    i. muscular atrophy
    i. neuralgia
    i. orbital pseudotumor
    i. scoliosis
idiophrenic
idioreflex
idiospasm
idiot
ignipedites
ikota

ileocolitis
    granulomatous i.
Ilhéus encephalitis
iliac
    i. artery injury
    i. crest bone graft stabilization
    i. crest resection
    i. crest syndrome
    i. fixation
    i. post
    i. screw
iliocostal muscle
iliofemoral thrombosis
iliohypogastric nerve
iliopsoas muscle
iliosacral
    i. and iliac fixation construct
    i. screw
illness
    mental i.
image
    accidental i.
    axial spin-echo i.
    B-mode i.
    body i.
    contrast-enhanced MR i.
    cross-sectional i.
    i. foldover
    i. formation principle
    ghost i.
    gradient-echo MR i.
    incidental i.
    in-phase i.
    i. integrated surgery treatment planning
    i. intensification
    i. intensifier
    long pulse repetition time/echo time i.
    motor i.
    out-of-phase i.
    phantom i.
    proton-weighted i.
    i. quality
    sagittal spin-echo i.
    sagittal T1-weighted SE i.
    sensory i.

image *(continued)*
    short pulse repetition time/echo time i.
    stereotactic PET i.
    tactile i.
    thin-section i.
    tilting of i.'s
    tilting of visual i.'s
    T1-weighted i.
    T2-weighted i.
    T1-weighted MR i.
    T2-weighted MR i.
    T1-weighted spin-echo i.
    T2-weighted spin-echo i.
image-guided stereotactic brain biopsy
imaging
    chemical-shift i.
    Chopper-Dixon hybrid i.
    color-flow i.
    computerized infrared telethermographic i.
    continuous-wave Doppler i.
    contrast-enhanced MR i.
    2DFT gradient-echo i.
    3DFT gradient-echo i.
    3DFT gradient-echo MR i.
    Diasonics magnetic resonance i.
    diffusion i.
    digital vascular i. (DVI)
    direct multiplanar i.
    Dixon method opposed i.
    Doppler i.
    echoplanar i.
    fast i.
    fat-suppression MR i.
    flow i.
    flow-sensitive MR i.
    fluoroscopic i.
    gadolinium-enhanced MR i.
    Gd-DTPA-enhanced cranial MR i.
    gradient-echo MR i.
    gradient-refocused i.
    half-Fourier i.
    half-NEX i.
    high-resolution 3DFT MR i.
    MAGNES magnetic source i.
    magnetic resonance i. (MRI)
    magnetic source i. (MSI)
    neurodiagnostic i.

    nonproton magnetic resonance i.
    oblique sagittal gradient-echo MR i.
    partial flip angle i.
    partial Fourier i.
    phase-sensitive gradient-echo MR i.
    proton i.
    pulsed Doppler i.
    quantitative i.
    radionuclide i.
    rapid acquisition radiofrequency-echo steady state i.
    real-time color Doppler i.
    short inversion recovery i. (STIR)
    spin-echo i.
    subtraction i.
    ^{99m}Tc-HMPAO SPECT i.
    Tc-99m HMPAO cerebral perfusion SPECT i.
    three-dimensional i.
    three-dimensional fast low-angle shot i.
    three-dimensional Fourier transform gradient-echo i.
    transcranial real-time color Doppler i.
    two-dimensional i.
    two-dimensional Fourier transform gradient-echo i.
imbalance
    acid-base i.
    autonomic i.
    sympathetic i.
    vasomotor i.
imbecile
imipenem-cilastin
imipramine
    i. hydrochloride
imitative tetanus
immaculate hemostasis
immediate
    i. posttraumatic automatism
    i. posttraumatic convulsion
immitis
    Coccidioides i.
immobility
immobilization
    i. method
    postoperative i.

sternal occipital
mandibular i. (SOMI)
immune
i. complex
i. system
immunoblot
immunocytochemistry
immunocytology
immunodeficiency
immunodiagnosis
immunoelectrotransfer blot
technique
immunoglobulin
immunohistochemistry
immunological paralysis
immunoperoxidase method
immunoreaction
immunosuppression
immunosuppressive therapy
immunotherapy
immunotoxin
immunoturbidimetry analyzer
impairment
mental i.
impedance
i. audiometry
i. method
imperception
impingement
anterior cord i.
implant
broken existing i.
Christoferson's disk bony i.
cochlear i.
custom i.
DTT i.
epilepsy i.
i. fatigue
ferromagnetic i.
ideal spinal i.
metallic otologic i.

otologic i.
i. removal
silicone i.
i. survival rate
TSRH i.
implantation
i. cone
nerve i.
screw i.
subdural grid i.
implanted infusion pump
impotence, impotency
atonic i.
paretic i.
symptomatic i.
impressio, pl. impressiones
i. petrosa pallii
impression
basilar i.
petrosal i. of the pallium
impressive aphasia
impulse
in
i. situ photocoagulation
i. situ spinal fusion
i. situ tricortical iliac-crest
block bone graft
i. vivo optical spectroscopy
(INVOS)
i. vivo stereological
assessment
inadequate stimulus
inattention
sensory i.
visual i.
incidence
myelopathy i.
nonunion i.
incidental
i. aneurysm
i. image

NOTES

incidental *(continued)*
    i. punctate white matter
       hyperintensity
incision
    Caldwell-Luc i.
    dural i.
    horseshoe i.
    Lynch i.
    posterolateral
       costotransversectomy i.
    right-sided submandibular
       transverse i.
    scalp i.
    skin i.
    standard retroperitoneal
       flank i.
    T-shaped i.
    vertical midline i.
incisura, pl. incisurae
    i. cerebelli anterior
    i. cerebelli posterior
    i. preoccipitalis
    tentorial i.
    i. tentorii
incisural
    i. dissection
    i. space
incisure
    Lanterman's i.'s
    Schmidt-Lanterman i.'s
inclusion
    i. body encephalitis
    i. lipoma
    i. tumor
incompatibility
    Rh i.
incomplete
    i. alexia
    i. band heterotopia
    i. neurofibromatosis
incontinence
    overflow i.
    paradoxical i.
    passive i.
    reflex i.
    urge i., urgency i.
incontinentia
incoordination
IND
    internodal distance
Inderal
index, gen. indicis, pl. indices,
  indexes

    cardiac i.
    cardiac risk i.
    cephalorrhachidian i.
    cerebrospinal i.
    hypothermic metabolic i.
    Klaus's height i.
    labeling i. (LI)
    pressure-volume i.
    pulsatility i. (PI)
    steal i.
    TCD pulsatility i.
indicator
    finger i.
indifference to pain syndrome
indigotin disulfonate sodium
indirect fracture
indium-111
Indocin
indomethacin
induction
    Faraday's law of i.
indusium, pl. indusia
    i. griseum
inertia time
infancy
    melanotic neuroectodermal
       tumor of i.
infantile
    i. convulsion
    i. diplegia
    i. ganglioglioma
    i. hemangioblastic
       hemangioma
    i. hemiplegia
    i. muscular atrophy
    i. myofibromatosis
    i. neuroaxonal dystrophy
    i. neuronal degeneration
    i. progressive spinal
       muscular atrophy
    i. Refsum disease
    i. spasm
    i. spastic paraplegia
    i. tetany
    i. X-linked ataxia
    i. X-linked deafness
infantilism
    static i.
infarct
    cystic lacunar i.
    lacunar i.
infarction
    borderzone i.

brain i.
calcarine cortex i.
cerebral i.
inferolateral i.
lacunar i.
myocardial i.
paramedian i.
striatocapsular i.
tuberothalamic i.
ventral pontine i.
vertebrobasilar i.
watershed i.
infection
Absidia i.
Candida i.
Coccidioides i.
Cryptococcus i.
cysticercal i.
dental i.
epidural i.
fungal i.
hepatitis B virus i.
Histoplasma i.
mucor i.
Mycoplasma i.
odontogenic i.
postoperative i.
i. prevention
Rhizopus i.
scalp i.
spinal i.
viral i.
infectious
i. aneurysm
i. ophthalmoplegia
i. polyneuritis
infective endocarditis
inferior
i. anastomotic vein
i. cerebellar peduncle
i. cerebral veins

i. cervical ganglion
i. choroid vein
i. colliculus
i. dental nerve
i. extradural approach
i. frontal convolution
i. frontal gyrus
i. frontal sulcus
i. ganglion of
glossopharyngeal nerve
i. ganglion of vagus
i. horn
i. horn of lateral ventricle
i. laryngeal nerve
i. longitudinal fasciculus
i. medullary velum
i. mesenteric ganglion
i. occipital gyrus
i. olivary nucleus
i. olive
i. parietal gyrus
i. parietal lobule
i. part of vestibulocochlear
nerve
i. polioencephalitis
i. quadrigeminal brachium
i. root of cervical loop
i. root of vestibulocochlear
nerve
i. salivary nucleus
i. semilunar lobule
i. surface of cerebellar
hemisphere
i. temporal convolution
i. temporal gyrus
i. temporal sulcus
i. thalamic peduncle
i. thalamostriate veins
i. transvermian approach
i. veins of cerebellar
hemisphere

NOTES

inferior *(continued)*
    i. vena cava
    i. vertebra
    i. vestibular area
    i. vestibular nucleus
inferior-lateral endonasal
    transsphenoidal approach
inferolateral infarction
infestation
    fluke i.
    guinea worm i.
infiltrate
    lymphocytic i.
infiltration
    paraneural i.
    perineural i.
infiltrative
inflammation
    i. bowel disease
    cartilage i.
    ear cartilage i.
    ischemic ocular i.
inflammatory lesion
inflow effect
influenzae
    Haemophilus i.
infracerebral
infraclinoid aneurysm
infragranular layer
infraorbital
    i. injection
    i. nerve
infraspinous fascia
infratemporal fossa
infratentorial
    i. approach
    i. supracerebellar approach
infundibula (*pl. of* infundibulum)
infundibular
    i. part of anterior lobe of
      hypophysis
    i. recess
    i. stalk
    i. stem
infundibuloma
infundibulum, pl. **infundibula**
    i. hypothalami
    hypothalamic i.
infusion
    i. computed tomography
    diastole-phased pulsatile i.
    i. pump
ingravescent apoplexy

ingrowth
    neuronal i.
inherent contrast
inheritance
    autosomal dominant i.
    autosomal recessive i.
inhibitor
    cyclooxygenase i.
    monoamine oxidase i.
    xanthine oxidase i.
inhibitory fibers
inhomogeneity
    field i.
iniencephaly
injection
    epidural i.
    epidural steroid i.
    etomidate i.
    infraorbital i.
    i. injury
    intraventricular i.
    paramagnetic contrast i.
    retrobulbar i.
    saline i.
injury
    acceleration i.
    acute burst i.
    avulsion i.
    brachial plexus avulsion i.
    brain i.
    burst i.
    cervical nerve root i.
    cervical spine i.
    chemical i.
    closed head i. (CHI)
    common iliac artery i.
    contrecoup i.
    contrecoup i. of brain
    coup i.
    coup i. of brain
    crush i.
    current of i.
    diffuse axonal i.
    diffuse brain i.
    endothelial i.
    extension i.
    extension-type cervical
      spine i.
    flexion-distraction i.
    flexion-extension i.
    head i.
    hemorrhagic shearing i.

hyperextension-
hyperflexion i.
iliac artery i.
injection i.
i. of intervertebral disk
laryngeal nerve i.
middle column i.
missile i.
neural i.
open head i.
operative i.
optic nerve i.
parasympathetic nerve i.
penetrating i.
peripheral nerve i.
i. potential
radiation i.
rotational i.
rotationally induced shear-
strain i.
shearing i.
soft tissue i.
spinal cord i.
spleen i.
stable cervical spine i.
suction i.
thoracic duct i.
thoracolumbar spinal i.
thoracolumbar spine flexion-
distraction i.
three-column cervical
spine i.
tracheal i.
traumatic brain i.
two-column cervical spine i.
unstable cervical spine i.
ureter i.
vascular i.
vena cava i.
vertebral artery i.

whiplash i.
Wilbrand's knee i.
injury-healing theory
Injury Severity Scale
innate reflex
inner cone fiber
innervation
adrenergic i.
i. apraxia
innominate
i. artery
i. substance
i. vein
Innovar
in-phase image
input
cerebral sensory i.
insensible
inserter
Texas Scottish Rite Hospital
hook i.
insertion
C-D rod i.
i. equipment
oblique screw i.
pedicle screw i.
screw i.
Syracuse anterior I-plate i.
insipidus
diabetes i.
inspiratory center
instability
atlantoaxial i.
lumbar spine i.
occipitoatlantoaxial i.
phase i.
postural i.
sagittal plane i.
vertebral cervical i.
installation procedure
instant scan

NOTES

Instat fibrin film
instrument
    Backlund's stereotactic i.
    Dwyer i.
    Malis bipolar i.
    i. migration
    pencil-grip i.
    pistol-grip i.
    Radionics bipolar i.
    solid-state i.
    spark-gap i.
    stereotactic i., stereotaxic i.
    Yasargil-Aesculap i.
    Zielke i.
instrumentation
    anterior distraction i.
    AO fixateur interne i.
    AO notched i.
    C-D i.
    compression i.
    compression U-rod i.
    Cotrel-Dubousset i.
    Cotrel-Dubousset pedicle
      screw i.
    Cotrel-Dubousset
      pedicular i.
    Cotrel-Dubousset spinal i.
    distraction i.
    double Zielke i.
    dynamic compression
      plate i.
    Edwards i.
    i. failure
    Harrington i.
    Harrington rod i.
    interspinous segmental
      spinal i. (ISSI)
    Jacobs locking hook spinal
      rod i.
    Jacobs locking spinal rod i.
    Kaneda anterior spinal i.
    Louis i.
    lumbar spine i.
    lumbosacral spine
      transpedicular i.
    Luque i.
    Luque II segmental
      spinal i.
    Luque segmental spinal i.
    Luque semirigid segmental
      spinal i.
    modular i.

    multiple hook assembly C-
      D i.
    posterior i.
    posterior cervical spinal i.
    posterior distraction i.
    posterior hook-rod spinal i.
    sacral spine modular i.
    sacral spine universal i.
    segmental i.
    segmental spinal i. (SSI)
    spinal i.
    Steffee i.
    stereotactic i.
    transpedicular spinal i.
    TSRH i.
    universal i.
    variable screw placement
      system i.
    VSP plate i.
    Zielke i.
insufficiency
    adrenal i.
    adrenocortical i.
    aortic i.
    i. of eyelids
    mechanical i.
    muscular i.
    vertebrobasilar i.
insula, gen. and pl. **insulae**
insular
    i. area
    i. cortex
    i. sclerosis
insulated electrode needle
Insulin
    Protamine Zinc I.
insulin
    i. coma treatment
    i. hypoglycemia test
insult
intact
    i. spinous lamina
    i. spinous process
intellectual aura
intensification
    image i.
intensifier
    image i.
    OEC-Diasonics mobile C-
      arm image i.
intensity
    signal i.

intention
    i. spasm
    i. tremor
interaction
    dipole-dipole i.
    electron-coupled nuclear
       spin-spin i.
    proton-electron dipole-
       dipole i.
interannular segment
interarticularis
    pars i.
interbody
    i. fusion
    i. graft
intercalary neuron
intercalated nucleus
intercavernous sinus
intercerebral
interclinoid ligament
intercostal neuralgia
intercostohumeralis
intercrural
    i. ganglion
interdural tumor
interest
    regions of i. (ROI)
interface
    long-term bone-
       instrumentation i.
interfacet wiring and fusion
interfascial approach
interfascicular fasciculus
interferon
interforniceal approach
interganglionic
intergemmal
intergyral
interhemicerebral
interhemispheric
    i. approach

    i. cyst
    i. fissure
    i. propagation time
interictal
    i. epileptiform spike
interlaminar
    i. clamp
    i. decompression
interleaved GRASS
interleukin
interlocking gyri
intermanual conflict
intermediate
    i. C-D hook
    i. ganglia
    i. layer
    i. nerve
    i. part
intermediate-acting insulin
  preparation
intermediolateral
    i. cell column of spinal
      cord
    i. mesencephalic syndrome
    i. nucleus
intermediomedial nucleus
intermedius
    ventralis i. (VIM)
intermeningeal
intermittent
    i. acute porphyria (IAP)
    i. cramp
    i. tetanus
    i. torticollis
interna
    hyperostosis frontalis i.
internal
    i. arcuate fibers
    i. auditory canal
    i. capsule
    i. capsule syndrome

NOTES

internal *(continued)*
    i. carotid artery (ICA)
    i. carotid artery balloon test occlusion
    i. carotid balloon test
    i. cerebral veins
    i. decompression
    i. fixation
    i. fixation plate-screw system
    i. fixation spring
    i. hydrocephalus
    i. jugular vein
    i. meningitis
    i. neurolysis
    i. pillar cells
    i. pulse generating unit
    i. pyocephalus
    i. respiration
    i. spinal fixation
interne
    AO/ASIF fixateur i.
    AO fixateur i.
    Dick AO fixateur i.
    fixateur i. (FI)
interneurons
internodal
    i. distance (IND)
    i. segment
internode
internuclear
    i. ophthalmoplegia
internuncial
    i. neuron
interoceptive
interoceptor
interofective system
interolivary
interparietal sulcus
interpedicular distance
interpeduncular
    i. cistern
    i. fossa
    i. fossa lesion
    i. ganglion
    i. nucleus
interpositi
    cavum veli i. (CVI)
interpositum
    velum i.
interscapular reflex
intersegmental fasciculi

interspace
    cervical i.
    lumbar i.
    thoracic i.
interspinous
    i. segmental spinal instrumentation (ISSI)
    i. segmental spinal instrumentation technique
interstitial
    i. brachytherapy
    i. neuritis
    i. nucleus of Cajal
    i. radiotherapy
interthalamic
    i. adhesion
interuncal distance
interventional
    i. materials
    i. neuroradiology
    i. radiology
interventricular foramen
intervertebral
    i. discitis
    i. disk
    i. ganglion
    i. osteochondrosis
intestinal trauma
intoxication
    water i.
intra-arterial
    i.-a. Amytal testing
    i.-a. drug delivery
intraarterial flow
intracapsular hemorrhage
intracarotid sodium Amytal memory testing
intracavernous
    i. aneurysm
    i. carotid aneurysm
    i. tumor
intracelial
intracellular deoxyhemoglobin
intracerebellar
intracerebral
    i. arteriovenous malformation
    i. ganglioma
    i. hematoma
    i. hemorrhage
    i. steal
intracisternal

intracranial
  i. abscess
  i. aneurysm
  i. cryptococcosis
  i. ganglion
  i. hematoma
  i. hemorrhage
  i. hypotension
  i. lesion
  i. mass lesion
  i. MR angiography
  i. neuroblastoma
  i. occlusion
  i. pneumatocele
  i. pneumocele
  i. pressure (ICP)
  i. rhizotomy
  i. steal phenomenon
  i. tumor
  i. vascular malformation
  i. venous sinus
intracranial-extracranial nerve graft
intracranial-intratemporal nerve graft
intractable
  i. epilepsy
  i. pain
intradural
  i. approach
  i. dissection
  i. inflammatory disease
  i. lipoma
  i. phase
  i. segment
  i. tumor
  i. tumor surgery
intrafascicular
intrafusal
  i. fibers
intragemmal
intragyral

intralaminar nuclei of thalamus
intramedullary
  i. nail
  i. toxoplasmosis
  i. tractotomy
intrameningeal
intramolecular
  i. dipole-dipole mechanism
  i. relaxation
intramural
intraneural
intranuclear
  i. ophthalmoplegia
intraocular
  i. hemorrhage
  i. neuritis
  i. pressure
intraoperative
  i. angiography
  i. balloon occlusion
  i. B-mode ultrasound
  i. cell saver
  i. dural tear
  i. facial nerve monitoring
  i. neck hyperextension
  i. rupture
  i. stress-relaxation
  i. ultrasonic probe
  i. ultrasound
  i. x-ray
intraorbital
  i. granular cell tumor
  i. lesion
  i. surgery
intraparenchymal
  i. cyst
  i. hematoma
  i. meningioma
intraparietal
  i. sulcus
  i. sulcus of Turner

NOTES

intrapontine
Intrascan ultrasound
intrasellar extension
intraspinal herniated disk
intraspinous muscle
intratentorial supracerebellar
   approach
intrathecal
   i. antibiotic
   i. morphine analgesia
intratumoral hypervascularity
intrauterine sonographic diagnosis
intravascular
   i. balloon occlusion
   i. device
   i. ligature
   i. streaming
intravenous oxygen-15 water bolus
   technique
intraventricular (I-V)
   i. catheter
   i. endoscopy
   i. hemorrhage
   i. injection
   i. meningioma
   i. tumor
intravoxel phase dispersion
intrinsic
   i. disease
   i. fibers
   i. reflex
   i. transverse connector
   i. transverse connector role
Intropin
intubation
   aqueductal i.
   nasogastric i.
   oral i.
intumescence
   tympanic i.
intumescent
intumescentia
   i. cervicalis
   i. ganglioformis
   i. lumbalis
   i. tympanica
invagination
   basilar i.
invasive tumor
inverse
   i. Anton's syndrome
   i. ocular bobbing
   i. square rule

inversed jaw-winking syndrome
inversion
   inversion recovery imaging
      with short-time i.
   i. recovery
   visual image i.
inverted
   i. radial reflex
   i. reflex
investigatory reflex
involuntary
   i. nervous system
involvement
   extraocular muscle i.
   tumorous i.
INVOS
   in vivo optical spectroscopy
iodine
   isotopic i.
iohexol
   i. CT ventriculogram
   i. myelography
iopamidol
iophendylate
iothalamate
   meglumine i.
ioversol
ioxaglate
   i. meglumine
   i. sodium
I-plate
   Syracuse anterior I-p.
ipsilateral
   i. reflex
I/Q imbalance ghost
iridis
   rubeosis i.
iridium-192
iridocyclitis
iridoparalysis
iridoplegia
   complete i.
   reflex i.
   sympathetic i.
iris neovascularization
iritis
   white i.
iron deficiency anemia
irradiation
   convergent beam i. (CBI)
   gamma i.
   hyperfractionated i.
irreversible shock

Irrigant
    Neosporin GU I.
irritable
    i. heart
    i. testis
irritation
ischemia
    cerebral i.
ischemic
    i. disease
    i. lumbago
    i. muscular atrophy
    i. ocular inflammation
    i. optic neuropathy
    i. stroke
ischialgia
ischiodynia
ischioneuralgia
^{125}**I seeds**
I-shaped scalp flap
Ishihara plate
island
    i.'s of Calleja
    i. pedicle scalp flap
    i. of Reil
isobutyl-2-cyanoacrylate
Isocal
isocentric linear accelerator
isocortex
isodense subdural hematoma
isoelectric electroencephalogram
isoetharine hydrochloride
isoflurane
    i. anesthesia
Isola
    I. spinal implant system
    I. spinal implant system
        accessory
    I. spinal implant system
        anchor

I. spinal implant system
    application
I. spinal implant system
    complication
I. spinal implant system
    component
I. spinal implant system
    design
I. spinal implant system
    dimensions
I. spinal implant system
    eye rod
I. spinal implant system
    hook
I. spinal implant system
    iliac post
I. spinal implant system
    iliac screw
I. spinal implant system
    longitudinal member
    contouring
I. spinal implant system
    plate-rod combination
isolated
    i. angiitis
    i. granulomatous angiitis of
        the central nervous system
        (GANS)
isomeric function
isometheptene
isomorphous gliosis
isoniazid
    i. neuropathy
isophane
isopropyl alcohol
isopropylparaiodoamphetamine
Isoproterenol
    Mucomyst with I.
isoproterenol
Isordil
isosorbide dinitrate

NOTES

isotope
isotopic iodine
isotrophic three-dimensional
  Fourier transform
isotropic 3DFT
isovolemic hemodilution
IsoVue
ISSI
    interspinous segmental spinal
      instrumentation
isthmi (*pl. of* isthmus)
isthmoparalysis
isthmoplegia
isthmus, pl. isthmi, isthmuses
    i. of cingular gyrus
    i. gyri cinguli
    i. of gyrus fornicatus
    i. of His

    i. of limbic lobe
    i. rhombencephali
    rhombencephalic i.
Isuprel
iter
    i. a tertio ad quartum
      ventriculum
ithykyphosis, ithycyphosis
ithylordosis
I-V
    intraventricular
Ivalon
    I. embolic sponge
    I. particle
    I. sponge
    I. wire coil
Iwabuchi clip
ixomyelitis

jack
    turnbuckle j.
jacket
    Minerva j.
jacksonian
    j. epilepsy
Jackson-Pratt drain
Jackson's
    J. law
    J. rule
    J. sign
    J. vagoaccessory hypoglossal
      paralysis
Jacobs
    J. locking hook spinal rod
    J. locking hook spinal rod
      instrumentation
    J. locking hook spinal rod
      instrumentation
      modification
    J. locking hook spinal rod
      technique
    J. locking spinal rod
      instrumentation
Jacobson's
    J. nerve
    J. reflex
Jadassohn's nevus sebaceus
Jaeger-Hamby procedure
Jahnke's syndrome
jake paralysis
Jakob-Creutzfeldt disease
Janet's test
Jannetta
    J. forceps
    J. microvascular
      decompression procedure
Jansen-Middleton
    J.-M. forceps
    J.-M. rongeur
    J.-M. scissors
Jansky-Bielschowsky disease
Japanese
    J. B encephalitis
    J. suction tip
jar
    heel j.
jargon
    j. aphasia
Jarit periosteal elevator

jaundice
    nuclear j.
Javid shunt
jaw
    j. jerk
    lock-j.
    j. reflex
jaw-winking
    j.-w. phenomenon
    j.-w. syndrome
jaw-working reflex
Jefferson's fracture
jejunostomy
Jendrassik's maneuver
Jerald forceps
jerk
    ankle j.
    chin j.
    crossed j.
    crossed adductor j.
    crossed knee j.
    elbow j.
    j. finger
    jaw j.
    knee j.
    supinator j.
jeweler's
    j. bipolar forceps
    j. forceps
jig
    Ace Hershey halo j.
Joffroy's
    J. reflex
    J. sign
joint
    atlantoaxial j.
    atlanto-occipital j.
    Charcot's j.
    j. disorder
    facet j.
    neuropathic j.
    sacroiliac j.
    j. sense
    temporomandibular j.
    zygapophyseal j.
Jolly's reaction
Jolly test
Joubert's syndrome
joule
J-sella deformity

J-tipped guidewire
jugular
- j. bulb
- j. bulb venous oxygen saturation
- j. foramen
- j. foramen syndrome
- j. ganglion
- j. vein
- j. vein dissection

jugulocephalic vein
jugulotympanicum
- glomus j

jumper
- j. disease
- j. disease of Maine

junction
- cervical medullary j.
- cervicothoracic j.
- craniocervical j.
- craniovertebral j.
- electrotonic j.
- gap j.
- liponeural j.
- lumbosacral j.
- myoneural j.
- neuromuscular j.
- thoracolumbar j.

junctional
- j. dilation
- j. kyphosis

juvenile
- j. amyotrophy
- j. angiofibroma
- j. chorea
- j. fibromatosis
- j. muscular atrophy
- j. myoclonic epilepsy
- j. pilocytic astrocytoma
- j. rheumatoid arthritis

juxtallocortex
juxtarestiform body

kakké
Kallmann's syndrome
kanamycin
Kandel stereotactic apparatus
Kaneda anterior spinal
   instrumentation
kaolin
Kap
      Hypotherm Gel K.
kappa opiate receptor
Karlin Microknife
Karnofsky
      K. Performance Scale
      K. Rating Scale
karyochrome
      k. cell
Kasabach-Merritt syndrome
Katzman test
Kayser-Fleischer rings
K complex
Kearns-Sayre syndrome
Keeler
      K. panoramic loupe
      K. video headlamp
Keen's
      K. operation
      K. point
keirospasm
Kelly stereotactic system
Kelvin body
Kenalog 40
Kennedy's syndrome
Kerandel's symptom
kerasin histiocytosis
keratitis
      neuroparalytic k.
keratoacanthoma
keratoconjunctivitis
      k. sicca
keratoderma blennorrhagicum
keratopathy
      band k.
      exposure k.
keratosis
      actinic k.
      k. obturans
      seborrheic k.
kernicterus
Kernig's sign
Kernig test

Kernohan's notch
Kerohan system of glioma
   classification
Kerr clip
Kerrison
      K. bone punch
      K. microronguer
      K. punch
      K. rongeur
ketamine
ketoacidosis
ketoconazole
ketoprofen
Keystone graft
kidney disease
Kiloh-Nevin syndrome
kinanesthesia
kindling
kinesioneurosis
kinesipathy
kinesogenic choreoathetosis
kinesthesia
kinesthesiometer
kinesthetic
      k. aura
      k. sense
kinetic
      k. ataxia
      k. drive
      k. tremor
kinetics
      cellular k.
King
      K. type I curve
      K. type II curve
      K. type III curve
      K. type II scoliosis
      K. type II thoracic and
      lumbar curves
      K. type IV curve
      K. type IV curve posterior
      correction
      K. type V curve
      K. type V scoliosis
kink
      cervicomedullary k.
kinky-hair disease
kinohapt
Kirby-Bauer disk diffusion method

Kirschner
    K. pin
    K. wire
    K. wire placement
Kisch's reflex
kit
    Laserscope discography k.
    Radiofocus introducer B k.
    Shiley distention k.
Klaus's height index
kleeblattschädel
Klippel-Feil syndrome
Klippel's disease
Klippel-Trenaunay syndrome
Klippel-Trenaunay-Weber syndrome
Klonopin
Klumpke-Dejerine syndrome
Klumpke's paralysis
Klüver-Bucy syndrome
knee
    k. jerk
    k. phenomenon
    k. reflex
knee-chest position
knee-jerk reflex
knife
    canal k.
    Cottle k.
    diamond k.
    electric k.
    gamma k.
    hot k.
    Leksell gamma k.
Knight forceps
knismogenic
Knochenschädel
Knodt rod
knot
    primitive k.
    vital k.
knuckle
    cervical aortic k.
Koala Pad graphics tablet
Kobayashi retractor
Kocher clamp
Kocher's point
Koerber-Salus-Elschnig syndrome
Koerte-Ballance operation
Kohnstamm's phenomenon
Kojewnikoff's epilepsy
Kölliker's reticulum
koniocortex

Korsakoff's
    K. psychosis
    K. syndrome
Kostuik
    K. rod
    K. screw
Kostuik-Harrington
    K.-H. device
    K.-H. distraction system
Krabbe's
    K. disease
    K. syndrome
Krause denervation
Krause's
    K. end bulbs
    K. respiratory bundle
Krimsky test
k-space
KTP/532 surgical laser
kubisagari, kubisagaru
Kufs disease
Kugelberg-Welander disease
Kühne's
    K. phenomenon
    K. spindle
Kümmell's spondylitis
Küntscher nail
kuru
Kussmaul-Landry paralysis
Kussmaul's
    K. aphasia
    K. coma
K-wire
    K-w. placement
kymatism
kynurenic acid
kyphoscoliosis
    neurofibromatosis k.
    k. secondary to
        neurofibromatosis
    severe k.
    thoracolumbar k.
kyphosis
    acute angular k.
    congenital k.
    k. correction
    k. creation
    iatrogenic lumbar k.
    junctional k.
    lumbar k.
    postlaminectomy k.
    posttraumatic k.

right thoracic curve with
  junctional k.
Scheuermann's k.
thoracic k.
thoracolumbar k.

kyphotic
  k. deformity
  k. deformity pathomechanics

NOTES

L

L4-5 disk disease
Labbé
    vein of L.
Labbé's
    L. neurocirculatory
      syndrome
    L. vein
labeling index (LI)
labetalol
labial paralysis
labiochorea
labioglossolaryngeal
labioglossomandibular approach
labioglossopharyngeal
labiomandibular
    l. approach
    l. glossotomy
labyrinth
    vestibular l.
labyrinthectomy
labyrinthine
    l. concussion syndrome
    l. disease
    l. fistula test
    l. reflexes
    l. righting reflexes
    l. torticollis
labyrinthitis
laceration
    brain l.
    scalp l.
Lacrilube
lacrimal
    l. duct
    l. gland
    l. gland dysfunction
    l. nerve
    l. reflex
lacrimation
lacrimo-gustatory reflex
lactate
    Ringer's l.
lactation
lactic acidosis
lactotroph cell
lacuna, pl. lacunae, lacunas
    l. cerebri
    lacunae laterales
lacunaire
    etat l.

lacunar
    l. infarct
    l. infarction
lacunas (pl. of lacuna)
Ladd fiberoptic system
Lafora
    L. body
    L. body disease
Lafora's
    L. disease
    L. familial myoclonic
      epilepsy
lagophthalmos
Lahey score
Laitinen Stereoadapter
lake
    lateral l.'s
    venous l.
lalognosis
laloplegia
Lamaze technique
lamella, pl. lamellae
    triangular l.
lamellated corpuscles
lamina, pl. laminae
    l. affixa
    l. alaris
    alar l. of neural tube
    laminae albae cerebelli
    l. arcus vertebrae
    l. basalis
    basal l. of neural tube
    basilar l.
    l. basilaris cochleae
    l. choroidea
    l. choroidea epithelialis
    l. cinerea
    l. dorsalis
    epithelial l.
    l. epithelialis
    intact spinous l.
    lateral medullary l. of
      corpus striatum
    medial medullary l. of
      corpus striatum
    laminae medullares cerebelli
    laminae medullares thalami
    l. medullaris lateralis
      corporis striati

lamina *(continued)*
    l. medullaris medialis
      corporis striati
    periclaustral l.
    l. quadrigemina
    Rexed l.
    rostral l.
    l. rostralis
    l. septi pellucidi
    l. of septum pellucidum
    l. spreader
    l. supraneuroporica
    l. tecti mesencephali
    l. terminalis cerebri
    l. ventralis
    l. of vertebral arch
laminar
    l. C-D hook
    l. cortex posterior aspect
    l. cortical necrosis
    l. cortical sclerosis
    l. hook
laminated cortex
laminectomized spine
laminectomy
    cervical l.
    cervical spine l.
    decompression l.
    decompressive l.
    Gill l.
    Girdlestone l.
    multilevel l.
    4-place l.
laminoplasty
laminotomy
lancinating
Landau-Kleffner syndrome
landmark
    pedicle l.
    surface l.
Landouzy-Dejerine dystrophy
Landouzy-Grasset law
Landry-Guillain-Barré syndrome
Landry's paralysis
Landry syndrome
Langenbach elevator
Langerhans cell granulomastosis
Langerhans' cells
language
    l. disorder
    l. zone
Lanoxin

Lanterman's
    L. incisures
    L. segments
lanthanide
Lapras catheter
large ball nerve hook
Larmor
    L. equation
    L. frequency
    L. precession
Larodopa
laryngeal
    l. chorea
    l. crisis
    l. epilepsy
    l. nerve injury
    l. syncope
    l. vertigo
laryngoparalysis
laryngoplegia
laryngospasm
laryngospastic reflex
Lasègue's
    L. sign
    L. test
laser
    argon l.
    carbon dioxide l.
    Cavitron l.
    l. disk decompression
      (LDD)
    KTP/532 surgical l.
    Nd:YAG l.
    Sharplan l.
    l. surgery
Laserflow blood perfusion monitor
Laserscope discography kit
Lasix
latah
late epilepsy
latent
    l. period
    l. reflex
    l. tetany
    l. zone
lateral
    l. aperture of the fourth
      ventricle
    l. approach
    l. cerebral fissure
    l. cerebral fossa
    l. cerebral sulcus
    l. column of spinal cord

l. corticospinal tract
l. cuneate nucleus
l. extracavitary approach
l. femoral cutaneous nerve
l. fillet
l. fossa of brain
l. funiculus of spinal cord
l. geniculate body
l. ground bundle
l. horn
l. inferior pontine syndrome
l. intradural approach
l. lakes
l. listhesis
l. longitudinal stria
l. medullary lamina of corpus striatum
l. medullary syndrome
l. nucleus of medulla oblongata
l. nucleus of thalamus
l. occipital sulcus
l. occipitotemporal gyrus
l. preoptic nucleus
l. projection
l. pyramidal tract
l. recess of fourth ventricle
l. recess stenosis
l. rectus palsy
l. reticular nucleus
l. roentgenogram
l. root of median nerve
l. root of optic tract
l. sinus
l. spinal sclerosis
l. spinothalamic tract
l. superior pontine syndrome
l. tarsorrhaphy
l. temporal resection
l. thalamic peduncle

l. thoracic meningocele
l. tuberal nuclei
l. ventricle
l. vertigo
l. vestibular nucleus
lateralis
ventralis l. (VL)
laterality
crossed l.
lateropulsion
l. of body movement
l. of eye movement
latex
l. balloon
l. covered pledget
lathyrism
latissimus dorsi muscle
latticed layer
lattice field
laughing sickness
laughter reflex
Laumonier's ganglion
Laurence-Biedl syndrome
Laurence-Moon-Bardet-Biedl syndrome
Laurence-Moon syndrome
law
l. of average localization
Bell-Magendie l.
Bell's l.
Broadbent's l.
l. of denervation
Flatau's l.
Gerhardt-Semon l.
Grasset's l.
Hagen-Poiseuille l.
Hilton's l.
l. of initial value
l. of isochronism
Jackson's l.
Landouzy-Grasset l.

NOTES

law *(continued)*
    Magendie's l.
    Müller's l.
    Poiseuille's l.
    l. of referred pain
    Ritter's l.
    Rosenbach's l.
    Semon's l.
    Sherrington's l.
    Stokes' l.
    van der Kolk's l.
    wallerian l.
    Wilder's l. of initial value
Lawford's syndrome
layer
    bacillary l.
    l. of Bechterew
    l.'s of cerebellar cortex
    l.'s of cerebral cortex
    cerebral l. of retina
    claustral l.
    ependymal l.
    epithelial choroid l.
    fillet l.
    fusiform l.
    ganglionic l. of cerebellar
      cortex
    ganglionic l. of cerebral
      cortex
    ganglionic l. of optic nerve
    ganglionic l. of retina
    granular l.'s of cerebral
      cortex
    granular l.'s of retina
    gray l. of superior colliculus
    Henle's fiber l.
    Henle's nervous l.
    infragranular l.
    intermediate l.
    latticed l.
    mantle l.
    marginal l.
    medullary l.'s of thalamus
    Meynert's l.
    molecular l.
    molecular l. of cerebellar
      cortex
    molecular l. of cerebral
      cortex
    molecular l.'s of olfactory
      bulb
    molecular l. of retina
    multiform l.

    neural l. of retina
    neuroepithelial l. of retina
    nuclear l.'s of retina
    optic l.
    pigmented l. of retina
    l. of piriform neurons
    plexiform l.
    plexiform l. of cerebral
      cortex
    plexiform l.'s of retina
    polymorphous l.
    Purkinje's l.
    pyramidal cell l.
    l. of rods and cones
    rostral l.
    spindle-celled l.
    ventricular l.
    Waldeyer's zonal l.
    zonular l.
l-bolt
    Texas Scottish Rite
      Hospital l-b.
LDD
    laser disk decompression
    LDD delivery system
lead
    l. encephalitis
    l. encephalopathy
    l. neuropathy
    l. palsy
    l. paralysis
lead-pipe rigidity
leakage
    cerebrospinal fluid l.
    chylous l.
Leatherman hook
Lee's ganglion
LeFort
    L. classification
    L. osteotomy
left
    l. common carotid artery
    l. thoracolumbar major
      curve pattern
left-footed
left-handed
left-sided thoracotomy
leg
    l. phenomenon
    restless l.'s
Legendre function
Legendre's sign
leg-raising test

Leibinger titanium mini-Würzburg implant system
Leichtenstern's
    L. phenomenon
    L. sign
Leigh's
    L. disease
    L. syndrome
Leksell
    L. frame
    L. gamma knife
    L. Micro-Stereotactic system
    L. rongeur
    L. selector
    L. stereotactic frame
    L. stereotactic gamma unit
    L. technique
lemniscus, pl. lemnisci
    acoustic l.
    auditory l.
    gustatory l.
    l. lateralis
    medial l.
    l. medialis
    l. spinalis
    trigeminal l.
    l. trigeminalis
length
    chord l.
    crown-rump l.
    pedicle screw chord l.
    pedicle screw path l.
lengthening
    distal catheter l.
    l. reaction
Lenhossék's processes
Lennox-Gastaut syndrome
Lennox syndrome
lens
    275mm objective l.

Lente
    L. Iletin I
lenticula
lenticular
    l. ansa
    l. ganglion
    l. loop
    l. nucleus
    l. progressive degeneration
lenticulo-optic
lenticulostriate
    l. arteries
lenticulothalamic
lentiform nucleus
leprosy
    anesthetic l.
    articular l.
    dry l.
    mutilating l.
    trophoneurotic l.
leprous neuropathy
leptomeningeal
    l. carcinoma
    l. carcinomatosis
    l. cyst
    l. fibrosis
    l. metastasis
    l. tumor
leptomeninges
leptomeningitis
    basilar l.
leptomeninx
leptomyelolipoma
Leriche's
    L. operation
    L. syndrome
Leriche sympathectomy
Leri's sign
Leroy-Raney scalp clip
Lesch-Nyhan syndrome

NOTES

Leser-Trélat sign
lesion
    basal ganglionic l.
    chiasmal l.
    demyelinating l.
    discoid skin l.
    dorsal root entry zone l.
    Duret's l.
    entry zone l.
    extracranial mass l.
    l. generation
    high-intensity l.
    inflammatory l.
    interpeduncular fossa l.
    intracranial l.
    intracranial mass l.
    intraorbital l.
    mass l.
    mucous membrane l.
    nail l.
    nonmeningiomatous
      malignant l.
    optic nerve l.
    paraorbital l.
    parasagittal l.
    periventricular l.
    periventricular
      hyperintense l.
    periventricular white
      matter l.
    pigment epithelial l.
    pseudomedial longitudinal
      fasciculus l.
    radiofrequency l.
    regurgitant l.
    retrochiasmal l.
    ring-wall l.
    rotationally induced shear-
      strain l.
    skin l.
    space-occupying brain l.
    spinal l.
    subtentorial l.
    supranuclear l.
    supratentorial l.
    upper motor neuron l.
lesioning
    dorsal root entry zone l.
    DREZ l.
    nucleus caudalis-nucleus
      solitarius DREZ l.
    radiofrequency l.

    trigeminal nucleus
      caudalis l.
LET
    linear energy transfer
lethal midline granuloma
lethargy
letter blindness
Letterer-Siwe disease
letters
    Snellen l.
leucotomy
leucovorin
leukocyte scintigraphy
leukocytoclastic vasculitides
leukocytosis
leukodystrophia
    l. cerebri progressiva
leukodystrophy
    globoid cell l.
    metachromatic l.
    Pelizaeus-Merzbacher l.
    sudanophilic l.
leukoencephalitis
    acute epidemic l.
    subacute sclerosing l.
leukoencephalopathy
    diffuse necrotizing l.
    progressive multifocal l.
      (PML)
leukokoria
leukomalacia
leukomyelopathy
leukopenia
leukotome
leukotomy
    prefrontal l.
    transorbital l.
leukotriene
levallorphan tartrate
levator
    l. palpebrae muscle
level
    spinal l.
    vertebral l.
leverage
levodopa
levothyroxine sodium
Lewy bodies
Leyden-Möbius muscular dystrophy
Leyden's
    L. ataxia
    L. neuritis
Leyla self-retaining tractor bar

Lhermitte-Duclos disease
Lhermitte's sign
LI
  labeling index
Librium
Lichtheim's sign
Liddell-Sherrington reflex
lidocaine
  l. test
lift
  brow l.
  pneumatic chair l.
Ligaclip
  Ethicon L.
Liga clip applier
ligament
  axial-occipital l.
  cruciate l.
  dentate l.
  denticulate l.
  fracture-dislocation with
    anterior l.
  interclinoid l.
  longitudinal l.
  posterior longitudinal l.
  Struthers' l.
  yellow l.
ligamentum, pl. ligamenta
  l. denticulatum
ligation
  hunterian l.
  sigmoid sinus l.
ligature
  intravascular l.
light sleep
Liliequist
  membrane of L.
lilliputian hallucination
limb
  ampullary l.'s of
    semicircular ducts

  anterior l. of internal
    capsule
  l.'s of bony semicircular
    canals
  common l. of membranous
    semicircular ducts
  phantom l.
  posterior l. of internal
    capsule
  retrolenticular l. of internal
    capsule
  simple membranous l. of
    semicircular duct
  sublenticular l. of internal
    capsule
limb-girdle muscular dystrophy
limbic
  l. lobe
  l. system
Limbitrol
limb-kinetic apraxia
limen, pl. limina
  l. insulae
liminal
  l. stimulus
liminometer
limit
  extreme narrowing l.
limitation
  receiver l.
limiting
  l. sulcus of Reil
  l. sulcus of rhomboid fossa
LINAC
  linear accelerator
  LINAC radiosurgery
  LINAC system
LINAC-based radiosurgical system
Lindau's
  L. disease
  L. tumor

NOTES

Linde XeScan
line
    AC-PC l.
      anterior commissure-
        posterior commissure line
    anterior commissure-
      posterior commissure l.
      (AC-PC line, AC-PC line)
    l. artifact
    Baillarger's l.'s
    basal l.
    l. of Bechterew
    bimastoid l.
    Chamberlain's l.
    Chamberlain's palato-
      occipital l.
    Chaussier's l.
    clivus canal l.
    diagastric l.
    Fishgold's l.
    foramen magnum l.
    l. frequency noise dot
    Garrett l.
    Garrett orientation l.
    l. of Gennari
    Gubler's l.
    Head's l.'s
    l. of Kaes
    McGregor's basal l.
    McRae's foramen
      magnum l.
    midpoint to meatal l.
    Obersteiner-Redlich l.
    palato-occipital l.
    posterior canal l.
    radio signal l.
    Reid's base l.
    Rolandic l.
    simian l.
    spinolamellar l.
    spinous interlaminar l.
    sylvian l.
    tender l.'s
    Ullmann's l.
    Voigt's l.'s
    Wackenheim's clivus
      canal l.
linear
    l. accelerator (LINAC)
    l. accelerator system
      (LINAC system)
    l. craniectomy
    l. energy transfer (LET)

    l. fracture
    l. skull fracture
linear accelerator (LINAC)
    isocentric l. a.
liner
    Teflon l.
lingua, gen. and pl. linguae
    l. cerebelli
lingual
    l. gyrus
    l. trophoneurosis
    l. vein
lingula, pl. lingulae
    l. cerebelli
lingular
linguofacial vein
linkage
    l. analysis
    rod l.
Lioresal
liothyronine sodium
lipase
    acid l.
lipid
    l. hypothesis
    l. metabolism disorder
lipidosis, pl. lipidoses
    cerebral l.
    cerebroside l.
    ganglioside l.
    sulfatide l.
lipofuscinosis
    ceroid l.
lipogranulomatosis
    Farber's l.
lipohyalinosis
lipoma
    epidermoid l.
    hamartomatous l.
    inclusion l.
    intradural l.
    spinal l.
    subarachnoid l.
lipomatosis
lipomeningocele
lipomyelocele
lipomyelomeningocele
lipomyeloschisis
liponeural junction
lipoprotein
    low-density l.
liposarcoma
lip reflex

liquid
    ethylene vinyl alcohol copolymer l.
liquor, gen. **liquoris**, pl. **liquores**
    l. cerebrospinalis
Lissauer's
    L. bundle
    L. fasciculus
    L. marginal zone
    L. tract
lissencephalia
lissencephalic
    l. syndrome
lissencephaly
Listeria monocytogenes
listhesis
    lateral l.
lisuride
literal agraphia
lithium
Little's disease
liver
    l. disease
    l. flap
load
    axial l.
loading
    axial l.
    Edwards modular system dynamic l.
lobar
    l. atrophy
    l. hemorrhage
    l. sclerosis
lobe
    anterior l. of hypophysis
    l.'s of cerebrum
    cuneiform l.
    falciform l.
    flocculonodular l.
    frontal l.

    limbic l.
    occipital l.
    parietal l.
    posterior l. of hypophysis
    quadrate l.
    temporal l.
lobectomy
    anterior temporal l.
    anteromesial temporal l.
    Falconer l.
    temporal l.
lobi (*gen. and pl. of* lobus)
lobotomy
    prefrontal l.
    radical prefrontal l.
    transorbital l.
Lobstein's ganglion
lobule
    ansiform l.
    anterior lunate l.
    biventral l.
    central l.
    crescentic l.'s of the cerebellum
    inferior parietal l.
    inferior semilunar l.
    paracentral l.
    posterior lunate l.
    quadrangular l.
    quadrate l.
    simple l.
    slender l.
    superior parietal l.
    superior semilunar l.
lobulet, lobulette
lobulus, gen. and pl. **lobuli**
    l. biventer
    l. biventralis
    l. centralis cerebelli
    l. clivi
    l. culminis

NOTES

lobulus *(continued)*
  l. cuneiformis
  l. folii
  l. fusiformis
  l. gracilis
  l. paracentralis
  l. parietalis inferior
  l. parietalis superior
  l. quadrangularis
  l. quadratus
  l. semilunaris inferior
  l. semilunaris superior
  l. simplex
lobus, gen. and pl. **lobi**
  l. anterior hypophyseos
  lobi cerebri
  l. clivi
  l. falciformis
  l. frontalis cerebri
  l. glandularis hypophyseos
  l. nervosus
  l. occipitalis cerebri
  l. parietalis cerebri
  l. posterior hypophyseos
  l. temporalis
local
  l. anesthesia
  l. epilepsy
  l. excitatory state
  l. field distortion
  l. sign
  l. syncope
  l. tetanus
  l. tic
localization
  l. agnosia
  cerebral l.
  2D graphic l.
  frame fixation-scanner
    assisted target l.
  manual target l.
  pedicle l.
  pneumotaxic l.
  scanner assisted target l.
  spatial l.
  stereotactic anatomic
    target l.
  stereotaxic l.
  target l.
  ultrasonographic l.

localizer
  Suetens-Gybels-Vandermeulen
    angiographic l.
  ultrasonic l.
location
  cervical sympathetic chain l.
  pedicle l.
locator
  Gill Thomas l.
loci (*pl. of* locus)
lock
  l. finger
  l. nut
locked facets
locked-in syndrome
lockjaw
locomotor ataxia
loculation syndrome
locus, pl. loci
  l. ceruleus
  l. cinereus
  l. ferrugineus
  l. niger
  l. perforatus anticus
  l. perforatus posticus
Loewenthal's
  L. bundle
  L. tract
logagnosia
logagraphia
logamnesia
logaphasia
logasthenia
**Logical Memory and Visual
  Reproduction subtest (Russell's
  revised)**
logopathy
logoplegia
logospasm
lomustine (CCNU)
long
  l. gyrus of insula
  l. pulse repetition time
  l. pulse repetition time/echo
    time image
  l. pulse repetition time/long
    echo time
  l. pulse repetition time/long
    echo time spin-echo
  l. root of ciliary ganglion
  l. segment fusion
  l. segment spinal fusion
  l. thoracic nerve

long-acting insulin preparation
longitudinal
    l. fissure of cerebrum
    l. ligament
    l. ligament rupture
    l. member to anchor
      connector
    l. pontine bundles
    l. spinal bar
long-term
    l.-t. bone-instrumentation
      interface
    l.-t. memory (LTM)
longus
    l. capitis muscle
    l. cervicis colli muscle
loop
    Blair-Ivy l.
    gamma l.
    Granit's l.
    Hartshill Ransford l.
    lenticular l.
    Meyer-Archambault l.
    Meyer's l.
    peduncular l.
    Ransford l.
    l.'s of spinal nerves
    subclavian l.
    unipolar cutting l.
    Vieussens' l.
loosening
    screw l.
Lopressor
lorazepam
lordosis
    l. creation
    lumbar spine l.
    l. preservation
    thoracic spine l.
Lorenz 1 mm micro osteosynthesis
  system

Lorfan
loss
    blood l.
    color vision l.
    gag reflex l.
    gaze-evoked visual l.
    hair l.
    heat l.
    lumbar lordosis iatrogenic l.
    signal l.
    transient monocular
      visual l.
    visual l.
    visual acuity l.
    weight l.
Louis-Bar syndrome
Louis instrumentation
loupe
    Keeler panoramic l.
Love-Gruenwald
    L.-G. cranial rongeur
    L.-G. disk rongeur
    L.-G. pituitary rongeur
Lovén reflex
Love pituitary rongeur
low
    l. cervical approach
    l. current monopolar
      coagulation
    l. delirium
    l. lumbar fracture
    l. lumbar spine fracture
    l. single thoracic curve
    l. tension glaucoma
low-density lipoprotein
Löwenberg's
    L. canal
    L. scala
lower
    l. abdominal periosteal
    reflex

NOTES

lower *(continued)*
  l. basilar aneurysm
  l. cervical spine
  l. cervical spine fusion
  l. cervical spine posterior
    stabilization
  l. cervical spine procedure
  l. cervical spine stabilization
  l. hook trial
  l. lumbar spine
  l. motor neuron
  l. motor neuron syndrome
  l. posterior lumbar spine
    and sacrum surgery
  l. thoracic pedicle
  l. thoracic spine
low-grade astrocytoma
low-pass filter
Low Profile Valve
loxia
L5-S1
  L5-S1 disk disease
  L5-S1 disk space
LTM
  long-term memory
Luc ethmoid forceps
Ludwig's
  L. ganglion
  L. nerve
luetic aneurysm
Luft's disease
lumbago
  ischemic l.
lumbar
  l. catheter
  l. curve
  l. discectomy
  l. disk disease
  l. disk herniation
  l. drainage
  l. enlargement of spinal
    cord
  l. facet disease
  l. flat back syndrome
  l. fusion
  l. ganglia
  l. hemilaminectomy
  l. interbody fusion
  l. interspace
  l. kyphosis
  l. lordosis iatrogenic loss
  l. lordosis preservation

  l. meningocele
  l. pedicle
  l. pedicle fixation
  l. pedicle marker
  l. pedicle screw
  l. port
  l. puncture
  l. puncture needle
  l. rheumatism
  l. scoliosis
  l. spinal fusion
  l. spinal stenosis
  l. spine
  l. spine biopsy
  l. spine burst fracture
  l. spine decompression
  l. spine fixation
  l. spine fusion
  l. spine instability
  l. spine instrumentation
  l. spine kyphotic deformity
  l. spine lordosis
  l. spine model
  l. spine pedicle diameter
  l. spine rotational stability
  l. spine segmental fixation
  l. spine stabilization
  l. spine transpedicular
    fixation
  l. spine trauma
  l. spine vertebral
    osteosynthesis
  l. spondylosis
  l. sympathectomy
  l. synovial cyst
  l. tumor
  l. vertebra
lumbarization
lumbar-peritoneal
  l.-p. shunt
  l.-p. shunting
lumboperitoneal shunt
lumbosacral
  l. corsette
  l. fusion
  l. junction
  l. junction bone density
  l. junction cortical thickness
  l. junction fracture
  l. plexus
  l. radiculopathy
  l. spine

l. spine transpedicular instrumentation
l. vertebra
Luminal
Lumsden
pneumotaxic center of L.
lunate
l. fissure
l. sulcus
lung disorder
lupinosis
lupus
l. anticoagulant
l. cerebritis
l. erythematosus
Luque
L. II segmental spinal instrumentation
L. instrumentation
L. instrumentation concave technique
L. instrumentation convex technique
L. loop fixation
L. rectangle
L. ring
L. rod
L. rod migration
L. segmental spinal instrumentation
L. semirigid segmental spinal instrumentation
L. sublaminar wiring technique
Luque-Galveston
L.-G. fixation
L.-G. post
lura

lural
Luschka
foramen of L.
luteinizing hormone-releasing hormone
luxation
rotatory l.
luxury perfusion
Luys' body
Lyme
L. borreliosis
L. disease
lymphadenopathy
lymphangioma
lymphocytes
tumor-infiltrating l. (TIL)
lymphocytic
l. adenohypophysitis
l. choriomeningitis
l. hypophysitis
l. infiltrate
lymphocytopenia
lymphocytosis
lymphoepithelial parotid tumor
lymphoid hypophysitis
lymphokine-activated killer cells
lymphoma
cerebral l.
malignant l.
lymphomatoid granulomatosis
lymphomatous tumor
Lynch incision
lyophilized dura
lypressin
lyra
l. davidis, lyre of David
lyssa

NOTES

M

Maalox
MacCarty forceps
Macewen's
    M. sign
    M. symptom
Machado-Joseph disease
macrencephaly, macrencephalia
macroadenoma
macroaneurysm
macrocephalic, macrocephalous
macrocephaly, macrocephalia
macrocranium
macroelectrode technique
macroencephalon
macroglia
    m. cell
macroglobulinemia of Waldenstrom
macrogyria
macroinstrument
macrophage
macrophthalmos
macropsia
macula, pl. maculae
    m. communicans
    m. cribrosa, pl. maculae
      cribrosae
    m. cribrosa inferior
    m. cribrosa media
    m. cribrosa quarta
    m. cribrosa superior
    m. densa
    m. lutea
    m. retinae
    m. sacculi
    m. utriculi
maculocerebral
Mad Hatter syndrome
Maffucci's syndrome
magaldrate
Magendie
    foramen of M.
Magendie-Hertwig
    M.-H. sign
    M.-H. syndrome
Magendie's
    M. foramen
    M. law
Magerl
    M. hook-plate system
    M. plate-screw system

    M. posterior C1-C2 screw
      fixation
    M. system
MAGIC syndrome
magna
    cisterna m.
    mega cisterna m.
Magnacal
magnae
    cisterna venae m.
Magnan's
    M. sign
    M. trombone movement
magnesia
    milk of m.
magnesium
    m. aluminum hydroxide
    m. hydroxide suspension
MAGNES magnetic source
  imaging
magnet
    cobalt samarium m.
    field m.
    main field m.
    m. quench
    m. reaction
    m. reflex
    m. shielding
    superconducting m.
    0.5-T superconducting m.
magnetic
    m. disk
    m. field vector
    m. moment
    m. resonance (MR)
    m. resonance angiography
    m. resonance imaging
      (MRI)
    m. resonance spectroscopy
    m. source imaging (MSI)
    m. stimulator
    m. susceptibility
    m. susceptibility artifact
magnetization
    spatial modulation of m.
      (SPAMM)
    spin m.
    transverse m.
magnetoelectric stimulation
magnetoencephalogram (MEG)

magnetoencephalography
magnetohydrodynamic effect
magnetometer
magnetophosphene
Magnevist
magnocellular
magnum
    foramen m.
Magstim 200
main
    m. d'accoucheur
    m. en crochet
    m. field
    m. field magnet
    m. sensory nucleus of the
      trigeminus
major
    m. epilepsy
    m. hysteria
mal
    grand m.
    petit m.
Malacarne's
    M. pyramid
    M. space
malar eminence
malaria
    cerebral m.
    therapeutic m.
maleate
    chlorpheniramine m.
    methysergide m.
    prochlorperazine m.
    timolol m.
malformation
    angiographically occult
      intracranial vascular m.
      (AOIVM)
    Arnold-Chiari m.
    arteriovenous m. (AVM)
    cavernous m.
    cerebrovascular m.
    Chiari m.
    Chiari I m.
    Chiari II m.
    Chiari III m.
    congenital m.
    craniofacial m.
    Dandy-Walker m.
    dural arteriovenous m.
    flocculonodular
      arteriovenous m.
    glomus arteriovenous m.

    intracerebral
      arteriovenous m.
    intracranial vascular m.
    medial hemispheric
      arteriovenous m.
    occipital m.
    occult cerebrovascular m.
    radiculomeningeal spinal
      vascular m.
    split-cord m. (SCM)
    thalamocaudate
      arteriovenous m.
    vascular m.
    vein of Galen m.
malignancy
    nasopharyngeal m.
malignant
    m. astrocytoma
    m. atrophic papulosis
    m. germ cell tumor
    m. glioma
    m. hyperthermia
    m. lymphoma
    m. melanoma
    m. stupor
    m. teratoma
malingering
Malis
    M. angled bayonet forceps
    M. bipolar instrument
    M. CMC-III electrosurgical
      system
    M. electrocoagulation unit
    M. irrigating bipolar CMC
      III
    M. solid state coagulator
malleable
    m. multipore suction tube
    m. sucker
malleation
mallet
malocclusion
malum
    m. vertebrale suboccipitale
mamillary
    m. body
    m. tubercle of
      hypothalamus
mamillotegmental fasciculus
mamillothalamic
    m. fasciculus
    m. tract
mammalian

mammary neuralgia
MaMT
    Maudsley Mentation Test
mandible
    osteotomy of m.
mandibular
    m. condylectomy
    m. fixation
    m. nerve
    m. osteotomy
    m. reflex
    m. retraction
    m. swing technique
mandibulotomy
Mandol
maneuver
    Bielschowsky's m.
    Buzzard's m.
    Dandy m.
    doll's eye m.
    Jendrassik's m.
    Phalen's m.
    Spurling's m.
    Valsalva m.
mania
manifestation
    behavioral m.
    neurotic m.
    psychophysiologic m.
    psychotic m.
manifest tetany
manipulation
    cranial nerve m.
mannitol
Mannkopf's sign
manometry
    anal sphincter m.
mantle
    brain m.
    m. layer
    m. sclerosis

Manual of Internal Fixation
manual target localization
manubrium
map
    phase-contrast m.
maplike skull
mapping
    brain m.
    brain electrical activity m.
    (BEAM)
    brainstem diencephalic m.
    cortical m.
    electrophysiological m.
    phase m.
    Talairach whole brain m.
    two-dimensional m.
marantic endocarditis
marasmus
Marcaine
Marchac forehead template
Marchant's zone
Marchiafava-Bignami disease
Marchi's tract
Marcus
    M. Gunn phenomenon
    M. Gunn syndrome
Marfan's syndrome
marginal
    m. gyrus
    m. layer
    m. sinus
margins
    dural m.
Marie's ataxia
Marie-Strümpell disease
Marinesco-Garland syndrome
Marinesco-Sjögren syndrome
Marinesco's succulent hand
marker
    biochemical tumor m.'s
    fiducial m.

NOTES

marker *(continued)*
    lumbar pedicle m.
    pedicle m.
    roentgenographic opaque m.
    thoracic pedicle m.
    tumor m.
Marlex
Maroteaux-Lamy disease
marsupial notch
Martin-Gruber anastomosis
Martinotti's cell
Masini's sign
mask
    m. facies
    Hutchinson's m.
masked epilepsy
masking
masklike face
mass
    m. action theory
    congenital nasal m.
    m. lesion
    m. reflex
    m. spectrometer
massa, gen. and pl. **massae**
    m. intermedia
massage
    carotid sinus m.
    digital temple m.
    nerve-point m.
masseter reflex
master gland
mastication disorder
masticatory
    m. diplegia
    m. nucleus
    m. spasm
mastoid
    m. complex
    m. process
mastoidectomy
mastoiditis
Matas'
    M. operation
    M. test
matching and tuning network
mater
    dura m.
material
    alloplastic m.
    ballistic m.'s
    Elgiloy clip m.
    interventional m.'s

    MP-35 clip m.
    nonferrous m.
    Phynox Cobalt Alloy
     clip m.
matrix
    germinal m.
matter
    gray m.
    periventricular white m.
    pontine gray m.
    white m.
mattress
    eggcrate m.
Matulane
matutinal epilepsy
Maudsley Mentation Test
  (MaMT)
Mauthner's
    M. cell
    M. sheath
Maxicamera
    Gamma M.
maxilla
maxillary
    m. antrum
    m. artery
    m. osteotomy
    m. sinus
    m. vein
maxillofacial
    m. fracture
    m. trauma
maxillomandibular artery
maxillotomy
maximal
    m. stimulus
    m. voluntary contraction
     (MVC)
Maxwell pairs
Mayer's reflex
Mayfield
    M. aneurysm clip
    M. clip
    M. head clamp
    M. headholder
    M. headrest system
    M. surgical system
Mayfield-Kees
    M.-K. skull fixation
     apparatus
    M.-K. table attachment
Mayo scissors
May-White syndrome

maze
Mazzoni's corpuscle
MCA
    middle cerebral artery
McCarthy's reflexes
McFadden
    M. clip
    M. cross-legged clip
McFadden-Kees clip
McGill
    M. forceps
    M. Pain Questionnaire
McGregor's basal line
McLone and Knepper etiological
    theory
McRae's foramen magnum line
measured stress
measurement
    blood flow m.
    vasodilator-stimulated rCBF
      single photon emission
      computed tomographic m.
    xenon CT m.
MeCCNU
    semustine
mechanical
    m. anosmia
    m. insufficiency
    m. plate design
    m. vertigo
mechanicoreceptor
mechanics
    quantum m.
mechanism
    association m.
    clamping m.
    m. of correction
    disengagement m.
    gating m.
    intramolecular dipole-
      dipole m.

    one-way flow m.
    rotating m.
    spring m.
    sunburst m.
mechanoreceptor
mechanoreflex
Meckel's
    M. cave
    M. ganglion
    M. sphenopalatine
      ganglionectomy
meclizine
medazepam
media
    contrast m.
    otitis m.
medial
    m. accessory olivary nucleus
    m. central nucleus of
      thalamus
    m. eminence
    m. epicondylectomy
    m. extradural approach
    m. fillet
    m. forebrain bundle
    m. geniculate body
    m. hemispheric
      arteriovenous malformation
    m. inferior pontine
      syndrome
    m. lemniscus
    m. longitudinal bundle
    m. longitudinal fasciculus
    m. longitudinal stria
    m. medullary lamina of
      corpus striatum
    m. medullary syndrome
    m. midpontine syndrome
    m. nucleus of thalamus
    m. occipitotemporal gyrus
    m. planter nerve

NOTES

medial *(continued)*
    m. pontine syndrome
    m. preoptic nucleus
    m. root of median nerve
    m. root of optic tract
    m. striate arteries
    m. superior pontine
    syndrome
    m. surface of cerebral
    hemisphere
    m. triangle of Hakuba
    m. vestibular nucleus
median
    m. aperture of the fourth
    ventricle
    m. corpectomy
    m. eminence
    m. frontal sulcus
    m. nerve
    m. nerve entrapment
    m. sulcus of fourth
    ventricle
medication cardex
mediodorsal nucleus
mediopubic reflex
medium
    Eagle's minimum
    essential m.
Medpacific LD 5000 Laser-
  Doppler perfusion monitor
Medrol
Medtronic SynchroMed implantable
  pump
medulla, pl. medullae
    m. oblongata
    m. spinalis
medullar
medullaris
    conus m.
medullary
    m. arteries of brain
    m. artery
    m. center
    m. chemoreceptor
    m. cone
    m. glioma
    m. layers of thalamus
    m. plate
    m. protrusion
    m. pyramidotomy
    m. sheath
    m. sign

    m. striae of the fourth
    ventricle
    m. stria of the thalamus
    m. substance
    m. teniae
    m. tube
    m. tumor
medullated
    m. nerve fiber
medullation
medullectomy
medulloblastoma
medullocell
medulloepithelioma
medullomyoblastoma
Mefoxin
MEG
    magnetoencephalogram
megacephalia
megacephalic
megacephalous
megacephaly
mega cisterna magna
megadolichovertebrobasilar anomaly
megalencephaly
    unilateral m.
megalgia
megaloblastic anemia
megalocephaly, megalocephalia
megaloencephalic
megaloencephalon
megaloencephaly
megalopapilla
meglumine
    m. iothalamate
    ioxaglate m.
megrim
Meige syndrome
Meissner's corpuscle
melanocytoma
    meningeal m.
melanoma
    malignant m.
    ocular m.
melanosis
    neurocutaneous m.
melanotic
    m. neuroectodermal tumor
    m. neuroectodermal tumor
    of infancy
MELAS syndrome
melatonin
Melkersson-Rosenthal syndrome

Mellaril
mellitus
    diabetes m.
melphalan
membrana, gen. and pl. **membranae**
    m. basilaris
    m. cerebri
    m. limitans gliae
    m. versicolor
membrane
    arachnoid m.
    basilar m.
    Fielding's m.
    m. of Liliequist
    pial-glial m.
    postsynaptic m.
    m. potential
    presynaptic m.
    spiral m.
    vestibular m.
membranectomy
membranous cochlea
memory
    anterograde m.
    m. deficit
    long-term m. (LTM)
    remote m.
    retrograde m.
    selective m.
    senile m.
    short-term m. (STM)
    m. trace
Mendel-Bechterew reflex
Mendel's instep reflex
Mengo encephalitis
Ménière's
    M. disease
    M. syndrome
meningeal
    m. angiomatosis
    m. artery

    m. carcinoma
    m. carcinomatosis
    m. hernia
    m. melanocytoma
    m. plexus
    m. tumor
    m. vein
meningeocortical
meningeorrhaphy
meninges (*pl. of* meninx)
meningioangiomatosis
meningioma
    angioblastic m.
    angle m.
    clinoidal m.
    convexity m.
    craniospinal m.
    cutaneous m.
    cystic intraparenchymal m.
    en plaque m.
    intraparenchymal m.
    intraventricular m.
    parasellar tentorial m.
    perioptic m.
    peritorcular m.
    petroclinoclival m.
    petroclival m.
    petroclivotentorial m.
    pineal m.
    psammomatous m.
    sphenoid m.
    sphenoid ridge m.
    sphenoid wing m.
    spinocranial m.
    tentorial apex m.
    tentorial leaf m.
    thoracic m.
    torcular m.
meningiomatosis
meningis (*gen. of* meninx)
meningism

NOTES

meningismus
meningitic
    m. streak
meningitidis
    Neisseria m.
meningitis, pl. meningitides
    aseptic m.
    bacterial m.
    basal m.
    basilar m.
    cerebrospinal m.
    coccidioidal m.
    epidemic cerebrospinal m.
    epidural m.
    external m.
    Haemophilus influenzae m.
    internal m.
    meningococcal m.
    Mollaret's m.
    neoplastic m.
    occlusive m.
    otitic m.
    serous m.
    m. serous spinalis
    tuberculous m.
meningocele
    lateral thoracic m.
    lumbar m.
    sacral m.
    spurious m.
    traumatic m.
meningocerebral cicatrix
meningococcal meningitis
meningocortical
meningocyte
meningoencephalitis
    acute primary
      hemorrhagic m.
    biundulant m.
    eosinophilic m.
    herpetic m.
    mumps m.
    primary amebic m.
    syphilitic m.
meningoencephalocele
meningoencephalomyelitis
meningoencephalopathy
meningohypohyseal trunk
meningomyelitis
meningomyelocele
meningorachidian vein
meningoradicular
meningoradiculitis

meningorrhachidian
meningorrhagia
meningotyphoid fever
meningovascular syphilis
meninx, gen. meningis, pl. meninges
    m. fibrosa
    m. primativa
    m. primitiva
    m. serosa
    m. tenuis
    m. vasculosa
meniscus, pl. menisci
    tactile m.
    m. tactus
Menkes'
    M. kinky hair syndrome
    M. syndrome
menstrual migraine
menstruation
mental
    m. agraphia
    m. chronometry
    m. dysfunction
    m. illness
    m. impairment
    m. retardation
mentality
mentation
MEP
    motor evoked potential
meperidine
    m. hydrochloride
meprobamate
meralgia
    m. paraesthetica
    m. paresthetica
merceline tape
mercurial tremor
Merkel's
    M. corpuscle
    M. tactile cell
    M. tactile disk
Merocel tampon
merorachischisis, merorrhachischisis
merosmia
MERRLA syndrome
Merzbacher-Pelizaeus disease
mesaxon
mesencephalic
    m. cistern
    m. flexure
    m. hemorrhage

m. nucleus of the
   trigeminus
m. sign
m. tegmentum
m. tractotomy
m. tract of trigeminal nerve
m. vein
mesencephalitis
mesencephalon
mesencephalo-oculofacial
   angiomatosis
mesencephalotomy
mesenchyme
   paraxial m.
mesenteric vasculitis
mesh
   Tantalum m.
   titanium micro m.
mesial temporal sclerosis
mesoblastic sensibility
mesoderm
mesoglia
mesoglial cells
mesolobus
mesoneuritis
   nodular m.
mesorrhachischisis
mesulergin
mesylate
   benztropine m.
metabolic
   m. acidosis
   m. alkalosis
   m. coma
   m. disturbance
   m. encephalopathy
metabolism
   cerebral m.
   nitrogen m.
   phosphate m.
metabolite

metacarpohypothenar reflex
metacarpothenar reflex
metachromatic leukodystrophy
metaiodobenzyl-guanidine (MIBG)
metal
   m. failure
   m. fatigue
   m. plate
metallic
   m. cranioplasty
   m. foreign body
   m. otologic implant
   m. tremor
metameric nervous system
metamorphopsia
Metamucil
metaplexus
metapore
Metaprel
metaproterenol sulfate
metaraminol bitartrate
metastasis, pl. metastases
   brain m.
   cerebral m.
   choroidal m.
   distant m.
   drop m.
   hemorrhagic m.
   leptomeningeal m.
   ocular m.
   retrobulbar orbital m.
   spinal m.
metastatic
   m. brain tumor
   m. breast cancer
   m. disease
   m. spinal tumor
   m. tumor
   m. tumor removal
metatarsalgia
metatarsal reflex

NOTES

195

metathalamus
metencephalic
metencephalon
meter
    electromagnetic flow m.
methadone hydrochloride
methamphetamine abuse
methanol
methantheline
methazolamide
methemoglobin
methicillin
    m. sodium
methocarbamol
method
    Anel's m.
    Antyllus' m.
    Brasdor's m.
    Hilton's m.
    hole preparation m.
    immobilization m.
    immunoperoxidase m.
    impedance m.
    Kirby-Bauer disk
     diffusion m.
    Moore's m.
    Pavlov m.
    Purmann's m.
    reduction m.
    Scarpa's m.
    Seldinger's m.
    Thane's m.
    Wardrop's m.
    Westergren m.
    Winston-Lutz m.
    Wintrobe m.
    xenon m.
    zeta m.
methodical chorea
methohexital
methotrexate
    m. sodium
methyldopa
methylglyoxal *bis*-guanylhydrazone
  (MGBG)
methylmalonic acidemia
methylmethacrylate
    m. block
    m. cranioplastic plug
    m. spacer
methylphenidate

methylprednisolone
    m. acetate
    m. and sodium succinate
methysergide
    m. maleate
metoclopramide
metopic
    m. suture
    m. synostosis
metopoplasty
metoprolol
    m. tartrate
metrizamide
    m. contrast study
    m. myelography
metrizamide-enhanced CT
metronidazole
metyrapone
    m. test
Mexate
mexiletine
Meyer-Archambault loop
Meyerding retractor
Meyer's loop
Meynert's
    M. cells
    M. commissures
    M. decussation
    M. fasciculus
    M. layer
    M. retroflex bundle
MGBG
    methylglyoxal *bis*-
    guanylhydrazone
MIBG
    metaiodobenzyl-guanidine
Michel scalp clip
micrencephalia
micrencephalous
micrencephaly
microadenoma
    cystic m.
microadenomectomy
    selective m.
microaneurysm
microangiopathy
microball hook
microcatheter
    m. system
    Tracker m.
microcephaly
    encephaloclastic m.
    schizencephalic m.

microcoil
>   endothelin-1 platinum-Dacron m.
>   Hilal m.
>   platinum m.
>   platinum-Dacron m.

microcrania
microcup forceps
microcurette
microcyst
microdiscectomy
microdissector
>   Rhoton m.

microdrill
>   high-speed m.

microdysgenesia
microelectrode
>   m. recording

microembolism
microencephaly
microfibrillar collagen
microforceps
microglia
>   m. cells

microgliacyte
microglial cells
microglioma
microgliomatosis
microgliosis
microglobulin
micrograph
>   electron m.

micrography
microguidewire
microgyria
Microknife
>   Karlin M.

microneurovascular anastomosis
micro-operative
>   m.-o. procedure
>   m.-o. treatment

microphthalmos
micropituitary rongeur
Micro-Plus titanium plating system
micropsia
microronguer
>   Kerrison m.

microscissors
>   curved conventional m.
>   straight m.

microscope
>   Hitachi scanning
>   electron m.
>   Moller m.
>   Omni 2 m.
>   operating m.
>   surgical m.
>   VARIMIC 900 m.
>   Zeiss-Contraves operating m.
>   Zeiss operating m.
>   Zeiss OpMi CS-NC2
>   surgical m.
>   zoom m.

microscopy
>   electron m.
>   scanning electron m. (SEM)

microseme
MicroSpan Capnometer 8800
Microsulfon
microsurgery
microsurgical procedure
microsuture
microsystem
>   SUN m.

microvascular
>   m. anastomosis
>   m. clip
>   m. decompression (MVD)

micrurgical
micturition
>   m. reflex
>   m. syncope

NOTES

Midas
 M. Rex craniotome
 M. Rex drill
 M. Rex instrumentation
  system
 M. Rex power system
midazolam
midbrain
 m. deafness
 m. tegmentum
 m. vesicle
middle
 m. cerebellar peduncle
 m. cerebral artery (MCA)
 m. cervical ganglion
 m. column injury
 m. cranial fossa
 m. fossa approach
 m. fossa exposure
 m. fossa floor/petrous
  dissection
 m. frontal convolution
 m. frontal gyrus
 m. frontal sulcus
 m. temporal convolution
 m. temporal gyrus
 m. temporal sulcus
midface
 m. degloving
 m. degloving technique
 m. retrusion
midget bipolar cells
midgracile
midline
 anatomical m.
 m. exposure
 m. fusion defect
 m. myelotomy
 m. shift
 m. spinal approach
 m. syndrome
midpoint to meatal line
**Midwest Regional Spinal Cord
 Injury Center Acute Care Unit**
migraine
 abdominal m.
 acephalgic m.
 basilar artery m.
 catastrophic m.
 classic m.
 common m.
 confusional m.

 familial hemiplegic m.
 fulgurating m.
 Harris' m.
 m. headache
 hemiplegic m.
 menstrual m.
 ophthalmic m.
 ophthalmoplegic m.
migration
 m. abnormalities
 electrode m.
 graft m.
 instrument m.
 Luque rod m.
 neuronal m.
 rod m.
Mikulicz' operation
Miles punch biopsy forceps
miliary aneurysm
milk-ejection reflex
milk of magnesia
Millard-Gubler syndrome
Mille
 M. Pattes screw
 M. Pattes technique
Miller-Dieker syndrome
Milles' syndrome
Millipore
Milton's disease
Miltown
Milwaukee brace
mimetic
 m. chorea
 m. paralysis
mimic
 m. convulsion
 m. spasm
 m. tic
Minamata disease
mind
 m. blindness
Minerin
miner's cramps
Minerva jacket
Mini
 M. Orbita plate
 M. Würzburg implant
  system
minilaparotomy
minimal brain dysfunction
mini-Sugita clip
minocycline

miosis
>paralytic m.
>spastic m.

mirabile
>rete m.

mirror
>Hardy 5 mm m.

mirror-writing
miryachit
misdirection phenomenon
Mishler valve
misonidazole
misregistration
>flow m.
>oblique flow m.

missile
>m. effect
>m. injury

Mitchell's disease
mitochondrial
>m. cytopathy
>m. encephalomyelopathy
>m. encephalomyopathy
>m. encephalopathy
>m. myopathy

mitotane
mitral
>m. cells
>m. valve disorder

mixed
>m. aphasia
>m. germ cell tumor
>m. glioma
>m. nerve
>m. paralysis

mixillectomy
mixture
>epinephrine-anesthetic m.
>thrombogenic ferrous m.

mneme
mnemenic, mnemic

mnemism
mobile spasm
Möbius disease
Möbius' syndrome
modality
model
>corpectomy m.
>lumbar spine m.

modification
>C-D screw m.
>Harriluque sublaminar wiring m.
>Jacobs locking hook spinal rod instrumentation m.

modified Harrington rod
modifier
>biological response m.

modular instrumentation
modulation
>pain m.

module
>CUSA electrosurgical m. (CEM)

Moe
>M. alar hook
>M. hook
>M. rod
>M. system

mogiarthria
mogigraphia
mogilalia
mogiphonia
molecular
>m. layer
>m. layer of cerebellar cortex
>m. layer of cerebral cortex
>m. layer of retina
>m. layers of olfactory bulb

Mollaret's meningitis
Moller microscope

NOTES

molluscum
    m. fibrosum
moment
    gradient m.
    magnetic m.
    three-point bending m.
Monakow's
    M. bundle
    M. nucleus
    M. syndrome
    M. tract
monathetosis
monaxonic
Mondonesi's reflex
monesthetic
mongol
mongolian
mongolism
mongoloid
monitor
    Doppler ultrasound m.
    Laserflow blood
      perfusion m.
    Medpacific LD 5000 Laser-
      Doppler perfusion m.
    Steritek ICP mini m.
monitor-2
    nerve integrity m. (NIM-2)
    Xomed nerve integrity m.
    Xomed-Treace nerve
      integrity m.
monitoring
    anesthetic m.
    cranial nerve m.
    Doppler m.
    Doppler precordial end-tidal
      carbon dioxide m.
    ECoG m.
    end-tidal nitrogen m.
    intraoperative facial
      nerve m.
    neurophysiological m.
    m. probe
    real-time m.
    scalp EEG m.
    screw position
      perioperative m.
    somatosensory evoked
      potential m.
    spinal cord function
      intraoperative m.
    subdural ICP m.
    video/EEG m.

monkey-paw
monoamine oxidase inhibitor
monoaminergic
monobactam
monobloc advancement
monochorea
monoclonal
    m. antibody
    m. gammopathy
monocyte
monocytogenes
    Listeria m.
monomelic amyotrophy
monomyoplegia
mononeural, mononeuric
mononeuralgia
mononeuritis
    m. multiplex
mononeuropathy
    m. multiplex
monoparesis
monoparesthesia
monophasia
monophasic
monoplegia
    m. masticatoria
monopolar
    m. coagulation
    m. electrode
monosodium glutamate
monospasm
monosynaptic
monotreme
Monro
    foramen of M.
Monro's
    M. foramen
    M. sulcus
monticulus, pl. monticuli
Moore's method
Morand's spur
Morgagni-Adams-Stokes syndrome
Morgagni's
    M. disease
    M. syndrome
Morganella morganii
morganii
    Morganella m.
morning glory syndrome
moron
Moro reflex
morphine sulfate

morphometry
    pedicle m.
morphosynthesis
Morquio's
    M. disease
    M. syndrome
Morscher plate
morselized
Morton's
    M. neuralgia
    M. neuroma
Morvan's
    M. chorea
    M. disease
mosquito forceps
mossy
    m. cell
    m. fibers
motion
    m. artifact
    brownian m.
    m. concentration
    higher order m.
    m. segment
    m. sickness
motoneuron
motor
    m. agraphia
    m. alexia
    m. aphasia
    m. apraxia
    m. area
    m. ataxia
    m. cell
    m. control
    m. cortex
    m. dapsone neuropathy
    m. decussation
    m. deficit
    m. disorder
    m. endplate

    m. evoked potential (MEP)
    m. fibers
    m. image
    m. nerve
    m. neuron
    m. neuron disease
    m. neuron paralysis
    m. nuclei
    m. nucleus of facial nerve
    m. nucleus of trigeminus
    m. paralysis
    m. point
    m. root of ciliary ganglion
    m. root of trigeminal nerve
    m. speech center
    m. unit
    vane-type m.
    m. zone
Motrin
mouse
    shiverer m.
mouth
    m. disorder
    dry m.
    tapir m.
movement
    after-m.
    associated m.
    choreic m.
    decomposition of m.
    m. disorder
    dysconjugate m.
    head m.
    lateropulsion of body m.
    lateropulsion of eye m.
    Magnan's trombone m.
    neurobiotactic m.
    non-rapid eye m. (NREM)
    pursuit m.'s
    pursuit eye m.
    rapid eye m. (REM)

NOTES

movement *(continued)*
    reflex m.
    saccadic eye m.
    vergence m.
moxalactam disodium
Moxam
moyamoya
    m. collateral enlargement
    m. disease
Moynihan forceps
MP-35 clip material
MR
    magnetic resonance
    MR imaging with
        gadolinium enhancement
    MR spectroscopy
MRI
    magnetic resonance imaging
    MRI compatibility
    gadolinium-enhanced MRI
    nonproton MRI
    MRI scan
    whole-spine MRI
MS
    multiple sclerosis
M segment
MSI
    magnetic source imaging
^{99}mTc-HMPAO
MTS electrohydraulic piston
mucin-secreting adenocarcinoma
mucocele
    paranasal m.
    sphenoid m.
mucolipidosis
Mucomyst with Isoproterenol
mucopolysaccharidosis VI
mucopyelocele
Mucor
Mucoraceae
mucor **infection**
mucormycosis
mucous membrane lesion
Mullan's
    M. triangle
    M. wire
Müller's
    M. fibers
    M. law
    M. muscle
    M. radial cells
    M. trigone
multiarc LINAC radiosurgery

multicore disease
multidimensional Fourier transform
multifocal
    m. glioma
    m. placoid pigment
    epitheliopathy
multiforme
    erythema m.
    glioblastoma m.
multiform layer
multi-infarct
    m.-i. dementia
    m.-i. progressive
    supranuclear palsy
multilevel laminectomy
multimodal adjuvant therapy
multiple
    m. hook assembly
    m. hook assembly C-D
    instrumentation
    m. mucosal neuroma
    syndrome
    m. myeloma
    m. neuritis
    m. sclerosis (MS)
    m. targeting
    m. trauma victim
multiple-point sacral fixation
multipolar
    m. cell
    m. neuron
multipore suction tip
multispan fracture hook
multisynaptic
mumps meningoencephalitis
mu opiate receptor
murmur
    brain m.
Murphy
    M. ball hook
    M. rake retractor
Murray Valley encephalitis
muscarinic effect
muscimol
muscle
    anterior serratus m.
    digastric m.
    m. dissection
    external intercostal m.
    greater rhomboid m.
    iliocostal m.
    iliopsoas m.
    intraspinous m.

latissimus dorsi m.
levator palpebrae m.
longus capitis m.
longus cervicis colli m.
Müller's m.
nuchal m.
omohyoid m.
paraspinal m.
pectoralis major m.
platysma m.
psoas m.
m. relaxant
m. rigidity
Rouget's m.
scalene m.
scalenus anticus m.
m. spasm
m. spindle
sternocleidomastoid m.
sternohyoid m.
sternomastoid m.
sternothyroid m.
strap m.
m. stretch reflex
teres major m.
m. tone
trapezius m.
muscular
    m. anesthesia
    m. atrophy
    m. dystrophy
    m. hyperesthesia
    m. insufficiency
    m. reflex
    m. sense
    m. trophoneurosis
musculocutaneous nerve
musculospiral paralysis
music
    m. ability sparing
    m. blindness

musical
    m. agraphia
    m. alexia
musician's cramp
mussitation
Mustargen
mutilating leprosy
mutism
    akinetic m.
    elective m.
    voluntary m.
muttering delirium
MVC
    maximal voluntary contraction
MVD
    microvascular decompression
M vector
myalgia
myasthenia
    m. gravis
myasthenic
    m. facies
    m. reaction
    m. syndrome
myatonia, myatony
    m. congenita
mycetism, mycetismus
    m. cerebralis
Mycobacterium tuberculosis
***Mycoplasma* infection**
mycosis
mycotic aneurysm
mydriasis
    alternating m.
    paralytic m.
    spasmodic m.
    spastic m.
    springing m.
mydriatic rigidity
myelapoplexy
myelatelia

NOTES

myelauxe
myelencephalic vein
myelencephalon
myelic
myelin
    m. basic protein
    m. body
    m. figure
    m. sheath
myelinated
    m. nerve fiber
myelination
myelinic
myelinization
myelinoclasis
myelinoclastic disease
myelinogenesis
myelinolysis
    central pontine m.
myelitic
myelitis
    acute transverse m.
    ascending m.
    bulbar m.
    concussion m.
    Foix-Alajouanine m.
    funicular m.
    subacute necrotizing m.
    systemic m.
    transverse m.
myeloarchitectonics
myelocele
myelocyst
myelocystic
myelocystocele
    terminal m.
myelocystomeningocele
myelocyte
myelodiastasis
myelodysplasia
myelogram
myelography
    computed tomographic m. (CTM)
    computed tomographic metrizamide m. (CTMM)
    delayed computed tomographic m.
    iohexol m.
    metrizamide m.
    water-soluble contrast m.
myeloid
myelolysis

myeloma
    multiple m.
myelomalacia
    angiodysgenetic m.
    cystic m.
myelomeningocele
myeloneuritis
myeloparalysis
myelopathic
myelopathy
    AIDS-related m.
    carcinomatous m.
    cervical spondylosis without m.
    cervical spondylotic m.
    compressive m.
    diabetic m.
    HTLV-1-associated m.
    m. incidence
    necrotizing m.
    paracarcinomatous m.
    radiation m.
    spondylotic m.
    subacute necrotizing m.
    m. syndrome
myelopetal
myelophthisic
myelophthisis
myeloplegia
myeloradiculitis
myeloradiculodysplasia
myeloradiculopathy
myeloradiculopolyneuronitis
myelorrhagia
myelorrhaphy
myeloschisis
myelosis
    funicular m.
myelosyphilis
myelosyringosis
myelotome
myelotomography
myelotomy
    Bischof's m.
    commissural m.
    midline m.
    T-m.
myenteric plexus
Myer's loop fibers
myesthesia
Mylanta
myoblastoma
    granular cell m.

myobradia
myocardial infarction
myocelialgia
myoclonia
    fibrillary m.
myoclonic
    m. absence
    m. astatic epilepsy
myoclonus
    m. epilepsy
    hereditary branchial m.
    m. multiplex
    nocturnal m.
    oculopalatal m.
    palatal m.
    palato-ocular m.
    stimulus sensitive m.
myocutaneous flap
myodynia
myodystony
myodystrophy, myodystrophia
myoesthesis, myoesthesia
myofascial
    m. pain
    m. syndrome
myofibromatosis
    infantile m.
myogenic paralysis
myoglobinuria
myoglobinuric renal failure
myogram
myography
myokymia
    facial m.
    hereditary m.
myomedulloblastoma
myoneural
    m. junction
myoneuralgia
    postural m.
myoneurasthenia

myoneuroma
myopalmus
myoparalysis
myoparesis
myopathic
    m. atrophy
    m. facies
myopathy
    mitochondrial m.
    proximal m.
myopia
    axial m.
myorhythmia
myosalgia
myoseism
myositis
    cervical m.
myospasm, myospasmus
    cervical m.
myotatic reflex
myotone
myotonia
    m. acquisita
    m. atrophica
    m. congenita
    m. dystrophica
    m. neonatorum
myotonic
    m. dystrophy
    m. muscular dystrophy
myotonoid
myotonus
myotony
myriachit
myringotomy
Mysoline
myxoma
    atrial m.
myxoneuroma
myxopapillary ependymoma

NOTES

N

NAA
   N-acetylaspartate
nadolol
nafate
   cefamandole n.
Nafcil
nafcillin
   n. sodium
Naffziger
   N. syndrome
Naffziger's test
Naftidrofuryl
Nageotte cells
nail
   intramedullary n.
   Küntscher n.
   n. lesion
nalbuphine hydrochloride
Nalfon
nalorphine
naloxone
   n. hydrochloride
naproxen
Narcan
narcohypnia
narcolepsy
narcolepsy-cataplexy syndrome
narcoleptic tetrad
narcosis
   nitrogen n.
narcotic
narrow AO dynamic compression
   plate
narrow-bite bone rongeur
narrowing
   degenerative n.
nasal
   n. chondritis
   n. dermoid
   n. dissection
   n. ganglion
   n. glioma
   n. sinus
   n. surgery
nascent motor unit potential
Nashold biopsy needle
nasociliary
   n. nerve
   n. root
nasoethmoidal encephalocele

nasofrontal encephalocele
nasofrontalis
   fonticulus n.
nasogastric
   n. intubation
   n. tube
nasomental reflex
naso-orbital encephalocele
nasopharyngeal
   n. blastomycosis
   n. cooling
   n. malignancy
   n. mucus retention cyst
nasopharynx
National Institute of Neurological
   Disorders and Stroke (NIDS)
NCV
   nerve conduction velocity
1505 NDSB occlusion balloon
   catheter
Nd:YAG
   neodymium:yttrium-aluminum-
      garnet
   Nd:YAG laser
near reflex spasm
Nebcin
neck
   buffalo n.
   n. dissection
   n. reflexes
   n. sign
   stiff n.
   wry n.
necrolysis
   epidermal n.
   toxic epidermal n.
necrosis
   acute tubular n.
   aseptic n.
   coagulative n.
   cystic n.
   cystic medial n.
   hemorrhagic n.
   laminar cortical n.
   pressure n.
   radiation n.
   tubular n.
   tumor n.
necrotizing
   n. angiitis

necrotizing *(continued)*
    n. encephalitis
    n. encephalomyelopathy
    n. myelopathy
needle
    angled n.
    n. aspiration
    brain biopsy n.
    butterfly n.
    n. dissector
    n. electrode
    n. electromyography
    Frazier's n.
    n. holder
    insulated electrode n.
    lumbar puncture n.
    Nashold biopsy n.
    spinal n.
    straight n.
    Thermistor n.
    Tuohy n.
    ventricular n.
neencephalon
Neftel's disease
negative feedback
negatively bathmotropic
Negro's phenomenon
Neisseria meningitidis
Nelson's syndrome
Nelson tumor
Nembutal
neocerebellum
neocortex
neodymium
neodymium:yttrium-aluminum-garnet
  (Nd:YAG)
neoencephalon
neoformans
    Cryptococcus n.
neokinetic
neomycin
neonatal
    n. apoplexy
    n. intraventricular
      hemorrhage
    n. tetany
neopallium
neoplasm
    cranial nerve n.
    extensive n.
    pearly n.
    trochlear nerve n.

neoplastic
    n. angioendotheliosis
    n. arachnoiditis
    n. disorder
    n. meningitis
Neosporin GU Irrigant
neostigmine
    n. test
neostriatum
neothalamus
neovascularization
    iris n.
nephritis
    shunt n.
Néri's sign
nerve
    abducent n.
    accelerator n.'s
    accessory n.
    acoustic n.
    afferent n.
    antebrachial cutaneous n.
    anterior interosseous n.
    aortic n.
    auditory n.
    augmentor n.'s
    autonomic n.
    n. avulsion
    axillary n.
    baroreceptor n.
    n. block
    carotid sinus n.
    n. cell
    n. cell body
    centrifugal n.
    centripetal n.
    cervical n.
    cochlear n.
    common peroneal n.
    n. conduction study
    n. conduction velocity
      (NCV)
    cranial n.'s
    Cyon's n.
    n. deafness
    n. decompression
    dental n.
    depressor n. of Ludwig
    digital n.
    dorsal scapular n.
    efferent n.
    eighth cranial n.
    eleventh cranial n.

n. ending
n. entrapment
esodic n.
excitor n.
excitoreflex n.
exodic n.
facial n.
n. fascicle
femoral n.
femoral cutaneous n.
n. fiber
n. field
fifth cranial n.
first cranial n.
fourth cranial n.
Galen's n.
n. ganglion
Gaskell's n.'s
genitofemoral n.
glossopharyngeal n.
gluteal n.
n. graft
greater occipital n.
greater superficial
 petrosal n.
Hering's sinus n.
n. hook
hypoglossal n.
iliohypogastric n.
n. implantation
inferior dental n.
inferior laryngeal n.
infraorbital n.
n. integrity monitor-2
 (NIM-2)
intermediate n.
Jacobson's n.
lacrimal n.
lateral femoral cutaneous n.
long thoracic n.
Ludwig's n.

mandibular n.
medial planter n.
median n.
mixed n.
motor n.
musculocutaneous n.
nasociliary n.
ninth cranial n.
occipital n.
oculomotor n.
olfactory n.
optic n.
n. pain
n. papilla
pathetic n.
peripheral n.
plantar n.
n. plexus
pneumogastric n.
posterior interosseous n.
posterior tibial n.
pressor n.
pressoreceptor n.
pudendal n.
radial n.
recurrent laryngeal n.
n. root
n. root avulsion
n. root block
n. root retractor
sacral n.
scapular n.
sciatic n.
second cervical n.
second cranial n.
secretory n.
sensory n.
seventh cranial n.
n. sheath tumor
sinus n. of Hering
sinuvertebral n.

NOTES

nerve *(continued)*
    sixth cranial n.
    n. of smell
    spinal n.
    spinal accessory n.
    n. stimulator
    superior laryngeal n.
    supraorbital n.
    suprascapular n.
    sural n.
    n. suture
    sympathetic n.
    tenth cranial n.
    third cranial n.
    thoracic n.
    tibial n.
    n. tract
    trifacial n.
    trigeminal n.
    trochlear n.
    twelfth cranial n.
    ulnar n.
    vagus n.
    vestibular n.
    vestibulocochlear n.
    n. of Wrisberg
    Wrisberg's n.
nerve-point massage
nervi (*gen. and pl. of* nervus)
nervimotility
nervimotion
nervimotor
nervine
nervosa
    anorexia n.
nervosism
nervous
    n. bladder
    n. distribution
    n. system
nervousness
nervus, gen. and pl. **nervi**
    n. abducens
    n. accessorius
    n. acusticus
    n. cochlearis
    nervi craniales
    n. facialis
    n. glossopharyngeus
    n. hypoglossus
    n. impar
    n. octavus
    n. oculomotorius

    nervi olfactorii
    n. opticus
    n. statoacusticus
    n. trigeminus
    n. trochlearis
    n. vagus
    n. vestibularis
    n. vestibulocochlearis
nest
    choristoma n.
net
    Neuro n.
netilmicin
network
    matching and tuning n.
    wide area n.
neuragmia
neural
    n. axis
    n. canal
    n. crest
    n. crest syndrome
    n. cyst
    n. deafness
    n. dissector
    n. ectoderm
    n. folds
    n. foramen remodeling
    n. ganglion
    n. groove
    n. imaging study
    n. injury
    n. layer of retina
    n. placode
    n. plate
    n. segment
    n. tube
    n. tube defect (NTD)
neuralgia
    atypical facial n.
    atypical trigeminal n.
    chronic migrainous n.
    epileptiform n.
    facial n.
    n. facialis vera
    Fothergill's n.
    geniculate n.
    glossopharyngeal n.
    hallucinatory n.
    Hunt's n.
    idiopathic n.
    intercostal n.
    mammary n.

Morton's n.
occipital n.
periodic migrainous n.
postherpetic n.
posttraumatic n.
Raeder's paratrigeminal n.
red n.
reminiscent n.
sciatic n.
stump n.
suboccipital n.
supraorbital n.
symptomatic n.
trifacial n.
trigeminal n.
vagoglossopharyngeal n.
neuralgic
n. amyotrophy
neuralgiform
neuramebimeter
neuranagenesis
neurapophysis
neurapraxia
neurasthenia
angiopathic n.,
angioparalytic n.
gastric n.
n. gravis
n. praecox
primary n.
pulsating n.
sexual n.
traumatic n.
neurasthenic
neurasthenic helmet
neuraxis
neuraxon, neuraxone
neurectasis, neurectasia, neurectasy
neurectomy
Cotte presacral n.
presacral n.

retrogasserian n.
Sonneberg n.
vestibular n.
neurectopia, neurectopy
neurepithelium
neurergic
neurexeresis
neuriatria, neuriatry
neurilemma
n. cells
neurilemoma
acoustic n.
Antoni type A n.
Antoni type B n.
neurility
neurimotility
neurimotor
neurinoma
acoustic n.
trigeminal n.
trigeminal nerve n.
neurit, neurite
neuritic
n. atrophy
n. plaque
neuritis, pl. **neuritides**
adventitial n.
ascending n.
axial n.
brachial n.
central n.
descending n.
Eichhorst's n.
eighth nerve n.
eighth nerve herpetic n.
endemic n.
fallopian n.
herpetic n.
interstitial n.
intraocular n.
Leyden's n.

NOTES

neuritis *(continued)*
    multiple n.
    occipital n.
    optic n.
    parenchymatous n.
    retrobulbar n.
    sciatic n.
    segmental n.
    suboccipital n.
    toxic n.
    traumatic n.
neuroadenolysis
neuroallergy
neuroanastomosis
    autogenous cable graft
      interposition VII-VII n.
neuroanatomy
neuroanesthesia
neuroarthropathy
neuroaugmentation
neuroaugmentive
neuroaxonal dystrophy
neuro-Behçet's disease
neurobiotactic movement
neurobiotaxis
neuroblastoma
    cerebral n.
    intracranial n.
    olfactory n.
neurocardiac
neurocele
neurochemistry
neurochitin
neurochorioretinitis
neurochoroiditis
neurocirculatory asthenia
neurocladism
neurocristopathy
neurocutaneous
    n. angiomatosis
    n. melanosis
    n. syndrome
neurocysticercosis
neurocyte
neurocytolysis
neurocytoma
neurodegenerative disease
neurodendrite
neurodendron
neurodiagnostic imaging
neurodynia
neuroectoderm

neuroectodermal
    n. tumor
neuroectomy
neuroencephalomyelopathy
neuroendocrine
    n. cell
    n. transducer cell
neuroendocrinology
neuroendoscope
neuroenteric cyst
neuroepithelial
    n. cells
    n. cyst
    n. layer of retina
    n. tumor
neuroepithelium
    n. of ampullary crest
    n. cristae ampullaris
    n. of macula
    n. maculae
neurofibril
neurofibrillar
neurofibrillary
    n. degeneration
    n. tangle
neurofibroma
    aryepiglottic fold n.
    plexiform n.
    spinal n.
neurofibromatosis
    n. 1
    n. 2
    abortive n.
    incomplete n.
    n. kyphoscoliosis
    kyphoscoliosis secondary
      to n.
    segmental n.
    von Recklinghausen's n.
neurofibrosarcoma
neurofilament
neuroganglion
neurogenic, neurogenetic
    n. atrophy
    n. bladder
    n. disorder
    n. fracture
neurogenous
neuroglia
    n. cells
neurogliacyte
neuroglial, neurogliar
neurogliomatosis

neurogram
neurography
neurohemal
neurohistology
neurohumor
neurohumoral transmission
neurohypophysial
neurohypophysis
neuroid
neuroimaging
    functional n.
    three-dimensional n.
neurokeratin
neurokinin
neurolemma
    n. cells
neuroleptic
    n. malignant syndrome
neurolinguistics
neurologic
    n. complication
    n. deficit
    n. evaluation
neurologist
neurology
    restorative n.
neurolymph
neurolymphomatosis
neurolysis
    internal n.
neurolytic
neuroma
    acoustic n.
    amputation n.
    n. cutis
    facial n.
    false n.
    fibrillary n.
    Morton's n.
    plexiform n.
    n. telangiectodes

    traumatic n.
    trigeminal n.
    Verneuil's n.
neuromalacia
neuromatosis
neuromere
neuromuscular
    n. blocking agent
    n. junction
    n. scoliosis
    n. scoliosis orthotic
      treatment
    n. scoliosis treatment
    n. spindle
    n. transmission
neuromusculoskeletal syndrome
neuromyasthenia
    epidemic n.
neuromyelitis
    n. optica
neuromyopathy
    carcinomatous n.
neuromyositis
neuromyotonia
neuron
    alpha motor n.
    autonomic motor n.
    bipolar n.
    gamma motor n.
    ganglionic motor n.
    Golgi type I n.
    Golgi type II n.
    intercalary n.
    internuncial n.
    lower motor n.
    motor n.
    multipolar n.
    postganglionic motor n.
    preganglionic motor n.
    pseudounipolar n.
    somatic motor n.

NOTES

neuron *(continued)*
  unipolar n.
  upper motor n.
  visceral motor n.
neuronal
  n. ingrowth
  n. migration
  n. pruning
  n. regeneration
  n. shrinkage
  n. sprouting
  n. tumor
neurone
Neuro net
neuronitis
neuronopathy
  sensory n.
neuronophage
neuronophagia, neuronophagy
neuronyxis
neuro-oncology
neuro-ophthalmology
neuro-otology
neuropapillitis
neuroparalysis
neuroparalytic
  n. keratitis
  n. ophthalmia
neuropath
neuropathic
  n. arthritis
  n. arthropathy
  n. hyperkyphoscoliosis
  n. joint
neuropathogenesis
neuropathology
neuropathy
  asymmetric motor n.
  brachial plexus n.
  cranial n.
  diabetic n.
  diphtheritic n.
  entrapment n.
  facial n.
  familial amyloid n.
  giant axonal n.
  glossopharyngeal n.
  hereditary n.
  hereditary hypertrophic n.
  hereditary sensory
   radicular n.
  hypertrophic interstitial n.
  hypoglossal n.

ischemic optic n.
isoniazid n.
lead n.
leprous n.
motor dapsone n.
oculomotor n.
onion bulb n.
optic n.
peripheral n.
segmental n.
symmetric distal n.
trigeminal n.
ulnar n.
vagus n.
vestibulocochlear n.
vitamin B_{12} n.
neuropeptide
neuropharmacology
neurophilic
neurophthalmology
neurophysins
neurophysiological monitoring
neurophysiology
neuropil, neuropile
neuroplasm
neuroplasty
neuroplegic
neuropodia
neuropore
  caudal n.
  rostral n.
neuropsychiatry
neuropsychologic,
  neuropsychological
  n. disorder
neuropsychology
neuropsychopathic
neuropsychopathy
neuroradiology
  interventional n.
  pediatric n.
neuroreceptor
neurorecidive
neurorecurrence
neurorelapse
neuroretinal angiomatosis
neuroretinitis
neurorrhaphy
neurosarcocleisis
neurosarcoidosis
neuroschisis
neuroschwannoma
neurosciences

neurosecretion
neurosecretory
    n. cells
    n. substance
neurosis, pl. neuroses
    accident n.
    obsessional n.
    occupational n.
    postconcussion n.
    posttraumatic n.
    professional n.
    n. tarda
    torsion n.
    traumatic n.
neurospasm
neurosplanchnic
neurospongium
Neurostation One
neurosthenia
neurostimulation
neurostimulator
neurosurgeon
neurosurgery
    functional n.
    stereotactic n.
neurosuture
neurosyphilis
neurotabes
    Dejerine's peripheral n.
neurotendinous
    n. organ
    n. spindle
neurotensin
neurotension
neurothekeoma
neurothele
neurotherapeutics, neurotherapy
neurothlipsis, neurothlipsia
neurotic
    n. manifestation
neuroticism

neurotization
neurotize
neurotmesis
neurotology
neurotome
neurotomy
    retrogasserian n.
neurotonic
neurotony
neurotoxic
neurotoxicity
neurotransmission
neurotransmitter
    amino acid n.
neurotrauma
neurotripsy
neurotrophic
    n. atrophy
neurotrophy
neurotropic
neurotropy, neurotropism
neurotrosis
neurotubule
neurovaricosis, neurovaricosity
neurovascular
    n. flap
neurovegetative
NEUROVIEW integrated
  visualization system
neurovisceral
neurula, pl. neurulae
neurulation
neutralization
    anterior n.
nevoid amentia
nevus, pl. nevi
    basal cell n.
    blue n.
    Ota's n.
    port wine n.
    Spitz n.

NOTES

newer-generation device
newtonian body
NEX
  number of excitations
nexus, pl. nexus
niacin
nicardipine
Nicolet Pathfinder I
Nicolet Viking II
  electrophysiologic system
nictation
nictitate
nictitating spasm
nictitation
nidal
NIDS
  National Institute of
    Neurological Disorders and
    Stroke
nidus, pl. nidi
    n. avis
    n. hirundinis
Niemann-Pick disease
nifedipine
night
    n. pain
    n. palsy
nigra
    fetal substantia n.
nigrostriatal
NIM-2
  nerve integrity monitor-2
nimodipine
Nimotop
nimustine (ACNU)
ninth cranial nerve
niobium-titanium
Nipride
Nishizaki-Wakabayashi suction
  tube
Nissl
    N. bodies
    N. degeneration
    N. granules
    N. substance
nitrate
nitrite
    amyl n.
Nitro-Bid
nitrogen
    blood urea n. (BUN)
    n. metabolism

n. narcosis
n. wasting
nitroglycerin
nitroprusside
    sodium n.
nitrosourea
Nitrostat
nitrous oxide
nizofenone
Nocardia asteroides
nocardiosis
nociceptive
    n. reflex
nociceptor
nocifensor
    n. reflex
noci-influence
nociperception
nocturnal
    n. diarrhea
    n. enuresis
    n. epilepsy
    n. myoclonus
    n. vertigo
nodding spasm
node
    Dürck's n.'s
    flocculonodular n.
    Hensen's n.
    primitive n.
    Ranvier's n.
    Schmorl's n.
    vital n.
nodosa
    periarteritis n.
    polyarteritis n. (PAN)
nodose ganglion
nodular
    n. enhancement
    n. headache
    n. mesoneuritis
    n. panencephalitis
nodule
    Schmorl's n.
nodulus, pl. noduli
noeud vital
noise
    acoustic n.
    n. reduction device
Nolvadex
nominal aphasia

nonaneurysmal perimesencephalic
  subarachnoid hemorrhage
nonchromaffin paraganglioma
noncommunicating hydrocephalus
nondetachable
    n. balloon
    n. endovascular balloon
    n. occlusive balloon
    n. silicone balloon catheter
nonferrous material
noninvasive diagnosis
nonionic
nonketotic hyperglycemia
nonmedullated
    n. fibers
nonmeningiomatous malignant
  lesion
nonmyelinated
nonneoplastic disease
nonpenetrating trauma
nonproton
    n. magnetic resonance
     imaging
    n. MRI
non-rapid eye movement (NREM)
nonspecific
    n. encephalomyeloneuropathy
    n. system
nonsteroidal anti-inflammatory drug
  (NSAID)
nonunion
    n. incidence
    n. rate
no-reflow phenomenon
norepinephrine
Norland digital oscilloscope
normal perfusion pressure
  breakthrough (NPPB)
normal-pressure hydrocephalus
normokalemic periodic paralysis

normotensive
normotonic
Norpramin
nortriptyline
nose-bridge-lid reflex
nose-eye reflex
notanencephalia
notch
       anterior n. of cerebellum
       Kernohan's n.
       marsupial n.
       posterior n. of cerebellum
       preoccipital n.
       semilunar n.
       n. of tentorium
notched
note blindness
Nothnagel's syndrome
notochord
Novo-10a CBF measuring device
NPH Iletin I
NPPB
    normal perfusion pressure
    breakthrough
NREM
    non-rapid eye movement
NSAID
    nonsteroidal anti-inflammatory
    drug
NTD
    neural tube defect
Nubain
nuchal
    n. muscle
    n. rigidity
nuclear
    n. bag
    n. jaundice
    n. layers of retina

NOTES

nuclear *(continued)*
    n. magnetic relaxation
      dispersion
    n. magnetic resonance
    n. magnetization vector
    n. MR scan
    n. ophthalmoplegia
    n. relaxation
nuclei (*pl. of* nucleus)
nucleofugal
nucleolysis
    percutaneous laser n.
nucleopetal
nucleotome
nucleus, pl. **nuclei**
    abducens n., n. abducentis,
      n. of abducent nerve
    accessory cuneate n.
    accessory olivary nuclei
    n. accumbens septi
    n. acusticus
    n. alae cinereae
    almond n.
    ambiguous n.
    n. ambiguus
    n. amygdalae
    amygdaloid n.
    nuclei anteriores thalami
    anterior nuclei of thalamus
    n. anterodorsalis,
      anterodorsal thalamic n.
    n. anteromedialis,
      anteromedial thalamic n.
    n. anteroventralis,
      anteroventral thalamic n.
    arcuate nuclei
    arcuate n.
    nuclei arcuati
    n. arcuatus
    n. arcuatus thalami
    auditory n.
    n. basalis of Ganser
    Bechterew's n.
    Blumenau's n.
    branchiomotor nuclei
    Burdach's n.
    n. caudalis
    n. caudalis-nucleus solitarius
      DREZ lesioning
    caudate n.
    n. caudatus
    n. centralis lateralis thalami

    n. centralis tegmenti
      superior
    centromedian n.
    n. centromedianus
    Clarke's n.
    cochlear nuclei
    nuclei cochleares
    n. colliculi inferioris
    convergence n. of Perlia
    n. corporis geniculati
      medialis
    nuclei corporis mamillaris
    nuclei of cranial nerves
    cuneate n.
    n. cuneatus
    n. cuneatus accessorius
    n. of Darkschewitsch
    deep cerebellar nuclei
    Deiters' n.
    dentate n.
    dentate n. of cerebellum
    n. dentatus cerebelli
    descending n. of the
      trigeminus
    dorsal n.
    dorsal accessory olivary n.
    n. dorsalis
    n. dorsalis corporis
      trapezoidei
    n. dorsalis nervi vagi
    dorsal motor n. of vagus
    dorsal n. of vagus
    dorsomedial n.
    dorsomedial hypothalamic n.
    n. dorsomedialis
      hypothalami
    Edinger-Westphal n.
    emboliform n.
    n. emboliformis
    external cuneate n.
    extrapyramidal n.
    n. facialis
    facial motor n.
    n. fasciculi gracilis
    n. fastigii
    n. fibrosus linguae
    n. filiformis
    force n.
    n. funiculi cuneati
    n. funiculi gracilis
    n. gelatinosus
    geniculate n.

n. gigantocellularis medullae oblongatae
n. globosus
n. of Goll
n. gracilis
Gudden's tegmental nuclei
gustatory n.
n. habenulae
habenular n.
hypoglossal n.
n. of hypoglossal nerve
inferior olivary n.
inferior salivary n.
inferior vestibular n.
intercalated n.
n. intercalatus
intermediolateral n.
n. intermediolateralis
intermediomedial n.
n. intermediomedialis
interpeduncular n.
n. interpeduncularis
n. interpositus
interstitial n. of Cajal
n. interstitialis
nuclei intralaminares thalami
intralaminar nuclei of thalamus
lateral cuneate n.
n. lateralis medullae oblongatae
n. lateralis thalami
n. of lateral lemniscus
lateral n. of medulla oblongata
lateral preoptic n.
lateral reticular n.
lateral n. of thalamus
lateral tuberal nuclei
lateral vestibular n.

n. lemnisci lateralis
n. of lens
lenticular n., lentiform n.
n. lentiformis
n. lentis
n. of Luys
main sensory n. of the trigeminus
n. of the mamillary body
masticatory n., n. masticatorius
medial accessory olivary n.
medial central n. of thalamus
n. of medial geniculate body
n. medialis centralis thalami
n. medialis thalami
medial preoptic n.
medial n. of thalamus
medial vestibular n.
mediodorsal n.
mesencephalic n. of the trigeminus
Monakow's n.
motor nuclei
motor n. of facial nerve
n. motorius nervi trigemini
motor n. of trigeminus
n. nervi abducentis
nuclei nervi cochlearis
n. nervi facialis
n. nervi hypoglossi
n. nervi oculomotorii
n. nervi trochlearis
nuclei nervi vestibulocochlearis
nuclei nervorum cranialium
n. niger
n. of oculomotor nerve, oculomotor n.

NOTES

nucleus *(continued)*
n. olivaris
n. olivaris accessorius
  dorsalis
n. olivaris accessorius
  medialis
Onuf's n.
nuclei of origin
nuclei originis
parabrachial nuclei
nuclei parabrachiales
n. paracentralis thalami
paracentral n. of thalamus
paraventricular n.
n. paraventricularis
Perlia's n.
pontine nuclei
nuclei pontis
n. posterior hypothalami
posterior hypothalamic n.
posterior medial n. of
  thalamus (*var. of* n.
  ventralis posteromedialis
  thalami)
posterior periventricular n.
n. preopticus lateralis
n. preopticus medialis
prerubral n.
n. pulposus
n. pyramidalis
raphe nuclei
nuclei raphes
red n.
reticular nuclei of the
  brainstem
n. reticularis thalami
reticular n. of thalamus
rhombencephalic
  gustatory n.
Roller's n.
roof n.
rostral interstitial n.
n. ruber
n. salivatorius inferior
n. salivatorius superior
Schwalbe's n.
secondary sensory nuclei
semilunar n. of Flechsig
n. sensorius principalis
  nervi trigemini
n. sensorius superior nervi
  trigemini
sole nuclei

n. solitarius
n. of solitary tract
somatic motor nuclei
special visceral efferent
  nuclei
special visceral motor nuclei
spherical n.
spinal n. of accessory nerve
n. spinalis nervi accessorii
spinal n. of the trigeminus
Spitzka's n.
Staderini's n.
Stilling's n.
subthalamic n.
n. subthalamicus
superior olivary n.
superior salivary n.
superior vestibular n.
supraoptic n.
n. supraopticus hypothalami
n. tecti
nuclei tegmenti
n. tegmenti pontis caudalis
n. tegmenti pontis oralis
terminal nuclei, nuclei
  terminales
nuclei terminationis
thalamic gustatory n.
thoracic n.
n. thoracicus
n. tractus mesencephali
  nervi trigemini
n. tractus solitarii
n. tractus spinalis nervi
  trigemini
trochlear n., n. of trochlear
  nerve
tuberal nuclei
nuclei tuberales
ventral anterior n. of
  thalamus
ventral intermediate n. of
  thalamus
n. ventralis anterior thalami
n. ventralis corporis
  trapezoidei
n. ventralis intermedius
  thalami
n. ventralis lateralis
n. ventralis posterior
  intermedius thalami
n. ventralis posterior
  thalami

n. ventralis posterolateralis
thalami
n. ventralis posteromedialis
thalami, posterior medial n.
of thalamus
n. ventralis thalami
ventral lateral n. of
thalamus
ventral posterior
intermediate n. of
thalamus
ventral posterior n. of
thalamus
ventral posterolateral n. of
thalamus, ventral posterior
lateral n. of thalamus
ventral posteromedial n. of
thalamus
ventral n. of thalamus
ventral tier thalamic nuclei
ventral n. of trapezoid
body
ventrobasal n.
n. ventro-intermedius
ventromedial n. of
hypothalamus
n. ventromedialis
hypothalami
vestibular nuclei
nuclei vestibulares
null-cell adenoma
nulling
gradient moment n.

number
n. of excitations (NEX)
quantum n.
Reynolds n.
numbness
waking n.
nut
n. alignment guide
lock n.
nutans
spasmus n.
nutation
nutrient vessel
nutrition
parenteral n.
total parenteral n.
nutritional polyneuropathy
nutritional-type cerebellar atrophy
nyctalgia
nylon suture
Nyquist
N. frequency
N. sampling criteria
nystagmus
convergence-retraction n.
downbeat n.
palatal n.
retraction n.
seesaw n.
torsional n.

NOTES

obdormition
Obersteiner-Redlich
    O.-R. line
    O.-R. zone
obesity
    hypothalamic o.
obex
Obex plugging
object blindness
objective
    275mm o. lens
    o. sensation
    o. vertigo
oblique
    o. bundle of pons
    o. flow misregistration
    o. sagittal gradient-echo MR
      imaging
    o. screw insertion
obliquity
    pelvic o.
obliterans
    thromboangiitis o.
obliterative
    o. arachnoiditis
    o. arteritis
oblongata
    medulla o.
OBS
    organic brain syndrome
obsessional neurosis
obsessive-compulsive disorder
obstacle sense
obstetrical
    o. hand
    o. paralysis
obstruction
    venous outflow o.
obstructive
    o. apnea
    o. hydrocephalus
    o. sleep apnea
obtund
obtundation
obturans
    keratosis o.
occipital
    o. encephalocele
    o. glioblastoma
    o. gyri

o. horn
o. lobe
o. lobe tumor
o. malformation
o. nerve
o. neuralgia
o. neuritis
o. operculum
o. pole
occipito-atlanto-axial complex
occipitoatlantoaxial instability
occipitocervical
    o. fixation
    o. fusion
    o. stabilization
occipitocollicular tract
occipitofrontal
    o. fasciculus
occipitoparietal artery occlusion
occipitopontine tract
occipitotectal tract
occipitotemporal sulcus
occipitothalamic
    o. radiation
occiput
occluded sinus
occluder
    Heifetz carotid o.
occlusion
    balloon o.
    balloon test o.
    carotid o.
    carotid artery o.
    o. coil
    distal o.
    dural sinus o.
    endovascular balloon o.
    internal carotid artery
      balloon test o.
    intracranial o.
    intraoperative balloon o.
    intravascular balloon o.
    occipitoparietal artery o.
    posterotemporal artery o.
    pre-Rolandic artery o.
    proximal o.
    superior sagittal sinus o.
    transtorcular o.
    vascular o.
    vertebral artery o.

occlusive
  o. cerebrovascular disease
  o. disease
  o. meningitis
occult
  o. cerebrovascular
   malformation
  o. hydrocephalus
  o. spinal dysraphism
occulta
  spina bifida o.
occupational
  o. neurosis
  o. spasm
ochronosis
octavus
ocular
  o. bobbing
  o. cup
  o. deviation
  o. dipping
  o. dysmetria
  o. flutter
  o. ischemic syndrome
  o. melanoma
  o. metastasis
  o. motor apraxia
  o. motor nerve paresis
  o. pain
  o. paralysis
  o. pneumoplethysmography
  o. pulse
  o. tilt reaction
  o. torticollis
  o. vesicle
Oculinum
oculocephalic
  o. reflex
  o. test
oculocephalogyric reflex
oculocerebrovasculometry
oculoencephalic angiomatosis
oculogyric crises
oculomotor
  o. nerve
  o. nerve paresis
  o. neuropathy
  o. nucleus
  o. response
  o. system
oculopalatal myoclonus
oculoplethysmography
oculosympathetic dysfunction

oculovestibular
  o. reflex
od
odaxesmus
odaxetic
Oden's syndrome
odogenesis
odonterism
odontogenic infection
odontoid
  o. dysplasia
  o. fracture
  o. fracture internal fixation
  o. fracture stabilization
  o. process
  o. process osteosynthesis
odontoideum
  os o.
odontoneuralgia
odynometer
OEC-Diasonics mobile C-arm
  image intensifier
offset
  frequency o.
  o. frequency
Ogura operation
OHDA
  6-hydroxydopamine
Oil
  Pitressin Tannate in O.
Oldberg pituitary forceps
olecranon reflex
olfactory
  o. anesthesia
  o. area
  o. bulb
  o. bundle
  o. cortex
  o. esthesioneuroblastoma
  o. glomerulus
  o. groove
  o. hyperesthesia
  o. hypesthesia
  o. nerve
  o. neuroblastoma
  o. organ
  o. peduncle
  o. pyramid
  o. receptor cells
  o. roots
  o. striae
  o. sulcus
  o. tract

o. trigone
o. tubercle
oligemia
oligoclonal bands
oligodendria
oligodendroblast
oligodendroblastoma
oligodendrocyte
oligodendroglia
o. cells
oligodendroglioma
oligosynaptic
oliva, pl. **olivae**
o. inferior
o. superior
olivary
o. body
o. degeneration
o. eminence
olive
inferior o.
superior o.
Olivecrona
O. aneurysm clamp
O. clip
O. clip applier
O. dissector
O. dura scissors
Olivier-Bertrand-Tipal frame
olivifugal
olivipetal
olivocerebellar tract
olivocochlear
o. bundle
olivopontocerebellar
o. atrophy
o. degeneration
olivospinal tract
Ollier's disease
Omega 1400
Ommaya reservoir

Omni
O. clip gun
O. 2 microscope
Omnipaque
Omnipen-N
Omni-Vent
omohyoid muscle
OMS
organic mental syndrome
oncocytoma
oncogene
ras o.
Oncovin
Ondine's curse
One
Neurostation O.
one-and-a-half syndrome
one-way flow mechanism
onion bulb neuropathy
on-off phenomenon
ontogeny
Onuf's nucleus
Opalski cell
open
o. angiography
o. C-D hook
o. cordotomy
o. head injury
o. hook
o. skull fracture
o. stereotactic craniotomy
operating microscope
operation
Ball's o.
Cloward o.
Cotte's o.
Dana's o.
Dandy o.
decompression o.'s
floating-forehead o.
Frazier-Spiller o.

NOTES

operation *(continued)*
    Hunter's o.
    Keen's o.
    Koerte-Ballance o.
    Leriche's o.
    Matas' o.
    Mikulicz' o.
    Ogura o.
    Smith-Robinson o.
    stereotactic o.
    Stoffel's o.
    Stookey-Scarff o.
    synchrocyclotron o.
    tongue-in-groove o.
operative
    o. approach
    o. injury
    o. risk
    o. technique
    o. wedge frame
opercular
    o. cortex
operculum, gen. operculi,
  pl. opercula
    occipital o.
ophryosis
OphSeg
    ophthalmic segment
ophthalmia
    neuroparalytic o.
ophthalmic
    o. artery
    o. artery aneurysm
    o. migraine
    o. segment (OphSeg)
    o. segment aneurysm
    o. vein
ophthalmicus
    herpes zoster o.
ophthalmodynamometer
    Bailliart o.
    compression o.
ophthalmodynamometry
    compression o.
    suction o.
ophthalmoparesis
ophthalmopathy
    Graves' o.
ophthalmoplegia
    o. externa
    fascicular o.
    infectious o.
    o. interna

internuclear o.
    o. internuclearis
intranuclear o.
nuclear o.
orbital o.
Parinaud's o.
    o. partialis
    o. progressiva
    o. totalis
ophthalmoplegic
    o. migraine
ophthalmoscopy
opiate receptors
opisthoporeia
opisthotonic
opisthotonoid
opisthotonos, opisthotonus
Oppenheim's
    O. disease
    O. reflex
    O. syndrome
OpSite dressing
opsoclonus
optic
    o. agnosia
    o. aphasia
    o. ataxia
    o. atrophy
    o. canal
    o. chiasm
    o. chiasmal syndrome
    o. chiasm compression
    o. cup
    o. decussation
    o. disk
    o. fissure
    o. glioma
    o. layer
    o. nerve
    o. nerve astrocytoma
    o. nerve glioma
    o. nerve hypoplasia
    o. nerve injury
    o. nerve lesion
    o. neuritis
    o. neuropathy
    o. part of retina
    o. radiation
    o. recess
    o. tract
    o. tract compression
    o. tract syndrome
    o. vesicle

optical
    o. alexia
    o. device
    o. glass
    o. righting reflexes
opticocarotid triangle
opticocerebral syndrome
opticofacial reflex
opticopyramidal syndrome
optimization
Optiray
optokinetic disorder
oral
    o. cavity
    o. contraceptive
    o. intubation
    o. retraction
    o. ulceration
Orbeli effect
orbicularis
    o. oculi reflex
    o. pupillary reflex
Orbis-Sigma valve
orbital
    o. apex syndrome
    o. chemosis
    o. decompression
    o. dystopia
    o. encephalocele
    o. fracture
    o. granulocytic sarcoma
    o. gyri
    o. hypertelorism
    o. ophthalmoplegia
    o. part
    o. pseudotumor
    o. roof
    o. sulci
    o. tumor
    o. varices
    o. vein

orbitofrontal cortex
orbitopathy
    thyroid o.
orbitotomy
orbitozygomatic
    o. mandibular osteotomy
    o. osteotomy
    o. temporopolar approach
organ
    annulospiral o.
    circumventricular o.'s
    o. of Corti
    Corti's o.
    end o.
    flower-spray o. of Ruffini
    Golgi tendon o.
    gustatory o.
    o. of hearing
    neurotendinous o.
    olfactory o.
    sense o.'s
    o. of smell
    spiral o.
    subcommissural o.
    o. of taste
    o. of touch
    vestibular o.
    vestibulocochlear o.
    o. of vision
    o. of Zuckerkandl
organa (*pl. of* organum)
organic
    o. brain disorder
    o. brain syndrome (OBS)
    o. contracture
    o. headache
    o. mental disorder
    o. mental syndrome (OMS)
    o. pain
    o. vertigo
organism embolus

NOTES

organoleptic
organum, pl. organa
 o. auditus
 o. gustus
 o. olfactus
 organa sensuum
 o. spirale
 o. tactus
 o. vestibulocochleare
 o. visus
orienting
 o. reflex
 o. response
origin
 anomalous o.
 apparent o.
 deep o.
 ectal o.
 ental o.
 real o.
 superficial o.
Orinase
ornithinemia
oropharyngeal reflex
orphenadrine
orthochorea
orthogonal
 o. angiography
orthograde degeneration
orthosis
 cervicothoracic o.
 postoperative lumbosacral o.
 thoracolumbar standing o.
 thoracolumbosacral o.
 (TLSO)
orthostatic hypotension
orthosympathetic
orthotics
orthotonos, orthotonus
oscillopsia
oscilloscope
 Norland digital o.
Osmitrol
osmoceptor
osmophobia
osmoreceptor
osmosis
osmotherapy
osmotic demyelination syndrome
os odontoideum
ossification
 heterotopic o.

ossifying
 o. arachnoiditis
 o. fibroma
osteitis deformans
osteoblastoma
osteochondroma
osteochondrosis
 intervertebral o.
osteodiastasis
osteoid osteoma
osteolysis
osteoma
 osteoid o.
osteomyelitis
 cranial o.
 pyogenic o.
 spinal o.
osteopathic scoliosis
osteopetrosis
 cranial o.
osteophyte
osteoplastic
 o. bone flap
 o. craniotomy
osteoporosis
 o. circumscripta
 o. circumscripta cranii
 posttraumatic o.
 o. with vertebral collapse
  and neurologic deficit
osteoporotic spine
osteosarcoma
osteosynthesis
 anterior column o.
 cranial o.
 facial o.
 lumbar spine vertebral o.
 odontoid process o.
 plate-screw o.
 posterior column o.
 thoracic spine vertebral o.
 thoracolumbar spine
  vertebral o.
 vertebral o.
 wire o.
osteotome
osteotomy
 craniofacial o.
 ethmoidal o.
 frontonasomaxillary o.
 fronto-orbital o.
 glabellar exposure o.
 LeFort o.

o. of mandible
mandibular o.
maxillary o.
orbitozygomatic o.
orbitozygomatic
  mandibular o.
Tessier o.
otalgia
geniculate o.
Ota's nevus
otic
o. abscess
o. capsule
o. ganglion
oticus
herpes zoster o.
otitic
o. hydrocephalus
o. meningitis
otitis
o. media
otocerebritis
otoencephalitis
otoganglion
otologic implant
otoneuralgia
otorhinorrhea
otorrhea
cerebrospinal fluid o.
otosclerosis
outer cone fiber
outlet
thoracic o.
out-of-phase image
output
cardiac o.
oval
o. area of Flechsig
o. corpuscle
o. fasciculus

ovale
foramen o.
overdistraction
overdrainage syndrome
overflow
o. incontinence
receiver o.
overhang
bony o.
overload
receiver o.
overresponse
over-right hypertropia
ovulation
oxacillin
oxazepam
oxidation states
oxide
nitrous o.
superparamagnetic iron o.
oxidized
o. cellulose
o. cotton
o. regenerated cellulose
oxime
hexamethyl-
  propyleneamine o.
  (HMPAO)
^{99m}Tc-hexamethyl-
  propyleneamine o.
  (^{99m}Tc-HMPAO)
oximeter
pulse o.
Somanetics INVOS 3100
  cerebral o.
oximetry
continuous venous o.
pulse o.
oxolinic acid
oxyacoia, oxyakoia
oxyaphia

NOTES

oxyaphia
oxybutynin
Oxycel
oxycellulose
oxycephalia
oxycephalic, oxycephalous
oxycephaly
oxychlorosene
oxycodone
    o. and acetaminophen
    o. and aspirin
oxyesthesia
oxygen
    cerebral venous gas tension
     of o. (PvO2)

hyperbaric o.
    o. tension
    o. therapy
oxygenation
    extracorporeal membrane o.
oxygeusia
oxyhemoglobin
oxyosmia
oxyosphresia
oxytetracycline
oxytocin

P

pacchionian
    p. bodies
    p. corpuscles
    p. glands
    p. granulations
pacemaker
Pachon's test
pachygyria
pachyleptomeningitis
pachymeningitis
    p. externa
    hemorrhagic p.
    hypertrophic cervical p.
    p. interna
    pyogenic p.
pachymeningopathy
pachymeninx
pacinian corpuscles
packing
    Avitene p.
    Vaseline gauze p.
PaCO2
    cerebral arterial gas tension of carbon dioxide
pad
    Gelfoam p.
paddies
    cotton p.
PAE
    paradoxical air embolism
Paget's disease
pain
    abdominal p.
    affected p.
    back p.
    chronic intractable p.
    deafferentation p.
    p. drawing
    dream p.
    effected p.
    facial p.
    faciocephalic p.
    girdle p.
    growing p.'s
    hemicranial p.
    heterotopic p.
    homotopic p.
    intractable p.
    p. modulation
    myofascial p.

    nerve p.
    night p.
    ocular p.
    organic p.
    p. pathway
    phantom p.
    phantom limb p.
    phantom tooth p.
    psychogenic p.
    p. reaction
    recurrent p.
    referred p.
    p. relief
    rest p.
    retro-orbital p.
    sciatic p.
    somatic p.
    p. threshold
    p. threshold reduction
    throat p.
    p. tolerance
    p. transduction
    visceral p.
Paine retinaculatome
painful
    p. anesthesia
    p. paraplegia
    p. point
pairs
    Maxwell p.
palatal
    p. myoclonus
    p. nystagmus
    p. paresis
    p. reflex
    p. split
palatine reflex
palato-occipital line
palato-ocular myoclonus
palatoplasty
palatoplegia
paleencephalon
pale globe
paleocerebellum
paleocortex
paleokinetic
paleostriatal
    p. syndrome
paleostriatum
paleothalamus

palikinesia, palicinesia
palilalia
palindromic encephalopathy
palinopsia
palinoptic hallucination
paliphrasia
pallanesthesia
pallesthesia
pallesthetic
    p. sensibility
pallial
pallidal
    p. syndrome
pallidectomy
pallidoamygdalotomy
pallidoansotomy
pallidotomy
    posteroventral p.
    VPL p.
pallidum
    Treponema p.
pallidus
    globus p.
pallium
pallor
palmar reflex
palm-chin reflex
palmi (*pl. of* palmus)
palmic
palmitic acid
palmodic
palmomental
    p. reflex
    p. test
palmus, pl. palmi
palsy
    abducens p.
    Bell's p.
    birth p.
    brachial birth p.
    bulbar p.
    cerebral p.
    craft p.
    cranial nerve p.
    creeping p.
    crutch p.
    Erb's p.
    facial p.
    Féréol-Graux p.
    fourth nerve p.
    gaze p.
    lateral rectus p.
    lead p.

    multi-infarct progressive
      supranuclear p.
    night p.
    posticus p.
    pressure p.
    progressive bulbar p.
    progressive supranuclear p.
    pseudoabducens p.
    pseudobulbar p.
    scrivener's p.
    seventh nerve p.
    shaking p.
    supranuclear p.
    Tapia's vagohypoglossal p.
    third nerve p.
    trembling p.
    trochlear nerve p.
    wasting p.
pamoate
    hydroxyzine p.
PAN
    polyarteritis nodosa
Pancoast's syndrome
Pancoast tumor
pancreatic encephalopathy
pancreatitis
pancuronium bromide
pandiculation
panencephalitis
    nodular p.
    sclerosing p.
    subacute sclerosing p.
panesthesia
pang
panhypopituitarism
panneuritis
    p. endemica
panodic
panplegia
Pansch's fissure
pansynostosis
pantalgia
pantanencephaly, pantanencephalia
panthodic
Pantopaque
papaphysis
papaverine
Papaverine-soaked Gelfoam
Papez circuit
papilla, pl. papillae
    acoustic p.
    nerve p.
papilledema

papillitis
papilloma
    p. neuropathicum, p.
      neuroticum
papillophlebitis
papulosis
    malignant atrophic p.
par
paraballism
parabrachial nuclei
paracarcinomatous
    p. encephalomyelopathy
    p. myelopathy
paracenesthesia
paracentesis
paracentral
    p. fissure
    p. lobule
    p. nucleus of thalamus
paracetamol
parachiasmal epidermoid tumor
parachute reflex
paracinesia, paracinesis
paraclinoidal aneurysm
paradoxical
    p. air embolism (PAE)
    p. cerebral embolism
    p. extensor reflex
    p. flexor reflex
    p. incontinence
    p. patellar reflex
    p. pupil
    p. pupillary phenomenon
    p. pupillary reflex
    p. reflex
    p. sleep
    p. triceps reflex
paradoxic embolism
para-equilibrium
paraesthesia
Parafon Forte

paraganglioma
    nonchromaffin p.
parageusia
parageusic
paragonimiasis
paragrammatism
paragraphia
parahippocampal gyrus
parahypophysis
parainfluenzae
    Haemophilus p.
parakinesia, parakinesis
paraldehyde
paraleprosis
paralexia
paralgesia
paralgia
paralysis, pl. paralyses
    acute ascending p.
    acute atrophic p.
    p. agitans
    ascending p.
    Brown-Séquard's p.
    bulbar p.
    central p.
    compression p.
    conjugate p.
    crossed p.
    crutch p.
    decubitus p.
    diphtheritic p.
    Duchenne-Erb p.
    Duchenne's p.
    Erb's p.
    Erb's spinal p.
    facial p.
    familial periodic p.
    faucial p.
    gaze p.
    ginger p.
    global p.

NOTES

paralysis *(continued)*
 glossolabiolaryngeal p.
 glossolabiopharyngeal p.
 Gubler's p.
 hyperkalemic periodic p.
 hypokalemic periodic p.
 immunological p.
 Jackson's vagoaccessory hypoglossal p.
 jake p.
 Klumpke's p.
 Kussmaul-Landry p.
 labial p.
 Landry's p.
 lead p.
 mimetic p.
 mixed p.
 motor p.
 motor neuron p.
 musculospiral p.
 myogenic p.
 normokalemic periodic p.
 obstetrical p.
 ocular p.
 periodic p.
 postdiphtheritic p.
 posticus p.
 Pott's p.
 pressure p.
 progressive bulbar p.
 pseudobulbar p.
 pseudohypertrophic muscular p.
 residual p.
 sensory p.
 sleep p.
 sodium-responsive periodic p.
 spastic spinal p.
 spinal p.
 supranuclear p.
 tick p.
 Todd's p.
 Todd's postepileptic p.
 wasting p.
 Zenker's p.
paralytic
 p. chorea
 p. dementia
 p. miosis
 p. mydriasis
 p. pontine exotropia
 p. scoliosis

paralyzant
paralyze
paralyzing vertigo
paramagnetic
 p. contrast
 p. contrast enhancement
 p. contrast injection
 p. relaxation
paramagnetism
paramedian
 p. infarction
 p. mesencephalic syndrome
 p. pontine syndrome
 p. region
 p. triangle
parametrismus
paramimia
paramusia
paramyoclonus
paramyotonia
 ataxic p.
 congenital p., p. congenita
 symptomatic p.
paramyotonus
paranalgesia
paranasal
 p. mucocele
 p. sinus
paraneoplastic syndrome
paranesthesia
paraneural
 p. infiltration
paraneurone
paranomia
paraorbital lesion
paraparesis
 tropical spastic p.
 X-linked spastic p.
paraparetic
paraphasia
 thematic p.
paraphasic
paraphia
paraphrasia
paraphysial, paraphyseal
 p. cysts
paraphysis, pl. paraphyses
parapineal
paraplectic
paraplegia
 ataxic p.
 congenital spastic p.
 p. dolorosa

p. in extension
p. in flexion
hereditary spastic p.
infantile spastic p.
painful p.
postoperative p.
Pott's p.
senile p.
spastic p.
superior p.
tetanoid p.
paraplegic
p. spasm
parapoplexy
parapraxia
paraproteinemia
parapsia
parareflexia
parasagittal lesion
parasellar
p. tentorial meningioma
p. tumor
parasinoidal sinuses
parasitic brain abscess
parasomnia
paraspinal
p. muscle
p. rod application
parastriate
p. area
p. cortex
parasympathetic
p. ganglia
p. nerve injury
p. nervous system
p. part
parasympathotonia
paraterminal
p. body
p. gyrus
parathyroid tetany

parathyroprival tetany
paraventricular nucleus
paravertebral
p. ganglia
p. venous plexus
paraxial mesenchyme
paraxon
parchment crackling
parectropia
parencephalia
parencephalitis
parencephalocele
parencephalous
parenchymal granuloma
parenchymatous
p. cell of corpus pineale
p. neuritis
parent artery
parenteral
p. alimentation
p. nutrition
paresis
accessory nerve p.
downward gaze p.
elevation p.
gaze p.
horizontal gaze p.
ocular motor nerve p.
oculomotor nerve p.
palatal p.
postictal p.
pseudoabducens nerve p.
trochlear nerve p.
upward gaze p.
vertical gaze p.
paresthesia
Berger's p.
paresthetic
paresthetica
meralgia p.

NOTES

paretic
    p. dementia
    p. impotence
Pargonimus westermani
paries, gen. **parietis**, pl. **parietes**
    p. vestibularis ductus
      cochlearis
parietal
    p. encephalocele
    p. foramen
    p. lobe
    p. lobe syndrome
parieto-occipital
    p.-o. fissure
    p.-o. sulcus
parietopontine tract
Parinaud's
    P. ophthalmoplegia
    P. syndrome
park bench position
parkinsonian
parkinsonism
Parkinson's
    P. disease
    P. facies
    P. triangle
Parlodel
Parnate
parolfactory
    p. area
parotid
    p. dissection
    p. duct
    p. tumor
parotitis
paroxysm
paroxysmal
    p. atrial fibrillation
    p. cerebral dysrhythmia
    p. sleep
pars, pl. **partes**
    p. anterior
    p. anterior commissurae
      anterioris
    p. anterior commissurae
      rostralis
    p. anterior facies
      diaphragmatis
    p. anterior fornix vaginae
    p. autonomica
    p. basilaris pontis
    p. caudalis
    p. centralis

    p. centralis ventriculi
      lateralis
    p. cervicalis
    p. cervicalis arteriae carotis
      internae
    p. cervicalis esophagi
    p. cervicalis medullae
      spinalis
    p. coccygea medullae
      spinalis
    p. cochlearis
    p. cupularis
    p. distalis
    p. dorsalis pontis
    p. frontalis corporis callosi
    p. infundibularis
    p. insularis
    p. interarticularis
    p. intermedia
    p. intermedia commissura
      bulborum
    p. intermedia lobi anterioris
      hypophyseos
    p. lumbalis
    p. lumbalis diaphragmatis
    p. lumbalis medullae
      spinalis
    p. nervosa hypophyseos
    p. occipitalis corporis callosi
    p. opercularis
    p. optica retinae
    p. orbitalis
    p. orbitalis glandulae
      lacrimalis
    p. orbitalis musculi
      orbicularis oculi
    p. orbitalis nervi optici
    p. orbitalis ossis frontalis
    p. parasympathica
    p. peripherica
    p. pharyngea hypophyseos
    p. plana
    p. plicata
    p. posterior
    p. posterior commissurae
      anterioris
    p. posterior facies
      diaphragmatis hepatis
    p. posterior fornix vaginae
    p. postlaminalis nervi optici
      vaginae
    p. reticulata

p. retrolentiformis capsulae internae
p. sacralis medullae spinalis
p. sellaris
p. spinalis
p. sublentiformis capsulae internae
p. sympathica
p. thoracica
p. thoracica aortae
p. thoracica ductus thoracici
p. thoracica esophagi
p. thoracica medullae spinalis
p. triangularis
p. vagalis
p. ventralis pontis
p. vertebralis
p. vestibularis

Parsonage-Aldren-Turner syndrome
Parsonage-Turner syndrome
part

anterior p.
anterior p. of pons
autonomic p.
basilar p. of pons
coccygeal p. of spinal cord
cochlear p. of vestibulocochlear nerve
cupular p., cupulate p.
distal p. of anterior lobe of hypophysis
dorsal p. of pons
inferior p. of vestibulocochlear nerve
infundibular p. of anterior lobe of hypophysis
intermediate p.
optic p. of retina
orbital p.
parasympathetic p.

superior p. of vestibulocochlear nerve
sympathetic p.
vagal p. of accessory nerve
ventral p. of the pons
vertebral p.
vestibular p. of vestibulocochlear nerve
partes (*pl. of* pars)
parthenium
Tanacetum p.
partial

p. central hypophysectomy
p. complex seizure
p. epilepsy
p. facetectomy
p. flip angle imaging
p. Fourier imaging
p. hemilaminectomy
p. pressure
p. seizure
partial-thickness craniectomy
particle

p. domain
Ivalon p.
polyvinyl alcohol p.
particulate embolization
pas

petit p.
passage

wire p.
passive

p. incontinence
p. tremor
past-pointing
patellar

p. reflex
p. tendon reflex
patello-adductor reflex
patellometer

NOTES

patency
 valve p.
pathematic aphasia
pathergy phenomenon
pathetic
 p. nerve
pathognomonic
pathomechanics
 kyphotic deformity p.
 spinal fusion p.
pathway
 auditory p.
 biochemical p.
 pain p.
patient
 adult scoliosis p.
 p. positioning
 variable screw placement
 system-plated p.
Patil stereotactic system II
Patrick's test
pattern
 Antoni type A p.
 Antoni type B p.
 double major curve p.
 field p.
 left thoracolumbar major
 curve p.
 radiofrequency
 homogeneity p.
 right thoracic left lumbar
 curve p.
 right thoracic left
 thoracolumbar curve p.
 right thoracic minor
 curve p.
 p. sensitive epilepsy
 type II curve p.
patty
 polyclot p.
paucisynaptic
Pauli exclusion principle
pause
 apneic p.
 respiratory p.
Pavlov method
Pavulon
**PC-2048B positron emission
 tomograph**
PCA
 posterior cerebral artery
PCNU
PCV chemotherapy

peak
 Bragg p.
Péan forceps
pearl tumor
pearly neoplasm
pear-shaped nerve hook
pectoralgia
pectoralis major muscle
pectoral reflex
pedal system
pedes (*pl. of* pes)
pediatric
 p. C-D hook
 p. Cotrel-Dubousset rod
 p. hook
 p. neuroradiology
 p. supratentorial hemispheric
 tumor
 p. TSRH hook
pedicle
 adjoining p.
 p. anatomy
 p. angle
 p. axis angle
 p. C-D hook
 p. cortex disruption
 p. diameter
 p. dimensions
 p. entrance point
 p. evaluation
 p. fixation
 p. hook
 p. landmark
 p. localization
 p. location
 lower thoracic p.
 lumbar p.
 p. marker
 p. morphometry
 p. probe
 p. screw
 p. screw breakage
 p. screw chord length
 p. screw construct
 p. screw hardware
 prominence
 p. screw insertion
 p. screw linkage design
 p. screw path length
 p. screw plating
 p. screw pullout strength
 p. screw-rod fixation

p. sounding probe
thoracic p.
pedicular fixation
pedionalgia
pedioneuralgia
pedis (*gen. of* pes)
peduncle
    cerebellar p.
    cerebral p.
    p. of corpus callosum
    p. of flocculus
    inferior cerebellar p.
    inferior thalamic p.
    lateral thalamic p.
    p. of mamillary body
    middle cerebellar p.
    olfactory p.
    superior cerebellar p.
    ventral thalamic p.
peduncular
    p. ansa
    p. loop
pedunculotomy
pedunculus, pl. **pedunculi**
    p. cerebellaris inferior
    p. cerebellaris medius
    p. cerebellaris superior
    p. cerebri
    p. corporis callosi
    p. corporis mamillaris
    p. flocculi
    p. of pineal body
    p. thalami inferior
    p. thalami lateralis
    p. thalami ventralis
PEEP
    positive end-expiratory pressure
Peet splanchnic resection
peg
    fibular p.

Pelizaeus-Merzbacher
    P.-M. disease
    P.-M. leukodystrophy
pellucidi
    cavum septi p. (CSP)
pelopsia
Pelorus surgical system
pelvic
    p. fixation
    p. ganglia
    p. obliquity
    p. plexus
pelvofemoral muscular dystrophy
pemoline
pencil grip
pencil-grip instrument
pendemoma
penetrating
    p. injury
    p. trauma
penetration
    anterior cortex p.
    antibiotic p.
    vertebral body anterior
      cortex p.
Penfield dissector
penicillin
    benzathine p.
    p. G
    p. G benzathine suspension
    p. V
Penicillium
Penrose drain
pentastarch
pentazocine
    p. analgesia
pentobarbital
Pentothal
pentoxifylline
pentylenetetrazol
Pepper syndrome

NOTES

peptidergic
perception
perceptorium
Percodan
percutaneous
    p. balloon commissurotomy
    p. cabling
    p. cordotomy
    p. electrode array
    p. glycerol rhizolysis (PGR)
    p. intra-arterial embolization
    p. laser nucleolysis
    p. radiofrequency
      gangliolysis
    p. radiofrequency rhizolysis
      (PRF)
    p. radiofrequency rhizotomy
    p. retrogasserian glycerol
      chemoneurolysis
    p. retrogasserian glycerol
      rhizolysis
    p. stimulation
    p. thecoperitoneal shunt
    p. transluminal angioplasty
perencephaly
Perez reflex
perfluorocarbon
perforated space
perforation
    esophageal p.
    vascular p.'s
perforator
    Aseculap skull p.
    cranial p.
    Heifetz skull p.
    powered automatic skull p.
perfusion
    p. deficit
    luxury p.
    p. pressure breakthrough
pergolide
Periactin
perianeurysmal hemorrhage
periapical abscess
periaqueductal gray
periarterial sympathectomy
periarteritis nodosa
periatrial disease
periaxonal
pericardial reflex
pericarditis
perichrome
periclaustral lamina

pericorpuscular synapse
pericranial temporalis flap
pericranii
    sinus p.
pericranitis
pericranium
peridural
periencephalitis
perigemmal
perikaryon, pl. perikarya
perilymphatic duct
perimeningitis
perimetry
    Goldman p.
perineural
    p. anesthesia
    p. infiltration
perineuria (*pl. of* perineurium)
perineurial
    p. cyst
perineuritis
perineurium, pl. perineuria
period
    absolute refractory p.
    latent p.
    readout p.
    silent p.
periodic
    p. edema
    p. migrainous neuralgia
    p. paralysis
perioperative reduction
perioptic
    p. meningioma
    p. subarachnoid space
periorbita
periorbital ecchymosis
periosteal
    p. elevator
    p. reflex
peripachymeningitis
peripheral
    p. apnea
    p. chemoreceptor
    p. nerve
    p. nerve injury
    p. nerve sheath tumor
    p. nervous system
    p. neuropathy
    p. tabes
periphlebitis retinae
perispondylitis

peristriate
  p. area
  p. cortex
peritoneal catheter
peritoneum
peritorcular meningioma
Peritrode
perivascular space
periventricular
  p. disease
  p. fibers
  p. gray
  p. hyperintense lesion
  p. lesion
  p. white matter
  p. white matter lesion
Perlia's nucleus
Perls' stain
permanent vegetative state
permeability
peroneal
  p. muscular atrophy
  p. phenomenon
  p. somatosensory evoked
    potential
perpendicular fasciculus
perphenazine
  p. and amitriptyline
    hydrochloride
Persantine
perseveration
persistent tremor
personality change
pes, gen. pedis, pl. pedes
  p. hippocampi
  p. pedunculi
PET
  positron emission tomography
  PET-guided biopsy
  PET scan
petechial hemorrhage

PET-FDG
  positron emission tomography
    with [^{18}F]-labeled
    fluorodeoxyglucose
petit
  p. mal
  p. mal epilepsy
  p. pas
Petit's syndrome
petroclinoclival meningioma
petroclival
  p. cholesterol granuloma
  p. meningioma
  p. tumor
petroclivotentorial meningioma
petrosal
  p. approach
  p. ganglion
  p. impression of the
    pallium
  p. sinus
petrositis
petrosquamosal sinus
petrous
  p. apex
  p. carotid-to-intradural
    carotid saphenous vein
    graft
  p. ganglion
petrousitis
Pette-Döring disease
Pfeiffer's syndrome
Pfuhl's sign
PGR
  percutaneous glycerol rhizolysis
  psychogalvanic response
phacoma
phacomatosis
phagocytosis
phakoma
phakomatosis

NOTES

phalangeal cells
Phalen's
    P. maneuver
    P. sign
    P. test
phantom
    gelatin p.
    hot-spot p.
    p. image
    p. limb
    p. limb pain
    p. pain
    plexiglas p.
    three-dimensional SPECT p.
    p. tooth pain
pharyngeal
    p. anesthesia
    p. cleft
    p. hypophysis
    p. pouch
    p. reflex
    p. weakness
pharyngismus
pharyngoplegia
pharyngospasm
phase
    p. coherence
    p. cycling
    p. effect
    p. encoding
    extradural p.
    p. instability
    intradural p.
    p. mapping
    p. reversal
    p. reversal potential
    p. shift
    transverse magnetization p.
    vector p.
phase-contrast map
phased-array color-flow ultrasound
  system
phase-encoding
    p.-e. direction
    p.-e. gradient
phase-sensitive
    p.-s. detector
    p.-s. gradient-echo MR
      imaging
phase-shift effect
phasic reflex
phencyclidine
phenelzine

Phenergan
phenobarbital
phenol
phenomenon, pl. phenomena
    arm p.
    Babinski's p.
    Bell's p.
    breakthrough p.
    cervicolumbar p.
    clasp-knife p.
    cogwheel p.
    crossed phrenic p.
    Cushing p.
    Dejerine-Lichtheim p.
    Dejerine's hand p.
    Duckworth's p.
    escape p.
    extinction p.
    facialis p.
    finger p.
    Galassi's pupillary p.
    Gibbs p.
    Grasset-Gaussel p.
    Grasset's p.
    Gunn p.
    halo p.
    hip p.
    hip-flexion p.
    Hoffmann's p.
    Hunt's paradoxical p.
    intracranial steal p.
    jaw-winking p.
    knee p.
    Kohnstamm's p.
    Kühne's p.
    leg p.
    Leichtenstern's p.
    Marcus Gunn p.
    misdirection p.
    Negro's p.
    no-reflow p.
    on-off p.
    paradoxical pupillary p.
    pathergy p.
    peroneal p.
    Pool's p.
    radial p.
    Raynaud's p.
    rebound p.
    release p.
    Ritter-Rollet p.
    Rust's p.

Schiff-Sherrington p.
Schüller's p.
Sherrington p.
staircase p.
steal p.
Strümpell's p.
tibial p.
toe p.
tongue p.
Uhthoff's p.
Westphal-Piltz p.
Westphal's p.
Wever-Bray p.
phenoxybenzamine
phenylalanine
phenylbutazone
phenylketonuria (PKU)
phenylpropanolamine
phenytoin
pheochromocytoma
Philadelphia collar
Philippe's triangle
Philips
  P. Gyroscan S5
  P. Gyroscan S15
  P. linear accelerator
Phillipson's reflex
Philly Bolt
phlebitis
  sinus p.
phlebography
Phoenix
  P. ancillary valve
  P. Anti-Blok ventricular
    catheter
  P. cruciform valve
  P. fifth ventricle system
phonic spasm
phonism
phonoangiography
  quantitative spectral p.

phonomyoclonus
phonomyography
phonoreceptor
phosphate metabolism
phosphene
phosphocreatine
phosphorus-31
photalgia
photesthesia
photic
  p. driving
  p. stimulation
photism
photocoagulation
  in situ p.
photodynia
photodysphoria
photoesthetic
photogenic epilepsy
photomicrograph
photomyoclonus
  hereditary p.
photon beam radiosurgery
photophobia
photopsia
photoptarmosis
photoradiation therapy
photosensitivity
photosensitizer
phrenalgia
phrenectomy
phrenemphraxis
phrenicectomy
phrenic ganglia
phreniclasia
phrenicoexeresis
phreniconeurectomy
phrenicotomy
phrenicotripsy
phrenoglottic
phrenology

NOTES

phrenoplegia
phrenospasm
phrenotropic
phrictopathic
phthisis bulbi
Phycomycetes
phylogeny
Phynox Cobalt Alloy clip material
physaliphorous cell
physiopsychic
physocephaly
physostigmine
PI
    pulsatility index
pia
pia-arachnitis
pia-arachnoid
pial
    p. artery
    p. funnel
pial-glial membrane
pia mater
    p. m. encephali
    p. m. spinalis
pianist's cramp
piano-player's cramp
piarachnoid
PICA
    posterior inferior cerebellar
    artery
    posterior inferior
    communicating artery
Pick's
    P. atrophy
    P. bodies
    P. bundle
    P. disease
    P. syndrome
pictures
    Allen p.
pieds terminaux
piesesthesia
pigment
    acute posterior multifocal
    placoid p.
    p. epithelial lesion
pigmented layer of retina
pillar
    anterior p. of fornix
    p. cells
    p. cells of Corti
    Corti's p.'s

p.'s of fornix
    posterior p. of fornix
pillar-and-post microsurgical
    retractor
pill-rolling
pilocytic astrocytoma
piloid
    p. astrocytoma
    p. gliosis
pilojection
pilomatrixoma
pilomotor
    p. fibers
    p. reflex
pilonidal sinus
Piltz sign
pimozide
pin
    p. headholder
    Kirschner p.
    Steinmann p.
    Synthes guide p.
pincer grip
pineal
    p. body
    p. cells
    p. cell tumor
    p. cyst
    p. gland
    p. habenula
    p. meningioma
    p. recess
    p. tumor
pinealectomy
pinealoblastoma
pinealocyte
pinealocytoma
pinealoma
    ectopic p.
    extrapineal p.
pinealopathy
pineoblastoma
pineocytoma
ping-pong
    p.-p. appearance
    p.-p. fracture
    p.-p. gaze
piniform
pinion headholder
pinus
piperacillin

piriform
    p. area
    p. cortex
piriformis syndrome
pistol grip
pistol-grip instrument
piston
    MTS electrohydraulic p.
pit
    central p.
    primitive p.
pith
Pitres'
    P. area
    P. sign
Pitressin
    P. Tannate in Oil
pitressin
    p. tanate
Pittsburgh Gamma Knife group
pituicytoma
pituitary
    p. abscess
    p. adamantinoma
    p. adenoma
    p. apoplexy
    p. basophilia
    p. basophilism
    p. cachexia
    p. dwarfism
    p. dysfunction
    p. gland
    p. stalk
    p. stalk section
pixel
PKU
    phenylketonuria
placement
    bone graft p.
    clip p.

    Kirschner wire p., K-wire
     placement
    K-wire p.
    plate p.
    posterolateral bone graft p.
    rod p.
    sacral screw p.
    variable screw p. (VSP)
placode
    neural p.
placoid pigment epitheliopathy
plagiocephaly
plain
    p. forceps
    p. radiography
    p. tomography
plana
    pars p.
plane
    coronal p.
    sagittal p.
planning
    image integrated surgery
     treatment p.
    preoperative p.
planotopokinesia
plant
    feverfew p.
plantalgia
plantar
    p. muscle reflex
    p. nerve
    p. reflex
plaque
    fibrous p.
    Hollenhorst p.
    neuritic p.
    senile p.
plasma
    p. factor
    p. thromboplastin

NOTES

plasmacytoma
plasmapheresis
Plasmatein
plasmin
plastic
    p. collar
    p. scalp clip
    p. shell
plate
    alar p. of neural tube
    AO dynamic compression p.
    AO reconstruction p.
    ASIF broad dynamic
      compression bone p.
    ASIF T p.
    basal p. of neural tube
    bone p.
    broad AO dynamic
      compression p.
    butterfly-shaped monoblock
      vertebral p.
    cartilage p.'s
    cartilaginous p.
    cartilaginous end p.
    Caspar p.
    cervical p.
    commissural p.
    contoured anterior spinal p.
    cortical p.
    craniocervical p.
    cranioplasty p.
    cribriform p.
    dorsal p. of neural tube
    3-D titanium mini
      bone p.'s
    end p.
    p. fixation
    Hardy-Rand-Rittler p.
    Harm's posterior cervical p.
    Ishihara p.
    medullary p.
    metal p.
    Mini Orbita p.
    Morscher p.
    narrow AO dynamic
      compression p.
    neural p.
    p. placement
    prochordal p.
    quadrigeminal p.
    roof p.
    round hole p.
    Roy-Camille p.

    sole p.
    spinous process p.
    stainless steel p.
    Steffee p.
    symmetrical sacral p.
    symmetrical thoracic
      vertebral p.
    T-p.
    terminal p.
    thoracolumbosacral p.
    titanium p.
    TSRH p.
    ventral p. of neural tube
    vertebral p.
    Vitallium p.
    wing p.
platelet activating factor
platelet-derived growth factor
platelet-fibrin embolus
plate-screw
    p.-s. fixation
    p.-s. osteosynthesis
plate-spacer washer
platform
    positioning p.
plating
    anterior p.
    anterior spinal p.
    Caspar p.
    pedicle screw p.
    posterior p.
    posterior spinal p.
    Steffee p.
Platinol
platinum
    p. coil
    p. microcoil
platinum-Dacron microcoil
platybasia
platysma
    p. muscle
pledget
    cottonoid p.
    latex covered p.
pleocytosis
plethysmograph
plethysmography
pleura
pleurothotonos, pleurothotonus
plexectomy
plexiform
    p. layer
    p. layer of cerebral cortex

p. layers of retina
p. neurofibroma
p. neuroma
plexiglas phantom
plexitis
plexus, pl. **plexus, plexuses**
anterior p.
Auerbach's p.
p. autonomici
brachial p.
cavernous p.
celiac p.
p. celiacus
choroid p.
p. of choroid artery
p. choroideus
p. choroideus ventriculi lateralis
p. choroideus ventriculi quarti
p. choroideus ventriculi tertii
choroid p. of fourth ventricle
choroid p. of lateral ventricle
choroid p. of third ventricle
epidural venous p.
Exner's p.
lumbosacral p.
meningeal p.
p. meningeus
myenteric p.
p. myentericus
nerve p.
p. nervorum spinalium
p. nervosus
paravertebral venous p.
pelvic p.
posterior p.
sagittal p.
p. of spinal nerves

p. submucosus
sympathetic plexuses
tentorial p.
p. uterovaginalis
plica, gen. and pl. **plicae**
p. choroidea
plicata
pars p.
PLIF
posterior lumbar interbody fusion
plug
methylmethacrylate cranioplastic p.
plugging
Obex p.
PML
progressive multifocal leukoencephalopathy
PNET
primitive neuroectodermal tumor
pneumatic chair lift
extracranial p.
intracranial p.
pneumatorrhachis
pneumatosis
epidural p.
pneumobulbar
pneumocele
extracranial p.
intracranial p.
pneumocephalus
epidural p.
tension p.
pneumocranium
pneumoencephalogram
pneumoencephalography
pneumogastric nerve
pneumoniae
Streptococcus p.

NOTES

pneumo-orbitography
pneumoplethysmography
    ocular p.
pneumorrhachis
pneumotaxic
    p. center of Lumsden
    p. localization
pneumotonometry
pneumoventricle
podismus
podospasm, podospasmus
poikilothermia
point
    anchoring p.
    apophysary p., apophysial p.
    entry p.
    Erb's p.
    Keen's p.
    Kocher's p.
    motor p.
    painful p.
    pedicle entrance p.
    powered automatic stopping
      drill p.
    pressure p.
    sacral brim target p.
    self-stopping drill p.
    sylvian p.
    tender p.'s
    trigger p.
    Trousseau's p.
    Valleix's p.'s
Poiseuille equation
Poiseuille's law
poisoning
    carbon monoxide p.
poker
    p. back
    p. spine
polar
    p. artery
    p. coordinate system
polarity
pole
    frontal p.
    occipital p.
    temporal p.
poli (pl. of polus)
polio
    French p.
polioclastic

poliodystrophia
    p. cerebri progressiva
    infantilis
poliodystrophy
    progressive cerebral p.
polioencephalitis
    p. infectiva
    inferior p.
    superior p.
    superior hemorrhagic p.
polioencephalomeningomyelitis
polioencephalomyelitis
polioencephalopathy
poliomyelencephalitis
poliomyelitis
    acute anterior p.
    acute bulbar p.
    chronic anterior p.
    p. treatment
poliomyeloencephalitis
poliomyelopathy
pollodic
polus, pl. poli
    p. frontalis cerebri
    p. occipitalis cerebri
    p. temporalis cerebri
polyanhydride biodegradable
  polymer wafer
polyanhydroglucuronic acid
polyarteritis nodosa (PAN)
polychondritis
    relapsing p.
Polycillin-N
polycinematosomnography
polyclonia
polyclot
    p. patty
polycythemia
polyene thread
polyester
polyesthesia
polyethylene
    p. sleeve
polyganglionic
polygyria
polyleptic
polymer
    cellulose acetate p.
polymethylmethacrylate
polymicrogyria
polymorphism
    restriction fragment
    length p. (RFLP)

polymorphous layer
polymyalgia
        p. arteritica
        p. rheumatica
polymyoclonus
polymyositis
polymyxin
polyneural
polyneuralgia
polyneuritic psychosis
polyneuritis
        acute idiopathic p.
        chronic familial p.
        erythredema p.
        infectious p.
polyneuronitis
polyneuropathy
        buckthorn p.
        nutritional p.
        uremic p.
polyopia
polyplegia
polyradiculitis
polyradiculomyopathy
polyradiculoneuropathy
polyradiculopathy
polyserositis
polysomnogram
polysomnography
polysynaptic
polytetrafluoroethylene
        expanded p. (e-PTFE)
polytomography
polyvinyl
        p. alcohol (PVA)
        p. alcohol foam
        p. alcohol particle
Pompili
pond fracture
pons, pl. pontes

        p. cerebelli
        p. varolii
pontile, pontine
        p. apoplexy
pontis
        brachium p.
Pontocaine
pontocerebellar recess
pontomedullary
        p. groove
        p. separation
Pool-Schlesinger sign
Pool's phenomenon
popliteal artery
Poppen
porencephalia
porencephalic
porencephalitis
porencephalous
porencephaly
porosis, pl. poroses
        cerebral p.
porphyria
        acute intermittent p.,
          acute p.
        hepatic p.
        intermittent acute p. (IAP)
port
        lumbar p.
        p. wine nevus
porta, pl. portae
portal-systemic encephalopathy
porte manteau procedure
Portnoy DPV device
Portuguese-Azorean disease
porus acusticus
position
        p. agnosia
        angular p.
        knee-chest p.
        park bench p.

NOTES

position *(continued)*
    prone p.
    reverse Trendelenburg p.
    p. sense
    sitting p.
    translational p.
    Trendelenburg p.
    tuck p.
positional vertigo
positioning
    patient p.
    p. platform
    proper neck p.
positive
    p. end-expiratory pressure (PEEP)
    p. feedback
positively bathmotropic
positron
    p. emission tomography (PET)
    p. emission tomography with [^{18}F]-labeled fluorodeoxyglucose (PET-FDG)
post
    iliac p.
    Isola spinal implant system iliac p.
    Luque-Galveston p.
postadrenalectomy syndrome
postapoplectic
postbasic stare
postcentral
    p. area
    p. fissure
    p. gyrus
    p. sulcus
postconcussion
    p. neurosis
    p. syndrome
postconcussional syndrome
postdiphtheritic paralysis
postdormital
postdormitum
postencephalitic
postepileptic
posterior
    p. approach
    p. arthrodesis
    p. atlantoaxial arthrodesis
    p. bone graft
    p. callosal vein

p. canal line
p. central convolution
p. central gyrus
p. cerebellar artery
p. cerebral artery (PCA)
p. cerebral commissure
p. cervical fixation
p. cervical spinal instrumentation
p. cervical spine surgery
p. choroidal artery
p. column cordotomy
p. column osteosynthesis
p. column of spinal cord
p. communicating artery
p. construct
p. decompression
p. distraction instrumentation
p. fixation system biomechanics
p. fossa
p. fossa syndrome
p. funiculus
p. hook-rod spinal instrumentation
p. horn
p. hypothalamic nucleus
p. inferior cerebellar artery (PICA)
p. inferior cerebellar artery syndrome
p. inferior communicating artery (PICA)
p. instrumentation
p. intermediate groove
p. interosseous nerve
p. interspinous wiring
p. joint syndrome
p. limb of internal capsule
p. lobe of hypophysis
p. longitudinal bundle
p. longitudinal ligament
p. lower cervical spine stabilization
p. lower cervical spine surgery
p. lumbar interbody fusion (PLIF)
p. lumbar interbody fusion surgery
p. lumbar spine and sacrum surgery

p. lunate lobule
p. medial nucleus of thalamus
p. median fissure of the medulla oblongata
p. median fissure of spinal cord
p. median sulcus of medulla oblongata
p. median sulcus of spinal cord
p. medullary velum
p. notch of cerebellum
p. occipitocervical approach
p. parolfactory sulcus
p. perforated substance
p. periventricular nucleus
p. pillar of fornix
p. pituitary fossa
p. pituitary gland ectopia
p. plating
p. plexus
p. primary ramus
p. pyramid of the medulla
p. rachischisis
p. rhizotomy
p. rod system
p. root
p. sclerosis
p. segmental fixation
p. spinal artery
p. spinal fusion
p. spinal plating
p. spinal sclerosis
p. spinocerebellar tract
p. stabilization
p. surgical exposure of sacrum and coccyx
p. tibial nerve
p. upper cervical spine surgery

p. vein of septum pellucidum
posterior-interbody lumbar spinal fusion
posterior-lateral lumbar spinal fusion
posterolateral
p. approach
p. bone graft
p. bone grafting
p. bone graft placement
p. costotransversectomy incision
p. costotransversectomy technique
p. fissure
p. fusion
p. groove
p. lumbosacral fusion
p. sulcus
posteroparietal
posterotemporal
p. artery occlusion
posteroventral pallidotomy
postganglionic
p. motor neuron
posthemiplegic
p. athetosis
p. chorea
postherpetic neuralgia
posthippocampal fissure
postictal
p. paresis
posticus
p. palsy
p. paralysis
postlaminectomy
p. kyphosis
p. syndrome
p. two-level spondylolisthesis
postlingual fissure

NOTES

postlunate fissure
postmeningitic hydrocephalus
postneuritic
postoperative
    p. anemia
    p. bracing
    p. care
    p. casting
    p. corticosteroids
    p. extubation
    p. immobilization
    p. infection
    p. lumbosacral orthosis
    p. paraplegia
    p. regimen
    p. tetany
postparalytic
postpartum pituitary necrosis
  syndrome
postpyramidal fissure
postradiation fibrosis
postrhinal fissure
postrolandic
posts
    Caspar retraction p.
postsynaptic
    p. membrane
posttetanic potentiation
posttraumatic
    p. chronic cord syndrome
    p. delirium
    p. dementia
    p. epilepsy
    p. hydrocephalus
    p. intradiploic
      pseudomeningocele
    p. kyphosis
    p. leptomeningeal cyst
    p. neck syndrome
    p. neuralgia
    p. neurosis
    p. osteoporosis
    p. psychosis
    p. spinal deformity
    p. syndrome
postural
    p. instability
    p. myoneuralgia
    p. reflex
    p. syncope
    p. tremor
    p. vertigo
posture sense

posturing
    decerebrate p.
postvaccinal encephalitis
potato tumor of neck
potential
    action p.
    auditory compound
      actional p.
    auditory evoked p.
    brain p.
    brainstem auditory
      evoked p. (BAEP)
    cochlear microphonic p.
    demarcation p.
    dermatosensory evoked p.
    direct auditory compound
      actional p.
    evoked p.
    extreme somatosensory
      evoked p. (ESEP)
    fasciculation p.
    fibrillation p.
    giant motor unit action p.
    injury p.
    membrane p.
    motor evoked p. (MEP)
    nascent motor unit p.
    peroneal somatosensory
      evoked p.
    phase reversal p.
    pudendal somatosensory
      evoked p.
    somatosensory evoked p.
      (SEP, SSEP)
    spinal sensory evoked p.
    visual evoked p.
potentiation
    posttetanic p.
Pott's
    P. abscess
    P. disease
    P. paralysis
    P. paraplegia
    P. puffy tumor
pouch
    Blake's p.
    pharyngeal p.
    Rathke's p.
Pourfour du Petit's syndrome
povidone-iodine
    aqueous p.-i.
Powassan encephalitis

powder
    antibiotic p.
power
    p. amplifier
    p. drill
    processing p.
    resolving p.
    p. router
powered
    p. automatic skull
      perforator
    p. automatic stopping drill
      point
pragmatagnosia
pragmatamnesia
praxis
praziquantel
preataxic
precaution
    radiation p.
precentral
    p. area
    p. cerebellar vein
    p. gyrus
    p. sulcus
precession
    fast imaging with steady p.
    (FISP)
    Larmor p.
precessional frequency
precision
    coil p.
precommissural
    p. bundle
    p. septal area
    p. septum
precontoured unit rod
preconvulsive
precuneal
precuneate
precuneus

prednisolone
prednisone
predormital
predormitum
predorsal bundle
prefixed chiasm
prefrontal
    p. area
    p. cortex
    p. leukotomy
    p. lobotomy
preganglionic
    p. motor neuron
prehemiplegic
preictal
premature closure
premedication
premotor
    p. area
    p. cortex
    p. syndrome
prenodular fissure
preoccipital notch
preoperative
    p. angiography
    p. evaluation
    p. planning
    p. preparation
    p. tomography
preoptic
    p. area
    p. region
preparalytic
preparation
    facet joint p.
    intermediate-acting
      insulin p.
    long-acting insulin p.
    preoperative p.
    rod contour p.

NOTES

preparation *(continued)*
    short-acting insulin p.
    wire contour p.
prepiriform gyrus
prepyramidal tract
pre-Rolandic artery occlusion
prerubral
    p. field
    p. nucleus
presacral
    p. neurectomy
    p. sympathectomy
presaturation pulse
presenile dementia
presentation
    clinical p.
preservation
    carotid p.
    lordosis p.
    lumbar lordosis p.
    p. technique
presigmoid-transtransversarium
  intradural approach
pressor
    p. fibers
    p. nerve
pressoreceptor
    p. nerve
    p. reflex
    p. system
pressure
    p. anesthesia
    central venous p.
    cerebral perfusion p. (CPP)
    cerebrospinal p.
    closure p.
    continuous positive
     airway p.
    p. gauge
    intracranial p. (ICP)
    intraocular p.
    p. necrosis
    p. palsy
    p. paralysis
    partial p.
    p. point
    positive end-expiratory p.
     (PEEP)
    pulmonary capillary
     wedge p.
    p. sense
    tentorial p.
pressure-volume index

prestriate area
presynaptic
    p. membrane
pretectal
    p. area
    p. region
    p. syndrome
pretectum
prevention
    infection p.
    rod rotation p.
prevertebral ganglia
PRF
    percutaneous radiofrequency
    rhizolysis
primary
    p. amebic
     meningoencephalitis
    p. brain vesicle
    p. clip
    p. end-to-end anastomosis
    p. fissure of the cerebellum
    p. generalized epilepsy
    p. hydrocephalus
    p. neurasthenia
    p. neuronal degeneration
    p. progressive cerebellar
     degeneration
    p. senile dementia
    p. sensation
    p. shock
    p. tumor
    p. visual area
    p. visual cortex
    p. vitreous
primativa
    meninx p.
primidone
primitive
    p. knot
    p. lamina terminalis
    P. neuroectodermal tumor (PNET)
    p. node
    p. otic artery
    p. pit
    p. streak
    p. trigeminal artery
    p. trigeminal artery variant
principle
    image formation p.
    Pauli exclusion p.
Prinzmetal's angina
prion

proaccelerin
Pro-Banthine
probe
    Doppler p.
    electromagnetic flow p.
    extended sector
      ultrasonic p.
    fluoroptic thermometry p.
    "gearshift" p.
    intraoperative ultrasonic p.
    monitoring p.
    pedicle p.
    pedicle sounding p.
    right-angled blunt p.
    Spinestat p.
    ultrasonic p.
probenecid
procarbazine
    p. hydrochloride
procedure
    ablative p.
    anterior stabilization p.
    carotid ablative p.
    cervical spine
      stabilization p.
    Cloward p.
    debulking p.
    Dewar posterior cervical
      fixation p.
    DREZ p.
    Gill p.
    installation p.
    Jaeger-Hamby p.
    Jannetta microvascular
      decompression p.
    lower cervical spine p.
    micro-operative p.
    microsurgical p.
    porte manteau p.
    retrogasserian p.

    Smith-Robinson p.
    two-stage p.
    upper cervical spine p.
process
    absent spinous p.
    anterior clinoid p.
    apical p.
    axonal p.
    clinoid p.
    deficient spinous p.
    Deiters' p.
    dendritic p.
    intact spinous p.
    Lenhossék's p.'s
    mastoid p.
    odontoid p.
    spinous p.
processing
    p. power
    signal p.
processor
    array p.
prochlorperazine maleate
prochordal plate
proctalgia
    p. fugax
proctoparalysis
proctoplegia
proctospasm
procursive
    p. chorea
    p. epilepsy
procyclidine
prodynorphin
proencephalon
proenkephalin
professional
    p. neurosis
    p. spasm

NOTES

profile
    demyelinative spinal
      fluid p.
    velocity p.
progestin
prognosis
program
    standard bone algorithm p.
programmable pulse generator
progressive
    p. bulbar palsy
    p. bulbar paralysis
    p. cerebellar tremor
    p. cerebral poliodystrophy
    p. lingual hemiatrophy
    p. multifocal
      leukoencephalopathy (PML)
    p. muscular atrophy
    p. muscular dystrophy
    p. spinal amyotrophy
    p. spinal muscular atrophy
    p. subcortical
      encephalopathy
    p. supranuclear palsy
    p. torsion spasm
projection
    anteroposterior p.
    axial p.
    Caldwell p.
    p. fibers
    lateral p.
    sagittal p.
    p. system
prolactin
prolactinoma
prolactin-producing adenoma
Prolene suture
proliferation
    cell p.
    smooth muscle p.
Prolixin
Proloid
prolongation
    pulse repetition time p.
promethazine hydrochloride
prominence
    pedicle screw hardware p.
pronator
    p. reflex
    p. teres syndrome
prone position
propantheline
proparacaine hydrochloride

propentofylline
proper
    p. fasciculi
    p. neck positioning
prophylactic treatment
prophylaxis
    anticonvulsant p.
Propionibacterium acnes
Proplast
proplexus
proposagnosia
propoxyphene
    p. hydrochloride
    p. napsylate and
      acetaminophen
propranolol
    p. hydrochloride
proprioception deficit
proprioceptive
    p. reflexes
    p. sensibility
proprioceptor
propriospinal
proptosis
propulsion
prosencephalon
prosopagnosia
prosopalgia
prosopalgic
prosopodiplegia
prosoponeuralgia
prosopoplegia
prosopoplegic
prosopospasm
prostacyclin
prostaglandin
Prostaphlin
prosthesis
    acrylic p.
prosthetic heart valve
Prostigmin test
prostration
Protamine
    P. Zinc and Iletin I
    P. Zinc Insulin
protection
    airway p.
    cerebral p.
protective
    p. glasses
    p. laryngeal reflex
protein
    p. C deficiency

cerebrospinal fluid p.
C-reactive p.
glial fibrillary acidic p.
myelin basic p.
p. S deficiency
proteinuria
prothrombin
p. time (PT)
protirelin
protocol
fractionation p.
proton
p. density
p. density weighting
p. imaging
p. magnetic resonance
spectroscopy
p. nuclear magnetic
resonance spectroscopy
p. relaxation time
p. spectrum
proton-electron dipole-dipole
interaction
protoneuron
proton-weighted image
protopathic
p. sensibility
protoplasmic
p. astrocyte
p. astrocytoma
protoporphyrin IX
protospasm
protruded disk
protrusion
medullary p.
protuberans
dermatofibrosarcoma p.
Proventil
provocative testing
proximal
p. clipping

p. myopathy
p. occlusion
proximoataxia
Prozac
pruning
neuronal p.
psalterial
psalterium, pl. **psalteria**
psammocarcinoma
psammoma
p. bodies
Virchow's p.
psammomatoid ossifying fibroma
psammomatous
p. meningioma
psammous
P segment
pselaphesis, pselaphesia
pseudagraphia
pseudaphia
pseudarthrosis
documented p.
failed back syndrome with
documented p.
p. rate
p. repair
pseudesthesia
pseudoabducens
p. nerve paresis
p. palsy
pseudoagrammatism
pseudoagraphia
pseudoaneurysm
pseudoapoplexy
pseudoapraxia
pseudoarthritis
pseudoataxia
pseudobulbar
p. palsy
p. paralysis
pseudocele

NOTES

pseudocephalocele
pseudochorea
pseudochromesthesia
pseudoclonus
pseudocoma
pseudoesthesia
pseudoganglion
pseudogeusesthesia
pseudogeusia
pseudo-Graefe sign
pseudohydrocephaly
pseudohypertrophic
    p. muscular atrophy
    p. muscular dystrophy
    p. muscular paralysis
pseudomalignancy
pseudomedial longitudinal fasciculus
  lesion
pseudomembranous colitis
pseudomeningitis
pseudomeningocele
    posttraumatic intradiploic p.
    traumatic p.
Pseudomonas aeruginosa
pseudomuscular hypertrophy
pseudoneoplasm
pseudoneuroma
pseudoparalysis
    arthritic general p.
    congenital atonic p.
pseudoparaplegia
    Basedow's p.
pseudoparesis
pseudophotesthesia
pseudoplegia
pseudoptosis
pseudorosette
pseudosclerosis
    Westphal's p., Westphal-
      Strümpell p.
pseudosplenium
pseudotabes
    pupillotonic p.
pseudotumor
    p. cerebri
    idiopathic orbital p.
    orbital p.
pseudounipolar
    p. cell
    p. neuron
pseudoventricle
pseudoxanthoma elasticum

psoas
    p. abscess
    p. muscle
psoriasis
    p. spondylitica
psoriatic arthritis
psychalgia
psychanopsia
psychataxia
psychedelic
psychiatric
    p. disorder
    p. disturbance
psychic
    p. seizure
    p. tic
psychochrome
psychochromesthesia
psychogalvanic
    p. reaction
    p. reflex
    p. response (PGR)
    p. skin reaction
    p. skin reflex
    p. skin response
psychogenic
    p. pain
    p. torticollis
psychogeusic
psychometrics
psychomotor
    p. epilepsy
    p. retardation
    p. seizure
psychophysiologic
    p. disorder
    p. manifestation
psychosensory aphasia
psychosis, pl. psychoses
    amnestic p.
    arteriosclerotic p.
    bromide p.
    dysmnesic p.
    Korsakoff's p.
    polyneuritic p.
    posttraumatic p.
    senile p.
    traumatic p.
psychosocial function
psychosomatic disorder
psychosurgery
psychotherapy
psychotic manifestation

psychroalgia
psychroesthesia
psychrophobia
psyllium
PT
    prothrombin time
PTA
    pure tone average
pterion
pterional
    p. approach
    p. craniotomy
pterygopalatine ganglion
ptosis, pl. ptoses
    cerebral p.
    p. sympathetica
PTS-Ultrason
pudendal
    p. nerve
    p. SEP
    p. somatosensory evoked
     potential
Pudenz
    P. valve
    P. ventricular catheter
puerperal
    p. convulsions
    p. eclampsia
PUKA
    Cloward's PUKA
pullout
    screw p.
    p. strength
pulmonary
    p. arteriovenous shunt
    p. capillary wedge pressure
    p. embolism
    p. shunt
pulmonocoronary reflex
pulp
    vertebral p.

pulposus
    herniated nucleus p.
    nucleus p.
pulsatility
    Gosling p.
    p. index (PI)
pulsating neurasthenia
pulsation
    carotid p.
pulse
    p. flip angle
    p. generator
    ocular p.
    p. oximeter
    p. oximetry
    presaturation p.
    radiofrequency p.
    p. repetition time
    p. repetition time
     prolongation
    p. sequence
    p. timing diagram
    p. wave Doppler
pulsed
    p. Doppler
    p. Doppler imaging
    p. fluorography
pulseless disease
pulvinar
pump
    Cordis Secor implantable p.
    drug infusion p.
    implanted infusion p.
    infusion p.
    Medtronic SynchroMed
     implantable p.
    Shiley-Infusaid p.
    SynchroMed model 8611H
     prototype implantable p.
    volumetric infusion p.

NOTES

punch
> bone p.
> Ferris Smith-Kerrison p.
> Hardy sella p.
> Kerrison p.
> Kerrison bone p.
> p. rongeur

punchdrunk
> p. syndrome

puncta (*pl. of* punctum)

punctata
> rhizomelic
>   chondrodysplasia p.

punctate white matter hyperintensity

punctum, gen. **puncti**, pl. **puncta**
> p. dolorosum
> p. luteum
> p. vasculosum

puncture
> Bernard's p.
> brain p.
> cisternal p.
> diabetic p.
> lumbar p.
> Quincke's p.
> spinal p.
> stereotactic p.
> sternal p.
> ventricular p.

Puno-Winter-Byrd (PWB)
> P.-W.-B. system

pupil
> Adie's p.
> Argyll Robertson p.
> fixed p.
> Holmes-Adie p.
> Hutchinson's p.
> paradoxical p.
> rigid p.
> Robertson p.
> tonic p.

pupillary
> p. abnormality
> p. light reflex
> p. reflex

pupillary-skin reflex
pupillomotor
pupilloplegia
pupillotonic pseudotabes
purchase
> bony p.

pure
> p. absence
> p. aphasias
> p. motor hemiplegia
> p. sensory stroke
> p. tone audiogram
> p. tone average (PTA)
> p. tone discrimination

Purkinje's
> P. cells
> P. corpuscles
> P. layer

Purmann's method
purpura
> Henoch-Schönlein p.
> thrombotic
>   thrombocytopenic p.

pursuit
> p. defect
> p. eye movement
> p. movements
> saccadic p.

purulent encephalitis
putamen
Putnam-Dana syndrome
putty
> Bishop's p.

PVA
> polyvinyl alcohol

PV foam
PvO2
> cerebral venous gas tension of
>   oxygen

PWB
> Puno-Winter-Byrd

pyelography
pyencephalus
pyknoepilepsy, pyknolepsy
pyla
pylar
pyocephalus
> circumscribed p.
> external p.
> internal p.

pyogenes
> *Streptococcus p.*

pyogenic
> p. discitis
> p. osteomyelitis
> p. pachymeningitis

pyramid
> anterior p.
> cerebellar p.

Malacarne's p.
p. of medulla oblongata
olfactory p.
posterior p. of the medulla
p. sign
syndrome of the p.
pyramidal
    p. cell layer
    p. cells
    p. decussation
    p. fibers
    p. radiation
    p. sign

p. tract
p. tractotomy
pyramidotomy
    medullary p.
    spinal p.
pyramis, pl. **pyramides**
    p. medullae oblongatae
    p. vermis
Pyribenzamine
pyriform
pyrimethamine
pyruvate

NOTES

Q

quader
quadrangular lobule
quadrantanopia
quadrate
    q. lobe
    q. lobule
quadriceps reflex
quadrigeminal
    q. arachnoid cyst
    q. bodies
    q. cistern
    q. plate
quadrigeminum
quadriparesis
quadripedal extensor reflex
quadriplegia
quadriplegic
quality
    image q.
quantitative
    q. imaging

    q. spectral
      phonoangiography
quantum
    q. mechanics
    q. number
Queckenstedt-Stookey test
Queckenstedt test
quench
    magnet q.
quick
Quincke's
    Q. disease
    Q. edema
    Q. puncture
quinidine
quinolone
quinuclidinyl benzilate
quotient
    cognitive laterality q. (CLQ)

R

rabies
raccoon eyes
rachial
rachicentesis
rachidial
rachidian
rachigraph
rachilysis
rachiocentesis
rachiochysis
rachiometer
rachiopathy
rachioplegia
rachioscoliosis
rachiotome
rachiotomy
rachischisis
    r. partialis
    posterior r., r. posterior
    r. totalis
rachitome
rachitomy
radial
    r. artery
    r. nerve
    r. phenomenon
    r. reflex
radiate
    r. crown
radiatio, pl. radiationes
    r. acustica
    r. corporis callosi
    r. optica
    r. pyramidalis
radiation
    acoustic r.
    r. angiopathy
    r. of corpus callosum
    r. effects
    geniculocalcarine r.
    Gratiolet's r.
    r. injury
    r. myelopathy
    r. necrosis
    occipitothalamic r.
    optic r.
    r. precaution
    pyramidal r.
    r. retinopathy
    single-fraction r.

    temporal lobe r.
    r. therapy
    r. vasculitis
    Wernicke's r.
radical
    free r.
    r. prefrontal lobotomy
radices (*pl. of* radix)
radicis (*gen. of* radix)
radicotomy
radiculalgia
radicular syndrome
radiculectomy
radiculitis
    acute brachial r.
radiculoganglionitis
radiculomedullary
    r. fistula
    r. syndrome
radiculomeningeal spinal vascular
    malformation
radiculomeningomyelitis
radiculomyelopathy
radiculoneuropathy
radiculopathy
    cervical r.
    lumbosacral r.
radiculospinal artery
radii of angulation
radiobicipital reflex
radiofluoroscopy
    televised r.
Radiofocus introducer B kit
radiofrequency (RF)
    r. coil
    r. eddy current
    r. electromagnetic field
    r. field
    r. generator
    r. heating
    r. homogeneity pattern
    r. lesion
    r. lesioning
    r. magnetic field
    r. pulse
    r. rhizotomy
    r. spoiling
    r. thermocoagulation
    r. transmitter
radiofrequency-induced echo

radiograph
radiography
    plain r.
radioimmunoassay
radioimmunotherapy
radiology
    interventional r.
radiolucent operating room table
  extension
radioneuritis
Radionics
    R. bipolar coagulation unit
    R. bipolar instrument
    R. RF lesion generator
radionucleotide scanning (RN
  scanning)
radionuclide
    r. cisternography
    r. imaging
    r. study
radiopaque fiducial
radioperiosteal reflex
radioreceptor
radiosensitizer
radio signal line
radiosurgery
    gamma r.
    gamma knife r.
    LINAC r.
    multiarc LINAC r.
    photon beam r.
    repeat r.
    stereotactic r.
    stereotaxic r.
radiotherapy (RT)
    heavy particle r.
    hyperfractionated r.
    interstitial r.
    stereotactic linear
    accelerator r.
radius of angulation
radix, gen. radicis, pl. radices
    r. anterior
    r. brevis ganglii ciliaris
    r. cochlearis
    radices craniales
    r. dorsalis
    r. facialis
    r. inferior
    r. inferior ansae cervicalis
    r. inferior nervi
    vestibulocochlearis
    r. lateralis nervi mediani

    r. lateralis tractus optici
    r. longa ganglii ciliaris
    r. medialis nervi mediani
    r. medialis tractus optici
    r. motoria
    r. nasociliaris
    r. nervi facialis
    radices nervi trigemini
    r. oculomotoria ganglii
    ciliaris
    r. parasympathica ganglii
    ciliaris
    r. posterior
    r. sensoria
    r. sensoria nervi trigemini
    radices spinales
    r. superior
    r. superior ansae cervicalis
    r. superior nervi
    vestibulocochlearis
    r. sympathica ganglii ciliaris
    r. ventralis
    r. vestibularis
Raeder's
    R. paratrigeminal neuralgia
    R. paratrigeminal syndrome
rage
    sham r.
Raimondi
    R. low pressure shunt
    R. peritoneal catheter
rami (pl. of ramus)
ramicotomy
ramisection
ramitis
Ramsay Hunt syndrome
ramus, pl. rami
    rami ad pontem
    rami centrales
    anteromediales
    rami choroidei
    r. choroidei posteriores
    laterales
    r. choroidei posteriores
    mediales
    r. choroidei ventriculi
    lateralis
    r. choroidei ventriculi quarti
    r. choroidei ventriculi tertii
    r. communicans, pl. rami
    communicantes
    r. communicans cum nervo
    glossopharyngeo

dorsal rami
posterior primary r.
r. sinus carotici
random waves
Raney
R. clip
R. scalp clip
R. scalp clip applier
range
frequency r.
ranitidine
Ransford loop
Ranvier's
R. crosses
R. disks
R. node
R. segment
raphe
r. corporis callosi
r. nuclei
r. pontis
Stilling's r.
rapid
r. acquisition
radiofrequency-echo steady
state imaging
r. eye movement (REM)
r. eye movement sleep
RAS
reticular activating system
rash
butterfly r.
heliotrope r.
ras **oncogene**
rat
Brattleboro r.
rate
erythrocyte sedimentation r.
fusion nonunion r.
implant survival r.
nonunion r.

pseudarthrosis r.
specific absorption r.
transverse relaxation r.
T2 relaxation r.
vertebral osteosynthesis
fusion r.
Rathke's
R. cleft cyst
R. pouch
R. pouch cyst
R. pouch tumor
ratio
absolute terminal
innervation r.
bicaudate r.
Cho:NAA r.
contrast-to-noise r. (CNR)
functional terminal
innervation r.
gyromagnetic r.
signal-to-noise r.
T:C r.
tumor:cerebellum ratio
^{99m}Tc HMPAO T/C r.
tumor:cerebellum r. (T:C
ratio)
rationale
reduction r.
Raymond-Cestan syndrome
Raymond's syndrome
Raymond type of apoplexy
Raynaud's phenomenon
rayon
RBE
relative biological effectiveness
rCBF
regional cerebral blood flow
R.D.
reaction of degeneration
reaction
allergic r.

NOTES

reaction *(continued)*
    anaphylactoid r.
    arousal r.
    r. of degeneration (DR, R.D.)
    delayed hypersensitivity r.
    drug r.
    dystonic r.
    echo r.
    galvanic skin r.
    gemistocytic r.
    general-adaptation r.
    heel-tap r.
    Jolly's r.
    lengthening r.
    magnet r.
    myasthenic r.
    ocular tilt r.
    pain r.
    psychogalvanic r., psychogalvanic skin r.
    startle r.
    r. time
    Wernicke's r.
Reaction Level Scale (RLS)
reactive
    r. astrocyte
    r. cell
reading disorder
readout
    r. gradient
    r. period
real origin
real-time
    r.-t. color Doppler imaging
    r.-t. monitoring
reanimation
    facial r.
rebleeding
rebound phenomenon
recanalization
    TCD r.
receiver
    r. bandwidth
    r. limitation
    r. overflow
    r. overload
    r. saturation
receptive aphasia
receptoma
receptor
    adrenergic r.
    alpha-adrenergic r.

    epsilon opiate r.
    kappa opiate r.
    mu opiate r.
    opiate r.'s
    sensory r.'s
    stretch r.'s
recess
    cerebellopontine r.
    cochlear r.
    infundibular r.
    lateral r. of fourth ventricle
    optic r.
    pineal r.
    pontocerebellar r.
    Reichert's cochlear r.
    suprapineal r.
    triangular r.
recessus, pl. recessus
    r. anterior
    r. cochlearis
    r. infundibuli
    r. lateralis ventriculi quarti
    r. opticus
    r. pinealis
    r. posterior
    r. suprapinealis
    r. triangularis
recipiomotor
Recklinghausen's disease
recognition time
recombinant
    r. DNA technique
    r. human tumor necrosis factor-α
    r. tissue plasminogen activator
reconstruction
    craniofacial r.
    3-dimensional r. wand
    three-dimensional r.
recording
    continuous on-line r.
    depth r.
    microelectrode r.
    videocassette r.
recovery
    inversion r.
    short time inversion r.
recruiting response
recruitment
rectangle
    Hartshill r.
    Luque r.

rectangular brain spatula
rectocardiac reflex
rectolaryngeal reflex
recurrence
recurrent
    r. artery of Heubner
    r. encephalopathy
    r. enteric cyst
    r. laryngeal nerve
    r. pain
    r. perforating artery
    r. tumor
red
    r. man syndrome
    r. neck syndrome
    r. neuralgia
    r. nucleus
    r. rubber catheter
redness of eye
reduction
    contrast sensitivity r.
    fracture r.
    fracture-dislocation r.
    r. method
    pain threshold r.
    perioperative r.
    r. rationale
    spondylolisthesis r.
    swan neck deformity r.
    r. technique
    T12-L1 fracture-
      dislocation r.
reduction/fixation
    spondylolisthesis r.
reduction-stabilization
re-exploration
referred
    r. pain
    r. sensation
ReFix non-invasive fixation

reflex
    abdominal r.'s
    Achilles r., Achilles
      tendon r.
    acoustic r.
    acousticopalpebral r.
    acquired r.
    acromial r.
    adductor r.
    allied r.'s
    anal r.
    ankle r.
    r. anosmia
    antagonistic r.'s
    aponeurotic r.
    r. arc
    attitudinal r.'s
    auditory r.
    auditory oculogyric r.
    auriculopalpebral r.
    auropalpebral r.
    axon r.
    Babinski r.
    back of foot r., **dorsum of**
      foot r.
    Barkman's r.
    basal joint r.
    Bechterew-Mendel r.
    behavior r.
    Benedek's r.
    Bezold-Jarisch r.
    biceps r.
    biceps femoris r.
    Bing's r.
    bladder r.
    blink r.
    body righting r.'s
    bone r.
    brachioradial r.
    Brain's r.
    bregmocardiac r.

NOTES

reflex *(continued)*
Brissaud's r.
bulbocavernosus r.
bulbomimic r.
carotid sinus r.
cephalic r.'s
cephalopalpebral r.
cervicocollic r.
Chaddock r.
chain r.
chin r.
Chodzko's r.
ciliospinal r.
cochleo-orbicular r.
cochleopalpebral r.
cochleopupillary r.
cochleostapedial r.
conditioned r. (CR)
contralateral r.
r. control
convulsive r.
coordinated r.
corneal r.
costal arch r.
costopectoral r.
cough r.
craniocardiac r.
cremasteric r.
crossed r.
crossed adductor r.
crossed extension r.
crossed knee r.
crossed r. of pelvis
crossed spino-adductor r.
cry r.
cuboidodigital r.
cutaneous r.
cutaneous pupil r.,
  cutaneous-pupillary r.
darwinian r.
deep r.
deep abdominal r.'s
defense r.
deglutition r.
Dejerine's r.
delayed r.
detrusor r.
diffused r.
digital r.
r. disorder
diving r.
dorsal r.

dorsam of foot r. (*var. of*
  back of foot r.)
dorsum pedis r.
elbow r.
enterogastric r.
epigastric r.
r. epilepsy
erector-spinal r.
esophagosalivary r.
external oblique r.
eye-closure r.
facial r.
faucial r.
femoral r.
femoroabdominal r.
finger-thumb r.
flexor r.
forced grasping r.
front-tap r.
gag r.
Galant's r.
galvanic skin r.
gastrocolic r.
gastroileac r.
Geigel's r.
Gifford's r.
gluteal r.
Gordon r.
grasp r.
grasping r.
great-toe r.
Guillain-Barré r.
gustatory-sudorific r.
H r.
r. headache
heart r.
Hering-Breuer r.
Hoffmann's r.
hypochondrial r.
hypogastric r.
r. incontinence
innate r.
interscapular r.
intrinsic r.
inverted r.
inverted radial r.
investigatory r.
ipsilateral r.
r. iridoplegia
Jacobson's r.
jaw r.
jaw-working r.
Joffroy's r.

Kisch's r.
knee r.
knee-jerk r.
labyrinthine r.'s
labyrinthine righting r.'s
lacrimal r.
lacrimo-gustatory r.
laryngospastic r.
latent r.
laughter r.
Liddell-Sherrington r.
lip r.
Lovén r.
lower abdominal
 periosteal r.
magnet r.
mandibular r.
mass r.
masseter r.
Mayer's r.
McCarthy's r.'s
mediopubic r.
Mendel-Bechterew r.
Mendel's instep r.
metacarpohypothenar r.
metacarpothenar r.
metatarsal r.
micturition r.
milk-ejection r.
Mondonesi's r.
Moro r.
r. movement
muscle stretch r.
muscular r.
myotatic r.
nasomental r.
neck r.'s
r. neurogenic bladder
nociceptive r.
nocifensor r.
nose-bridge-lid r.

nose-eye r.
oculocephalic r.
oculocephalogyric r.
oculovestibular r.
olecranon r.
Oppenheim's r.
optical righting r.'s
opticofacial r.
orbicularis oculi r.
orbicularis pupillary r.
orienting r.
oropharyngeal r.
palatal r., palatine r.
palmar r.
palm-chin r.
palmomental r.
parachute r.
paradoxical r.
paradoxical extensor r.
paradoxical flexor r.
paradoxical patellar r.
paradoxical pupillary r.
paradoxical triceps r.
patellar r.
patellar tendon r.
patello-adductor r.
pectoral r.
Perez r.
pericardial r.
periosteal r.
pharyngeal r.
phasic r.
Phillipson's r.
pilomotor r.
plantar r.
plantar muscle r.
postural r.
pressoreceptor r.
pronator r.
proprioceptive r.'s
protective laryngeal r.

NOTES

reflex *(continued)*
psychogalvanic r.,
  psychogalvanic skin r.
pulmonocoronary r.
pupillary r.
pupillary light r.
pupillary-skin r.
quadriceps r.
quadripedal extensor r.
radial r.
radiobicipital r.
radioperiosteal r.
rectocardiac r.
rectolaryngeal r.
Remak's r.
respiratory r.
righting r.'s
Roger's r.
rooting r.
Rossolimo's r.
scapular r.
scapulohumeral r.
scapuloperiosteal r.
Schäffer's r.
semimembranosus r.
semitendinosus r.
r. sensation
sinus r.
skin r.'s
skin-muscle r.'s
skin-pupillary r.
snapping r.
snout r.
sole r.
sole tap r.
spinal r.
spino-adductor r.
Starling's r.
startle r.
static r.
statokinetic r.
statotonic r.'s
sternobrachial r.
stretch r.
Strümpell's r.
styloradial r.
superficial r.
supination r.
supinator r.
supinator longus r.
supraorbital r.
suprapatellar r.
supraumbilical r.

swallowing r.
r. sympathetic dystrophy
synchronous r.
tarsophalangeal r.
tendo Achillis r.
tendon r.
r. therapy
thumb r.
toe r.
tonic r.
trace conditioned r.
trained r.
triceps r.
triceps surae r.
trigeminofacial r.
trochanter r.
Trömner's r.
ulnar r.
unconditioned r.
upper abdominal
  periosteal r.
urinary r.
utricular r.'s
vasopressor r.
venorespiratory r.
vesical r.
vestibulo-ocular r.
vestibulospinal r.
viscerogenic r.
visceromotor r.
viscerosensory r.
visual orbicularis r.
vomiting r.
Weingrow's r.
Westphal's pupillary r.
wink r.
withdrawal r.
wrist clonus r.
reflexogenic
r. zone
reflexogenous
reflexograph
reflexology
reflexometer
reflexophil, reflexophile
reflexotherapy
refractory state
Refsum's
R. disease
R. syndrome
regeneration
aberrant r.

axonal r.
neuronal r.
regimen
postoperative r.
region
craniocervical r.
paramedian r.
preoptic r.
pretectal r.
watershed r.
Wernicke's r.
regional
r. cerebral blood flow (rCBF)
r. enteritis
r. hypothermia
regions of interest (ROI)
Registry
Acoustic Neuroma R.
Brain Tumor R.
regression
spontaneous r.
Regular Iletin I
regulation
volume r.
regulator
suction Regugauge r.
regurgitant lesion
Reichert-Mundinger
R.-M. stereotactic head frame
R.-M. syndrome
Reichert's cochlear recess
Reid's
R. base line
R. baseline
Reil's
R. ansa
R. band
R. ribbon
R. triangle

reinforcement
reinnervation
Reissner's fiber
Reiter's syndrome
relapsing polychondritis
relational threshold
relative biological effectiveness (RBE)
relaxant
muscle r.
relaxation
dipole-dipole r.
intramolecular r.
nuclear r.
paramagnetic r.
r. rate enhancement
spin-lattice r.
spin-spin r.
stress r.
T1 r.
T2 r.
r. theory
r. time
transverse r.
release phenomenon
Relefact-TRH
relief
pain r.
Relton-Hall frame
REM
rapid eye movement
REM sleep
Remak's
R. fibers
R. ganglia
R. reflex
R. sign
reminiscent
r. aura
r. neuralgia
remodeled forehead

NOTES

273

remodeling
    craniofacial r.
    neural foramen r.
remote memory
removal
    implant r.
    metastatic tumor r.
    rib r.
    transsphenoidal r.
renal
    r. failure
    r. ganglia
Rendu-Osler angiomatosis
Rendu-Osler-Weber disease
Renshaw cells
repair
    Gardner meningocele r.
    pseudarthrosis r.
    rod fracture r.
repeat radiosurgery
rephasing
    even-echo r.
replacement
    facet r.
    tile plate facet r.
representation
    Cartesian coordinate r.
    spherical coordinate r.
requirement
    energy r.
research
    construct r.
resection
    caudal lamina r.
    cesarean r.
    condyle r.
    iliac crest r.
    lateral temporal r.
    Peet splanchnic r.
    surgical r.
    transthoracic vertebral
      body r.
    tumor r.
    vertebral r.
resective surgery
reserpine
reservoir
    Ommaya r.
    retromastoid Ommaya r.
    Rickham r.
    side-port flat-bottomed
      Ommaya r.
    r. sign

    suboccipital Ommaya r.
    ventricular Ommaya r.
residual paralysis
resin
    Spurr's epoxy r.
resolution
    spatial r.
resolving power
resonance
    fast-scan magnetic r.
    magnetic r. (MR)
    nuclear magnetic r.
resonant frequency
resonator
    birdcage r.
respiration
    Biot's r.
    Cheyne-Stokes r.
    diffusion r.
    electrophrenic r.
    internal r.
    tissue r.
respirator brain
respiratory
    r. acidosis
    r. alkalosis
    r. anosmia
    r. center
    r. disorder
    r. pause
    r. reflex
response
    auditory brain stem r.
      (ABR)
    axon r.
    brainstem auditory
      evoked r. (BAER)
    Cushing r.
    electromyographic r.
    evoked r.
    galvanic skin r. (GSR)
    hyperadrenergic r.
    oculomotor r.
    orienting r.
    psychogalvanic r.,
      psychogalvanic skin r.
      (PGR)
    recruiting r.
    somatosensory evoked r.
      (SER)
    sonomotor r.
    unconditioned r.
    visual evoked r. (VER)

rest
    r. pain
    3-point head r.
restiform
    r. body
    r. eminence
restless
    r. legs
    r. legs syndrome
restorative neurology
restriction
    r. endonuclease
    r. fragment length
      polymorphism (RFLP)
retardation
    mental r.
    psychomotor r.
rete
    r. mirabile
    r. mirabile caroticum
retention
    brain r.
    fluid r.
reticula (*pl. of* reticulum)
reticular
    r. activating system (RAS)
    r. formation
    r. nuclei of the brainstem
    r. nucleus of thalamus
    r. substance
reticulata
    pars r.
reticulospinal
    r. tract
reticulotomy
reticulum, pl. reticula
    r. cell sarcoma
    Kölliker's r.
retina
    blood and thunder r.

retinaculatome
    Paine r.
retinae
    periphlebitis r.
retinal
    r. cones
    r. cyst
    r. detachment
    r. embolism
    r. pigment epitheliopathy
    r. pigment epithelium
    r. stroke
    r. vasculitis
retinitis
retinoblastoma
retinocerebral angiomatosis
retinocochleocerebral arteriolopathy
retinopathy
    hypotensive r.
    radiation r.
    stasis r.
    venous stasis r.
retracting suture
retraction
    brain r.
    cerebellar r.
    mandibular r.
    r. nystagmus
    oral r.
    sigmoid sinus r.
    soft palate r.
    temporal r.
    temporal lobe r.
retractor
    Beckman r.
    r. blade
    brain r.
    Budde halo ring r.
    Burford r.
    Caspar r.

NOTES

retractor *(continued)*
    Caspar cervical r.
    Cloward blade r.
    Cloward-Hoen r.
    Cottle-Neivert r.
    Crile r.
    Crockard r.
    Cushing r.
    Cushing bivalve r.
    Cushing decompressive r.
    Cushing subtemporal r.
    deep r.'s
    D'Errico r.
    double fishhook r.
    Finochietto r.
    flexible arm r.
    Gelpi r.
    Greenberg r.
    Greenberg and Sugita r.
    Hardy lip r.
    Kobayashi r.
    Meyerding r.
    Murphy rake r.
    nerve root r.
    pillar-and-post
      microsurgical r.
    self-retaining r.
    self-retaining brain r.
    Senn r.
    single hook r.
    Sugita r.
    Taylor r.
    Weitlaner r.
    Yasargil r.
    Yasargil-Leyla brain r.
retrieval
retroauricular edema
retrobulbar
    r. injection
    r. neuritis
    r. orbital metastasis
retrochiasmal lesion
retrocochlear deafness
retrocollic
    r. spasm
retrocollis
retrocursive absence
retroflex fasciculus
retrogasserian
    r. neurectomy
    r. neurotomy
    r. procedure

retrograde
    r. blood flow
    r. chromatolysis
    r. degeneration
    r. memory
retrography
retrogressive differentiation
retrolabyrinthine presigmoid
  approach
retrolental
retrolenticular
    r. limb of internal capsule
retrolisthesis
retromastoid
    r. Ommaya reservoir
    r. suboccipital craniectomy
retro-ocular
retro-orbital pain
retroperitoneal approach
retropharyngeal
    r. abscess
    r. approach
    r. hematoma
    r. space
retropulsed bone excision
retropulsion
retrovirus
retrusion
    midface r.
Rett's syndrome
Retzius'
    R. fibers
    R. foramen
    R. gyrus
revascularization
    brain r.
reverberating circuit
reversal
    phase r.
reverse
    r. ocular bobbing
    r. Trendelenburg position
reversible
    r. C-arm
    r. decortication
    r. ischemic neurological
      deficit (RIND)
    r. ischemic neurologic
      disability (RIND)
    r. shock
Revilliod's sign
rewinder gradient
Rexed lamina

Reye's syndrome
Reynolds number
RF
    radiofrequency
        RF electrocoagulation
RFLP
    restriction fragment length
    polymorphism
rhabdomyoma
rhabdomyosarcoma
rhenium-186
rheoencephalogram
rheoencephalography
rheumatic
    r. chorea
    r. disease
    r. heart disease
    r. tetany
    r. torticollis
rheumatica
    polymyalgia r.
rheumatism
    lumbar r.
rheumatoid
    r. arteritis
    r. arthritis
    r. disease
    r. disorder
    r. factor
    r. spondylitis
rhigosis
rhigotic
rhinal
    r. fissure
    r. sulcus
Rh incompatibility
rhinencephalic
rhinencephalon
rhinitis
    vasomotor r.
    viral r.

rhinoplasty
rhinorrhea
    cerebrospinal fluid r.
rhinoseptal approach
rhinosinusitis
rhizolysis
    percutaneous glycerol r.
    (PGR)
    percutaneous
    radiofrequency r. (PRF)
    percutaneous retrogasserian
    glycerol r.
rhizomelic chondrodysplasia
  punctata
rhizomeningomyelitis
rhizopathy
Rhizopus
    R. infection
rhizotomy
    anterior r.
    bilateral ventral r.
    Dana posterior r.
    dorsal r.
    facet r.
    Frazier-Spiller r.
    glycerol r.
    intracranial r.
    percutaneous
    radiofrequency r.
    posterior r.
    radiofrequency r.
    thermal r.
    trigeminal r.
Rhodesian trypanosomiasis
rhombencephalic
    r. gustatory nucleus
    r. isthmus
rhombencephalitis
rhombencephalon
rhombencephalosynapsis
rhombic

NOTES

rhombocele
rhomboidal sinus
rhomboid fossa
rhombomere
Rhoton
    R. blunt-ring curette
    R. forceps
    R. microdissector
Rhoton-Merz suction tube
rhythm
    alpha r.
    Berger r.
    beta r.
    delta r.
    fast r.
    theta r.
rhythmic chorea
rib
    r. fracture
    r. graft
    r. removal
ribavirin
ribbed hook
ribbon
    r. blade
    Reil's r.
Ribes' ganglion
Richards-Rundle syndrome
Richards tamp
Richmond bolt
ricin
rickets
Rickham reservoir
ridge
    supraorbital r.
Ridley's
    R. circle
    R. sinus
Riechert-Mundinger stereotactic
  frame
rifampin
right
    r. frontotemporal
      craniotomy
    r. temporoparietal
      craniotomy
    r. thoracic curve
    r. thoracic curve scoliosis
    r. thoracic curve with
      hypokyphosis
    r. thoracic curve with
      junctional kyphosis

    r. thoracic left lumbar
      curve pattern
    r. thoracic left lumbar
      scoliosis
    r. thoracic left
      thoracolumbar curve
      pattern
    r. thoracic left
      thoracolumbar scoliosis
    r. thoracic minor curve
      pattern
right-angle
    r.-a. booster clip
    r.-a. drill
right-angled blunt probe
right-footed
right-handed
righting reflexes
right-sided
    r.-s. submandibular
      transverse incision
    r.-s. thoracotomy
right-to-left shunt
rigid
    r. curve
    r. curve scoliosis
    r. internal fixation
    r. pedicle screw
    r. pupil
    r. round back
rigidity
    catatonic r.
    C-D instrumentation r.
    cerebellar r.
    clasp-knife r.
    cogwheel r.
    Cotrel pedicle screw r.
    decerebrate r.
    lead-pipe r.
    muscle r.
    mydriatic r.
    nuchal r.
    spinal fixation r.
Riley-Day syndrome
rim
    supraorbital r.
RIND
    reversible ischemic neurological
      deficit
    reversible ischemic neurologic
      disability
ring
    Brown-Roberts-Wells base r.

Budde halo r.
carotid r.'s
cricoid r.
dural r.
enhancing r.
halo r.
head r.
Kayser-Fleischer r.'s
Luque r.
tentorial r.
ringed formed forceps
Ringer's lactate
ring-wall lesion
Rinne test
Riopan
risk
operative r.
Risser-Cotrel body cast
risus caninus, risus sardonicus
Ritter-Rollet phenomenon
Ritter's
R. law
R. opening tetanus
RLS
Reaction Level Scale
RN scanning
Robaxin
Robertson pupil
rod
aluminum master r.
r. bending
r. cell of retina
compression r.
compressive r.
r. contour preparation
Corti's r.'s
distraction r.
double-L r.
double-L spinal r.
Edwards modular system
universal r.

r. fiber
r. fracture repair
Harrington r.
Isola spinal implant system
eye r.
Jacobs locking hook
spinal r.
Knodt r.
Kostuik r.
r. linkage
Luque r.
r. migration
modified Harrington r.
Moe r.
pediatric Cotrel-Dubousset r.
r. placement
precontoured unit r.
r. rotation prevention
screw alignment r.
spinal r.
unit spinal r.
Wiltse system aluminum
master r.
Wiltse system spinal r.
rod-hook construct
rodonalgia
rod-sleeve
Edwards modular system
spinal r.-s.
roentgenogram
biplane r.
lateral r.
roentgenographic opaque marker
Roger's reflex
Rogozinski spinal rod system
ROI
regions of interest
Rolandic
R. line

NOTES

rolandic
  r. epilepsy
  r. seizure
Rolando's
  R. angle
  R. area
  R. cells
  R. column
  R. gelatinous substance
  R. substance
  R. tubercle
role
  intrinsic transverse
    connector r.
Roller's nucleus
Romano-Ward syndrome
Romberg-Howship symptom
rombergism
Romberg's
  R. disease
  R. sign
  R. symptom
  R. syndrome
  R. trophoneurosis
Romberg test
rongeur
  Adson r.
  Beyer r.
  Beyer laminectomy r.
  bone-biting r.
  Cloward r.
  Cloward-Harper r.
  disk r.
  Ferris Smith-Kerrison r.
  Hoen intervertebral disk r.
  Hoen pituitary r.
  Horsley r.
  Jansen-Middleton r.
  Kerrison r.
  Leksell r.
  Love-Gruenwald cranial r.
  Love-Gruenwald disk r.
  Love-Gruenwald pituitary r.
  Love pituitary r.
  micropituitary r.
  narrow-bite bone r.
  punch r.
  Tiedmann r.
roof
  r. of fourth ventricle
  r. nucleus
  orbital r.
  r. plate

roof-patch graft
roofplate
root
  anterior r.
  cochlear r. of
    vestibulocochlear nerve
  conjoined nerve r.
  cranial r.'s
  dorsal r.
  entering r.'s
  facial r.
  r. of facial nerve
  r. filaments
  inferior r. of cervical loop
  inferior r. of
    vestibulocochlear nerve
  lateral r. of median nerve
  lateral r. of optic tract
  long r. of ciliary ganglion
  medial r. of median nerve
  medial r. of optic tract
  motor r. of ciliary ganglion
  motor r. of trigeminal
    nerve
  nasociliary r.
  nerve r.
  olfactory r.'s
  r.'s of olfactory tract,
    lateral and medial
  posterior r.
  sensory r. of ciliary
    ganglion
  sensory r. of trigeminal
    nerve
  short r. of ciliary ganglion
  spinal r.'s
  spinal nerve r.
  superior r. of cervical loop
  superior r. of
    vestibulocochlear nerve
  symptomatic r.
  transoral r.
  trigeminal r.
  r.'s of trigeminal nerve
  ventral r.
  vestibular r. of
    vestibulocochlear nerve
rooting reflex
rootlets
Rosenbach's law
Rosenthal fiber
Rosenthal's vein
Rose's cephalic tetanus

rosette
Rossolimo's
    R. reflex
    R. sign
rostra (*pl. of* rostrum)
rostrad
rostral
    r. basilar artery syndrome
    r. cingulotomy
    r. interstitial nucleus
    r. lamina
    r. layer
    r. neuropore
    r. transtentorial herniation
rostralis
rostrum, pl. **rostra, rostrums**
    r. corporis callosi
rotary vertigo
rotating mechanism
rotation
    gantry r.
rotational
    r. correction
    r. injury
rotationally
    r. induced shear-strain
      injury
    r. induced shear-strain
      lesion
rotatory
    r. luxation
    r. spasm
    r. tic
Roth-Bernhardt's disease
Roth's disease
Roth spot
rotoscoliosis
rotundum
    foramen r.
Rouget's muscle

round
    r. eminence
    r. hole plate
round-handled forceps
round-tipped periosteal elevator
Roussy-Lévy
    R.-L. disease
    R.-L. syndrome
router
    power r.
Roy-Camille
    R.-C. plate
    R.-C. posterior screw plate
      fixation
    R.-C. posterior screw plate
      fixation biomechanics
    R.-C. technique
RT
    radiotherapy
rubber
    r. sheeting
    silicone r.
rubeosis iridis
rubrobulbar tract
rubroreticular tract
rubrospinal
    r. decussation
    r. tract
rudimentum, pl. **rudimenta**
    r. hippocampi
Ruffini's corpuscles
rule
    inverse square r.
    Jackson's r.
    r. of two
running stitch
rupture
    aneurysmal r.
    intraoperative r.
    longitudinal ligament r.

NOTES

ruptured
r. aneurysm
r. disk
Russell's syndrome
Russian
R. autumn encephalitis
R. spring-summer
encephalitis (Eastern
subtype)

R. spring-summer
encephalitis (Western
subtype)
R. tick-borne encephalitis
Rust's
R. disease
R. phenomenon

sabulous
sac
　　endolymphatic s.
saccade
　　contrapulsion of s.'s
saccadic
　　s. abnormality
　　s. eye movement
　　s. pursuit
　　s. slowing
saccular
　　s. aneurysm
　　s. spot
sacculus, pl. **sacculi**
　　s. communis
sacral
　　s. alar screw
　　s. brim target point
　　s. cyst
　　s. decompression
　　s. fixation
　　s. foraminal approach
　　s. ganglia
　　s. meningocele
　　s. nerve
　　s. nerve root cyst
　　s. pedicle screw
　　s. pedicle screw fixation
　　s. plexus avulsion
　　s. screw
　　s. screw placement
　　s. spine
　　s. spine decompression
　　s. spine fixation
　　s. spine fusion
　　s. spine modular
　　　instrumentation
　　s. spine stabilization
　　s. spine universal
　　　instrumentation
sacrifice
sacrococcygeal
　　s. myxopapillary
　　　ependymoma
　　s. spine
　　s. teratoma
sacroiliac joint
sacroiliitis
sacrolisthesis

sacrum
　　s. fusion screw fixation
saddle
　　s. coil
　　s. nose deformity
Saenger's sign
Saethre-Chotzen syndrome
sagittal
　　s. anatomic alignment
　　s. deformity
　　s. pedicle angle
　　s. pedicle diameter
　　s. plane
　　s. plane instability
　　s. plexus
　　s. projection
　　s. sinus
　　s. slice fracture
　　s. spin-echo image
　　s. T1-weighted SE image
SAH
　　subarachnoid hemorrhage
Saint
　　S. Anthony's dance
　　S. John's dance
　　S. Vitus dance
salaam
　　s. attack
　　s. convulsions
　　s. spasm
salbutamol
salicylate
saline
　　s. injection
　　s. torch
salivary
　　s. gland
　　s. gland dysfunction
Salmonella
saltation
saltatory
　　s. chorea
　　s. spasm
salts
　　Earle's s.
samarium cobalt
Samuels-Weck Hemoclip
sand
　　s. bodies

sand *(continued)*
    brain s.
    s. tumor
Sandhoff's disease
sandwich
    fascia-muscle-fascia s.
Sanfilippo disease
Sansert
saphenous
    s. vein
    s. vein bypass graft
    s. vein graft
    s. vein patch graft
sarcoglia
sarcoidosis
sarcoma
    angiolithic s.
    Ewing's s.
    granulocytic s.
    orbital granulocytic s.
    reticulum cell s.
sarcomatous tumor
sardonic grin
satellite cells
satellitosis
satiety center
saturation
    arterial oxygen s.
    jugular bulb venous
      oxygen s.
    receiver s.
saturnine
    s. encephalopathy
    s. tremor
saver
    intraoperative cell s.
saw
    Gigli s.
    undercutting s.
scala, pl. scalae
    Löwenberg's s.
    s. media
Scale
    Edinburgh 2 Coma S.
     (E2CS)
    EVM grading of Glasgow
     Coma S.
    Glasgow Coma S. (GCS)
    Glasgow Outcome S. (GOS)
    Injury Severity S.
    Karnofsky Performance S.
    Karnofsky Rating S.

Reaction Level S. (RLS)
Wechsler Adult
  Intelligence S.
Wechsler Adult
  Intelligence S., Revised
Wechsler Intelligence S. for
  Children, Revised (WISC-
  R)
Wechsler Memory S.
scale
    Ashworth s.
    coma s.
scalenectomy
scalene muscle
scalenotomy
scalenus
    s. anterior syndrome
    s. anticus
    s. anticus muscle
scalloping
scalp
    s. clip
    s. closure
    s. contusion
    s. EEG monitoring
    s. flap
    s. incision
    s. infection
    s. laceration
    s. tenderness
scan
    bone-window CT s.
    contrast-enhanced CT s.
    CT s.
    instant s.
    MRI s.
    nuclear MR s.
    PET s.
    sequential computed
     tomographic s.
    s. time
    T1-weighted inversion
     recovery s.
scanner
    s. assisted target localization
    General Electric CT 9800 s.
    Siemens Magnetom s.
    SwiftLase s.
    Vista American Health 0.5
     Tesla MRI s.
scanning
    diffusion-weighted s.

duplex s.
s. electron microscopy
  (SEM)
functional activation PET s.
radionucleotide s. (RN
  scanning)
RN s.
    radionucleotide scanning
s. speech
xenon CT s.
scaphocephaly
scaphohydrocephalus,
  scaphohydrocephaly
scapular
    s. nerve
    s. reflex
scapulohumeral
    s. atrophy
    s. reflex
scapuloperiosteal reflex
scar
    hemosiderin s.
Scarpa's
    S. ganglion
    S. method
scattergram
scattering
    Compton s.
Scedosporium apiospermum
scelalgia
scelotyrbe
Sceratti arc
Schacher's ganglion
Schäffer's reflex
Schaltenbrand-Wahren stereotactic
  atlas
Schaumberg's disease
Scheie's disease
schema, pl. schemata
    body s.

Scheuermann's
    S. disease
    S. kyphosis
Schiff-Sherrington phenomenon
Schilder's disease
Schirmer's syndrome
Schirmer test
schistorrhachis
schistosomiasis
schizaxon
schizencephalic microcephaly
schizencephaly
schizogyria
schizotonia
Schlesinger's sign
Schlichter test
Schmidt-Fischer angle
Schmidt-Lanterman
    S.-L. clefts
    S.-L. incisures
Schmidt's
    S. syndrome
    S. vagoaccessory syndrome
Schmorl's
    S. node
    S. nodule
Scholz' disease
Schüller-Christian syndrome
Schüller's phenomenon
Schultze's
    S. cells
    S. sign
Schütz' bundle
Schwabach test
Schwalbe's nucleus
Schwann cells
schwannoma
    acoustic s.
    cerebellopontine angle s.
schwannosis
Schwann's white substance

NOTES

285

Schwartz tractotomy
sciatic
    s. nerve
    s. neuralgia
    s. neuritis
    s. notch syndrome
    s. pain
    s. scoliosis
sciatica
scintiangiography
scintigram
    ^{99m}Tc-HMPAO leukocyte s.
scintigraphy
    leukocyte s.
    ^{99m}Tc-HMPAO leukocyte s.
    ^{201}Tl s.
scintillating scotoma
scintillation camera
scintiphoto
scissor gait
scissoring
scissors
    alligator s.
    alligator MacCarty s.
    Codman s.
    Harrington s.
    Jansen-Middleton s.
    Mayo s.
    Olivecrona dura s.
    Smellie's s.
SCIWORA
    spinal cord injury without
    radiological abnormality
sclerencephaly, sclerencephalia
scleritis
sclerodactyly, sclerodactylia
scleroderma
sclerosing panencephalitis
sclerosis, pl. **scleroses**
    Alzheimer's s.
    amyotrophic lateral s. (ALS)
    Canavan's s.
    cerebral s.
    combined s.
    diffuse cerebral s.
    diffuse infantile familial s.
    discogenic s.
    disseminated s.
    focal s.
    hippocampal s.
    insular s.
    laminar cortical s.
    lateral spinal s.

    lobar s.
    mantle s.
    mesial temporal s.
    multiple s. (MS)
    posterior s.
    posterior spinal s.
    systemic s.
    tuberous s.
    s. of white matter
SCM
    split-cord malformation
scoliosis
    adult s.
    compensatory s.
    congenital s.
    degenerative lumbar s.
    double curve s.
    double major curve s.
    double thoracic curve s.
    fracture with s.
    idiopathic s.
    King type II s.
    King type V s.
    lumbar s.
    neuromuscular s.
    osteopathic s.
    paralytic s.
    right thoracic curve s.
    right thoracic left lumbar s.
    right thoracic left
     thoracolumbar s.
    rigid curve s.
    sciatic s.
    thoracic curve s.
    thoracolumbar s.
    thoracolumbar idiopathic s.
    thoracolumbar spine s.
Scoliosis Research Society
scoliotic
    s. curve fixation
scopolamine
Score
    Abbreviated Injury S. (AIS)
    Acute Physiology S.
    House-Brackmann S.
score
    ASA s.
    Hachinski ischemic s.
    Lahey s.
    speech discrimination s.
    (SDS)
scotoma, pl. **scotomata**
    flittering s.

hemianopic s.
scintillating s.
Scott cannula
Scoville clip
screen
    ether s.
screening
    genetic s.
screw
    alar s.
    s. alignment bar
    s. alignment rod
    s. angulation
    s. backout
    bone s.
    s. breakage
    cancellous s.
    Caspar s.
    Caspar cervical s.
    cortical s.
    Cotrel pedicle s.
    Edwards modular system
      spinal/sacral s.
    Edwards sacral s.
    Edwards spinal/sacral s.
    s. fixation
    iliac s.
    iliosacral s.
    s. implantation
    s. insertion
    s. insertion technique
    Isola spinal implant system
      iliac s.
    Kostuik s.
    s. loosening
    lumbar pedicle s.
    Mille Pattes s.
    pedicle s.
    s. plate approach
    s. position perioperative
      monitoring

    s. pullout
    rigid pedicle s.
    sacral s.
    sacral alar s.
    sacral pedicle s.
    set s.
    s. stabilization
    stainless steel s.
    s. stripout
    subarachnoid s.
    superior thoracic pedicle s.
    Texas Scottish Rite
      Hospital s.
    Texas Scottish Rite Hospital
      pedicle s.
    thoracolumbar pedicle s.
    transarticular s.
    transpedicular s.
    triangulated pedicle s.
    tulip pedicle s.
screwdriver
screw-to-screw compression
  construct
scriptorius
    calamus s.
scrivener's palsy
SCS
    spinal cord stimulation
SDS
    speech discrimination score
SE
    spin-echo
sealant
    tissue fibrin s.
seamstress's cramp
seatbelt fracture
sebaceous adenoma
sebaceus
    Jadassohn's nevus s.
seborrheic keratosis

NOTES

Sechrist monoplace hyperbaric
  chamber
second
  s. cervical nerve
  s. cranial nerve
  s. temporal convolution
secondary
  s. degeneration
  s. encephalitis
  s. fissure of the cerebellum
  s. generalized epilepsy
  s. hydrocephalus
  s. post-traumatic
    syringomyelia
  s. sensory cortex
  s. sensory nuclei
  s. visual area
  s. visual cortex
Secor system
secret curette
secretion
  syndrome of inappropriate
    antidiuretic hormone s.
secretory
  s. function
  s. nerve
sectio, pl. sectiones
section
  attached cranial s.
  coronal s.
  detached cranial s.
  frozen s.
  pituitary stalk s.
  vestibular nerve s.
sectoranopia
Sedan cannula
seed
  grass s.
  ^{125}I s.'s
seeding
  subarachnoid s.
  surgical s.
Seeligmüller's sign
seesaw nystagmus
segment
  clinoidal s. (ClinSeg)
  interannular s.
  internodal s.
  intradural s.
  Lanterman's s.'s
  M s.
  motion s.
  neural s.

ophthalmic s. (OphSeg)
P s.
Ranvier's s.
s.'s of spinal cord
sympathetic s.
segmenta (pl. of segmentum)
segmental
  s. anesthesia
  s. arterial disorganization
  s. compression construct
  s. fixation
  s. instrumentation
  s. neuritis
  s. neurofibromatosis
  s. neuropathy
  s. spinal instrumentation
    (SSI)
segmentation
  volume s.
segmentum, pl. segmenta
  s. internodale
  segmenta medullae spinalis
  s. medullae spinalis
    cervicalia
  s. medullae spinalis
    coccygea
  s. medullae spinalis
    lumbalis
  s. medullae spinalis sacralis
  s. medullae spinalis
    thoracica
Seitelberger's disease
seizure
  absence s.
  anosognosic s.
  complex partial s. (CPS)
  generalized tonic-clonic s.
  grand mal s.
  partial s.
  partial complex s.
  psychic s.
  psychomotor s.
  rolandic s.
  sylvian s.
  tonic-clonic s.
Sekhar
Seldinger
  S. retrograde wire/intubation
    technique
  S. technique
Seldinger's method
selection
  bone plate s.

Edwards modular system
   construct s.
slice s.
selective
   s. embolization
   s. memory
   s. microadenomectomy
   s. relaxation enhancement
   s. thoracic fusion
   s. thoracic spine fusion
   s. T2 shortening
selector
   Leksell s.
selegiline
self-hypnosis
self-retaining
   s.-r. brain retractor
   s.-r. brain retractor frame
   s.-r. retractor
self-stimulation
self-stopping drill point
sella
   diaphragma s.
   empty s.
   s. turcica
sellae
   diaphragma s.
   tuberculum s.
sellar
   s. aneurysm
   s. cyst
   s. tumor
Selter's disease
Selverstone
   S. clamp
   S. type clamp
SEM
   scanning electron microscopy
semantic aphasia
semialdehyde
   succinic s.

semicircular
   s. canal
   s. ducts
semicoma
semicomatose
semiconscious
Semilente
   S. Iletin I
semilunar
   s. fasciculus
   s. ganglion
   s. notch
   s. nucleus of Flechsig
semimembranosus reflex
seminoma
semioval center
semitendinosus reflex
Semmes curette
Semon-Hering theory
Semon's law
semustine (MeCCNU)
senile
   s. chorea
   s. delirium
   s. dementia
   s. memory
   s. paraplegia
   s. plaque
   s. psychosis
   s. tremor
Senn retractor
sensate
sensation
   cincture s.
   delayed s.
   general s.
   girdle s.
   objective s.
   primary s.
   referred s.
   reflex s.

NOTES

289

sensation *(continued)*
    special s.
    subjective s.
    transferred s.
sense
    s. of equilibrium
    joint s.
    kinesthetic s.
    muscular s.
    obstacle s.
    s. organs
    position s.
    posture s.
    pressure s.
    seventh s.
    sixth s.
    space s.
    special s.
    static s.
    tactile s.
    temperature s.
    thermal s.
    thermic s.
    time s.
    visceral s.
sensibility
    articular s.
    bone s.
    cortical s.
    deep s.
    dissociation s.
    electromuscular s.
    epicritic s.
    mesoblastic s.
    pallesthetic s.
    proprioceptive s.
    protopathic s.
    splanchnesthetic s.
    vibratory s.
sensible
sensiferous
sensigenous
sensimeter
sensitive
sensitivity
sensomobile
sensomobility
sensomotor
sensor
    CardioSearch s.
sensoria (*pl. of* sensorium)
sensorial
    s. areas

sensoriglandular
sensorimotor
    s. area
sensorimuscular
sensorineural
    s. deafness
sensorium, pl. sensoria, sensoriums
sensorivascular
sensorivasomotor
sensory
    s. alexia
    s. amusia
    s. aphasia
    s. areas
    s. cortex
    s. crossway
    s. decussation of medulla
      oblongata
    s. deficit
    s. distribution
    s. epilepsy
    s. ganglion
    s. image
    s. inattention
    s. nerve
    s. neuronopathy
    s. paralysis
    s. precipitated epilepsy
    s. receptors
    s. root of ciliary ganglion
    s. root of trigeminal nerve
    s. speech center
    s. tract
sensory-motor
    s.-m. strip
    s.-m. stroke
sentient
sentinel
    s. spinous process fracture
Sentinel system
SEP
    somatosensory evoked potential
      pudendal SEP
separation
    articular mass s.
    atlanto-occipital s.
    pontomedullary s.
separator
    Dorsey dural s.
    Woodson dural s.
septa (*pl. of* septum)
septal area
septi (*gen. of* septum)

septic
>s. embolus
>s. shock
>s. thrombosis
>s. venous vasculitis

septicemia
septomarginal
>s. fasciculus
>s. tract

septo-optic dysplasia
septum, gen. **septi**, pl. **septa**
>s. cervicale intermedium
>s. linguae
>s. lucidum
>s. pellucidum
>precommissural s.
>s. of tongue
>transparent s.
>transverse s.

sequence
>gradient-refocused s.
>pulse s.
>spin warp pulse s.
>stimulated spin echo s.
>(STEAM)
>STIR s.

sequential
>s. computed tomographic
>scan
>s. GRASS
>s. ultrasonography

sequential gradient-recalled
acquisition in the steady state
SER
>somatosensory evoked response

Serax
serial
>s. CT
>s. percutaneous needle
>drainage

seronegative spondyloarthropathy

serositis
serotonin
serous
>s. apoplexy
>s. meningitis

serpentine aneurysm
Serratia
serrations
>dentated s.

sertraline
serum
>antilymphocyte s. (ALS)

set
>aluminum contouring
>template s.
>Bremer halo crown
>traction s.
>Greenberg retractor s.
>s. screw

settling
>cranial s.

seventh
>s. cranial nerve
>s. cranial nerve
>transposition
>s. nerve palsy
>s. sense

severe
>s. degenerative disk disease
>s. kyphoscoliosis
>s. rigid right thoracic curve

sewing spasm
sexual neurasthenia
shaking palsy
sham-movement vertigo
shampoo
>chlorhexidine s.

sham rage
sharing
>Edwards modular system
>load s.

NOTES

Sharplan
    S. laser
    S. Ultra ultrasonic aspirator
shaving cramp
shearing injury
shear-strain deformation
shear stress
sheath
    carotid s.
    dural s.
    femoral introducer s.
    Henle's s.
    s. of Key and Retzius
    Mauthner's s.
    medullary s.
    myelin s.
    s. of Schwann
Sheehan's syndrome
sheeting
    rubber s.
Sheffield gamma unit
shell
    plastic s.
Sherrington phenomenon
Sherrington's law
shield
    AME PinSite s.
shielding
    magnet s.
shift
    brain s.
    chemical s.
    fat-water chemical s.
    field s.
    frequency s.
    midline s.
    phase s.
Shiley
    S. catheter
    S. catheter distention
      system
    S. distention kit
Shiley-Infusaid pump
shim coil
shimming
shiver
shiverer mouse
shivering
shock
    break s.
    cardiogenic s.
    deferred s.
    delayed s.

    delirious s.
    electric s.
    erethistic s.
    hypovolemic s.
    irreversible s.
    primary s.
    reversible s.
    septic s.
    spinal s.
    vasogenic s.
short
    s. gyri of the insula
    s. inversion recovery
      imaging (STIR)
    s. pulse repetition time
    s. pulse repetition time/echo
      time
    s. pulse repetition time/echo
      time image
    s. pulse repetition
      time/short echo time
    s. root of ciliary ganglion
    s. segment fusion
    s. segment spinal fusion
    s. time inversion recovery
short-acting insulin preparation
shortening
    selective T2 s.
    T2 s.
short-latency SSEP
short-term memory (STM)
shot
    fast low angle s. (FLASH)
shot-feel
shoulder-girdle syndrome
shoulder-hand syndrome
shredded Teflon felt
shrinkage
    neuronal s.
shudder
shunt
    s. blockage
    CSF s.
    s. filter
    Javid s.
    lumbar-peritoneal s.
    lumboperitoneal s.
    s. nephritis
    percutaneous
      thecoperitoneal s.
    pulmonary s.
    pulmonary arteriovenous s.
    Raimondi low pressure s.

right-to-left s.
subdural-pleural s.
syringoperitoneal s.
syringosubarachnoid s.
syrinx s.
s. tap
thecoperitoneal Pudenz-
Schulte s.
Torkildsen s.
T-shaped Edwards-Barbaro
syringeal s.
T-tube s.
ventriculoatrial s.
ventriculoperitoneal s.
VP s.
shunting
lumbar-peritoneal s.
ventricular peritoneal s.
ventriculoamniotic s.
ventriculoperitoneal s.
Shy-Drager syndrome
SIADH
syndrome of inappropriate
secretion of antidiuretic
hormone
sialidosis
sialorrhea
sicca
keratoconjunctivitis s.
sick
s. headache
s. sinus syndrome
sickle
s. cell anemia
s. cell disease
s. flap
sickness
acute African sleeping s.
African sleeping s.
chronic African sleeping s.
East African sleeping s.

falling s.
laughing s.
motion s.
sleeping s.
West African sleeping s.
side-cutting cannula
side effect
side-opening laminar hook
side-port flat-bottomed Ommaya
reservoir
sideration
siderosis
Siegert's sign
Siemens
S. couch
S. Magnetom scanner
S. Somatom Plus
Siemerling-Creutzfeldt disease
sigmoid
s. sinus
s. sinus ligation
s. sinus retraction
sign
Abadie's s. of tabes dorsalis
alien hand s.
Babinski's s.
Bamberger's s.
Barré's s.
Battle's s.
Bechterew's s.
Beevor's s.
Biernacki's s.
s. blindness
Bonhoeffer's s.
Brudzinski's s.
Cantelli's s.
Castellani-Low s.
Chaddock s.
Chvostek's s.
contralateral s.
Crichton-Browne's s.

NOTES

293

sign *(continued)*
    crossed adductor s.
    Dejerine's s.
    doll's eye s.
    double fragment s.
    Duchenne's s.
    empty delta s.
    empty sella s.
    empty triangle s.
    Erb's s.
    Erb-Westphal s.
    Escherich's s.
    external malleolar s.
    eyelash s.
    fan s.
    Froment's s.
    Goldstein's toe s.
    Gordon's s.
    Gorlin's s.
    Graefe's s.
    Grasset's s.
    Griesinger's s.
    Hoffmann's s.
    Homans' s.
    Hoover's s.'s
    Jackson's s.
    Joffroy's s.
    Kernig's s.
    Lasègue's s.
    Legendre's s.
    Leichtenstern's s.
    Leri's s.
    Leser-Trélat s.
    Lhermitte's s.
    Lichtheim's s.
    local s.
    Macewen's s.
    Magendie-Hertwig s.
    Magnan's s.
    Mannkopf's s.
    Masini's s.
    medullary s.
    mesencephalic s.
    neck s.
    Néri's s.
    s. of the orbicularis
    Pfuhl's s.
    Phalen's s.
    Piltz s.
    Pitres' s.
    pontine s.
    Pool-Schlesinger s.
    pseudo-Graefe s.

    pyramid s.
    pyramidal s.
    Remak's s.
    reservoir s.
    Revilliod's s.
    Romberg's s.
    Rossolimo's s.
    Saenger's s.
    Schlesinger's s.
    Schultze's s.
    Seeligmüller's s.
    Siegert's s.
    Signorelli's s.
    Simon's s.
    spine s.
    Stewart-Holmes s.
    Straus' s.
    string s.
    Tinel's s.
    tram track s.
    Trousseau's s.
    Uhthoff s.
    von Graefe's s.
    Weber's s.
    Weiss' s.
    Wernicke's s.
    Westphal's s., Westphal-
      Erb s.
signal
    s. filtering
    high-intensity s.
    s. intensity
    s. intensity curve
    s. loss
    s. processing
    s. strength
    s. voltage waveform
signal-to-noise
    s.-t.-n. ratio
    s.-t.-n. threshold
Signa 1.5 Tesla unit
significant displacement
Signorelli's sign
Silastic
    S. catheter
    S. device
    S. sponge
    S. wick
silent
    s. area
    s. period
silicone
    s. balloon

s. implant
s. rubber
s. sponge
simethicone
aluminum hydroxide with magnesium hydroxide and s.
simian
s. crease
s. fissure
s. line
Simmons plating system
Simon's sign
simple
s. absence
s. decompression
s. lobule
s. membranous limb of semicircular duct
s. skull fracture
simplex
herpes s.
simultagnosia
simultanagnosia
Sinemet
Sinequan
single
s. hook retractor
s. photon emission computed tomography (SPECT)
single-fraction radiation
single-level spinal fusion
single-rod construct
sinistral
sinistrality
sinistrocerebral
sinistromanual
sinistropedal
sinodural angle
sinography

sinonasal psammomatoid ossifying fibroma
sinus, pl. **sinus, sinuses**
s. cavernosus
cavernous s.
circular s.
s. circularis
confluence of sinuses
cranial dermal s.
dilated intercavernous s.
s. durae matris
dural s.
dural venous s.
sinuses of dura mater
endodermal s.
ethmoid s.
intercavernous s.
intracranial venous s.
lateral s.
marginal s.
maxillary s.
nasal s.
s. nerve of Hering
occluded s.
paranasal s.
parasinoidal sinuses
s. pericranii
petrosal s.
petrosquamosal s.
s. phlebitis
pilonidal s.
s. rectus
s. reflex
rhomboidal s., s. rhomboidalis
Ridley's s.
sagittal s.
sigmoid s.
sphenoid s.
sphenoidal s.
sphenotemporal s.

NOTES

sinus (continued)
    spinal dermal s.
    straight s.
    tentorial s.
    venous s.
sinusitis
sinuum
    confluens s.
sinuvertebral nerve
site
    graft s.
    hook s.
sitting position
sixth
    s. cranial nerve
    s. sense
    s. ventricle
Sjögren's syndrome
Sjöqvist tractotomy
skein
    choroid s.
skeletal deformity
skeletonize
skew deviation
skin
    s. flap
    glossy s.
    s. incision
    s. lesion
    s. reflexes
skin-muscle reflexes
skin-pupillary reflex
skull
    s. base
    cloverleaf s.
    s. fracture
    maplike s.
    steeple s., tower s.
SLE
    systemic lupus erythematosus
sleep
    s. apnea
    crescendo s.
    s. disorder
    s. dissociation
    electric s.
    electrotherapeutic s.
    s. epilepsy
    light s.
    paradoxical s.
    s. paralysis
    paroxysmal s.

    rapid eye movement s., REM s.
    s. spindle
sleep-induced apnea
sleepiness
sleeping sickness
sleeplessness
sleeve
    s. graft
    polyethylene s.
slender
    s. fasciculus
    s. lobule
slice
    s. fracture
    s. selection
slice-select encoding gradient
Slimline clip
sling
    clip-reinforced cotton s.
sling/wrapping technique
slit hemorrhage
slit-ventricle syndrome
slot fracture
slotted suction tip
slowing
    saccadic s.
Sly's disease
small-bowel carcinoid tumor
smell
    s. blindness
    s. disorder
smell-brain
Smellie's scissors
Smith-Robinson
    S.-R. operation
    S.-R. procedure
    S.-R. technique
Smithwick
    S. ganglion hook
    S. hook
    S. sympathectomy
smooth
    s. muscle proliferation
    s. pursuit defect
snap finger
snapping reflex
Sneddon's syndrome
Snellen letters
snout reflex
snuffbox
    anatomical s.

sodium
>ampicillin s.
>cefalothin s.
>cefoxitin s.
>dantrolene s.
>indigotin disulfonate s.
>ioxaglate s.
>levothyroxine s.
>liothyronine s.
>methicillin s.
>methotrexate s.
>nafcillin s.
>s. nitroprusside
>thiopental s.
>warfarin s.
>zomepirac s.

sodium-responsive periodic paralysis
Soemmering's
>S. ganglion
>S. spot

soft
>s. palate retraction
>s. tissue dissection
>s. tissue injury
>s. tissue stretching

SOF'WIRE spinal fixation
solar ganglia
soldier's heart
sole
>s. nuclei
>s. plate
>s. reflex
>s. tap reflex

sole-plate ending
solid state coagulator
solid-state instrument
solitarius
>nucleus s.

solitary
>s. bundle
>s. tract

solium
>*Taenia s.*

Solomon-Bloembergen equation
Solu-Cortef
Solu-Medrol
solution
>10% acetylcysteine 0.05%
>isoproterenol
>hydrochloride s.
>[^{18}F] fluoride s.
>hydroxyethyl methacrylate
>polymerizing s.
>Zenker's s.

soma
Somanetics INVOS 3100 cerebral oximeter
somatagnosia
somatalgia
somatesthesia
somatesthetic
somatic
>s. motor neuron
>s. motor nuclei
>s. pain
>s. sensory cortex

somatochrome
Somatom DR1
somatopathic
somatosensory
>s. cortex
>s. evoked potential (SEP, SSEP)
>s. evoked potential monitoring
>s. evoked response (SER)

somatotopagnosis
somatotopic
somatotopy
somatotroph cell
somatotropin
somesthesia

NOTES

somesthetic
    s. area
    s. system
SOMI
    sternal occipital mandibular
    immobilization
    SOMI brace
somite
    embryonic cervical s.
somnambulic epilepsy
somnambulism
somnocinematograph
somnocinematography
somnolence, somnolency
    s. syndrome
somnolent
somnolentia
Songer
    S. cable
    S. cable system
Sonneberg neurectomy
sonography
    color-flow Doppler s.
    Doppler s.
    transcranial color-coded real-
    time s. (TCCS)
    transcranial Doppler s.
    (TCD)
sonomotor
    s. response
sonophobia
sopor
soporose, soporous
Sotos syndrome
sound
    coconut s.
    contralateral routing of s.
    (CROS)
source
    Zeiss Super Lux 40 light s.
South African tick-bite fever
Southern blotting
space
    craniospinal s.
    dead s.
    disk s.
    epidural s.
    extradural s.
    His' perivascular s.
    incisural s.
    k-s.
    L5-S1 disk s.
    Malacarne's s.

    perforated s.
    perioptic subarachnoid s.
    perivascular s.
    retropharyngeal s.
    s. sense
    subarachnoid s.
    subdural s.
    Tarin's s.
    Virchow-Robin s.
space-occupying brain lesion
spacer
    ceramic vertebral s.
    methylmethacrylate s.
SPAMM
    spatial modulation of
    magnetization
sparing
    music ability s.
spark-gap instrument
spasm
    anorectal s.
    Bell's s.
    canine s.
    carpopedal s.
    clonic s.
    convergence s.
    cynic s.
    dancing s.
    facial s.
    facial habit s.
    functional s.
    habit s.
    hemifacial s.
    histrionic s.
    infantile s.
    intention s.
    masticatory s.
    mimic s.
    mobile s.
    muscle s.
    near reflex s.
    nictitating s.
    nodding s.
    occupational s.
    paraplegic s.
    phonic s.
    professional s.
    progressive torsion s.
    retrocollic s.
    rotatory s.
    salaam s.
    saltatory s.
    sewing s.

synclonic s.
tailor's s.
tonic s.
tonoclonic s.
tooth s.'s
torsion s.
vasomotor s.
winking s.
spasmodic
s. apoplexy
s. diathesis
s. mydriasis
s. tic
s. torticollis
spasmogenic
spasmology
spasmolygmus
spasmolysis
spasmolytic
spasmophilia
spasmophilic
s. diathesis
spasmus
s. agitans
s. caninus
s. coordinatus
s. nictitans
s. nutans
spastic
s. abasia
s. aphonia
s. diplegia
s. gait
s. hemiplegia
s. miosis
s. mydriasis
s. paraplegia
s. spinal paralysis
spasticity
clasp-knife s.

s. of conjugate gaze
sphincter s.
spatial
s. frequency
s. homogeneity
s. localization
s. modulation of
magnetization (SPAMM)
s. resolution
spatium, pl. **spatia**
s. subdurale
spatula
brain s.
curved-tipped s.
s. dissector
double-vector brain s.
duck-billed anodized s.
rectangular brain s.
tapered brain s.
special
s. sensation
s. sense
s. somatic afferent column
s. visceral column
s. visceral efferent nuclei
s. visceral motor nuclei
specific
s. absorption rate
s. curve
specimen staining
SPECT
single photon emission
computed tomography
SPECT analysis
dual-isotope SPECT
^{99m}Tc HMPAO SPECT
^{201}Tl SPECT
spectra (*pl. of* spectrum)
spectral
s. density

NOTES

spectral *(continued)*
 s. density function
 s. velocity
spectrometer
 mass s.
spectroscopy
 magnetic resonance s.
 MR s.
 proton magnetic
  resonance s.
 proton nuclear magnetic
  resonance s.
 in vivo optical s. (INVOS)
spectrum, pl. spectra, spectrums
 Doppler frequency s.
 fortification s.
 proton s.
speculum
 bivalved s.
 Cushing-Landolt s.
 Hardy s.
 Hardy bivalve s.
speech
 s. centers
 cerebellar s.
 s. discrimination score
  (SDS)
 s. disorder
 s. disturbance
 echo s.
 explosive s.
 s. reception threshold (SRT)
 scanning s.
 staccato s.
 subvocal s.
 syllabic s.
spelencephaly
Spencer biopsy forceps
Spens' syndrome
Spetzler-Martin classification
Spetzler's Microvac suction tube
Spetzler system
SPF Spinal Fusion Stimulators
S-phase fraction
sphenocavernous syndrome
sphenoethmoidectomy
sphenoid
 s. encephalocele
 s. meningioma
 s. mucocele
 s. ridge meningioma
 s. sinus

 s. wing
 s. wing meningioma
sphenoidal
 s. herniation
 s. sinus
sphenoidectomy
sphenoiditis
sphenoidostomy
sphenoidotomy
sphenopalatine
 s. ganglion
 s. ganglionectomy
sphenotemporal sinus
spheresthesia
spherical
 s. coordinate representation
 s. nucleus
sphincter
 anal s.
 s. spasticity
 urinary s.
sphingolipidosis
 cerebral s.
spider cell
Spielmeyer's acute swelling
Spielmeyer-Sjögren disease
Spielmeyer-Vogt disease
spike
 interictal epileptiform s.
 s. and wave complex
Spiller-Frazier technique
spin
 s. magnetization
 s. velocity
 s. warp pulse sequence
spina, gen. and pl. spinae
 s. bifida, s. bifida
 s. bifida aperta
 s. bifida cystica
 s. bifida manifesta
 s. bifida occulta
 s. dorsalis
spinal
 s. accessory nerve
 s. accessory nerve-facial
  nerve anastomosis
 s. anesthesia
 s. angiography
 s. apoplexy
 s. arteriography
 s. arteritis
 s. artery
 s. ataxia

s. atrophy
s. block
s. canal
s. catheter
s. column
s. concussion
s. cord
s. cord arachnoiditis
s. cord compression
s. cord function
  intraoperative monitoring
s. cord injury
s. cord injury without
  radiological abnormality
  (SCIWORA)
s. cord stimulation (SCS)
s. coronal plane deformity
s. decompression
s. deformity
s. deformity/instability
s. deformity treatment
s. dermal sinus
s. dermal sinus tract
s. drainage
s. dysraphism
s. ependymoma
s. epidural abscess
s. epidural angiolipoma
s. fixation
s. fixation rigidity
s. fusion
s. fusion pathomechanics
s. fusion technique
s. ganglion
s. headache
s. implant design
s. implant load to failure
s. infection
s. injury operative
  stabilization
s. instrumentation

s. lesion
s. level
s. lipoma
s. metastasis
s. metastatic disease
s. needle
s. nerve
s. nerve root
s. neurofibroma
s. nucleus of accessory
  nerve
s. nucleus of the trigeminus
s. osteomyelitis
s. osteotomy stabilization
s. paralysis
s. puncture
s. pyramidotomy
s. reflex
s. reflex arc
s. rod
s. rod cross-bracing
s. roots
s. sensory evoked potential
s. shock
s. stabilization
s. stenosis
s. stroke
s. tap
s. tract
s. tractotomy
s. tract of trigeminal nerve
s. tuberculosis
s. tumor
Spinal Fixation Study Group
spinalis
  meningitis serous s.
"spinal-tension-band"
spinant
spindle
  s. cell
  Kühne's s.

NOTES

spindle *(continued)*
    muscle s.
    neuromuscular s.
    neurotendinous s.
    sleep s.
spindle-celled layer
spindle-cell tumor
spine
    bamboo s.
    cervical s.
    cleft s.
    dendritic s.'s
    dorsal s.
    s. fusion
    laminectomized s.
    lower cervical s.
    lower lumbar s.
    lower thoracic s.
    lumbar s.
    lumbosacral s.
    osteoporotic s.
    poker s.
    sacral s.
    sacrococcygeal s.
    s. sign
    thoracic s.
    thoracolumbar s.
    tumor metastatic to s.
    upper thoracic s.
    variable screw placement
      system-instrumented
      lumbar s.
spin-echo (SE)
    s.-e. imaging
    long pulse repetition
      time/long echo time s.-e.
Spinestat probe
spinifugal
spinipetal
spin-lattice relaxation
spino-adductor reflex
spinobulbar
spinocerebellar
    s. ataxia
    s. tracts
spinocerebellum
spinocollicular
spinocranial meningioma
spinogalvanization
spinolamellar line
spino-olivary tract
spinopontine degeneration

spinotectal
    s. tract
spinothalamic
    s. cordotomy
    s. tract
    s. tractotomy
spinous
    s. interlaminar line
    s. process
    s. process fracture
    s. process plate
    s. process wire
    s. process wiring
spin-spin
    s.-s. coupling
    s.-s. relaxation
spiral
    s. foraminous tract
    s. ganglion of cochlea
    s. membrane
    s. organ
spirochetal aneurysm
spirochete
Spirohydantoin
spirometry
spiromustine
spironolactone
Spitzka's
    S. marginal tract
    S. marginal zone
    S. nucleus
Spitz nevus
splanchnesthesia
splanchnesthetic sensibility
splanchnic
    s. afferent column
    s. anesthesia
    s. efferent column
    s. ganglion
splanchnicectomy
splanchnicotomy
spleen injury
splenial gyrus
splenium, pl. splenia
    callosal s.
    s. corporis callosi
splenomegaly
split
    s. brain
    s. brain syndrome
    s. notochord syndrome

palatal s.
vermian s.
split-cord malformation (SCM)
spoiling
radiofrequency s.
spondylalgia
spondylarthritis
spondylarthrocace
spondylectomy
spondylitic
spondylitis
ankylosing s.
cryptococcal s.
s. deformans
Kümmell's s.
rheumatoid s.
tuberculous s.
spondyloarthropathy
seronegative s.
spondylocace
spondylo construct
spondylodesis
ventral derotation s. (VDS)
spondylolisthesis
degenerative s.
grade IV s.
high-grade s.
postlaminectomy two-level s.
s. reduction
s. reduction/fixation
symptomatic s.
s. with significant
displacement
spondylolisthetic
spondylolysis
spondylomalacia
spondylopathy
spondyloptosis
spondylopyosis
spondyloschisis

spondylosis
cervical s.
degenerative s.
hyperostotic s.
lumbar s.
thoracolumbar s.
spondylosyndesis
spondylotic myelopathy
spondylotomy
sponge
absorbable gelatin s.
gelatin s.
Ivalon s.
Ivalon embolic s.
Silastic s.
silicone s.
spongiform
s. encephalopathy
s. virus encephalopathy
spongioblast
spongioblastoma
spongiocyte
spongy degeneration
spontaneous
s. neuronal hyperactivity
s. regression
spoon
Hardy pituitary s.
spot
café au lait s.'s
central direct current
bright s.
cherry-red s.
cotton wool s.
Graefe's s.'s
hypnogenic s.
Roth s.
saccular s.
Soemmering's s.
temperature s.
Trousseau's s.

NOTES

303

spot *(continued)*
 utricular s.
 yellow s.
spotted fever
spreader
 Blount s.
 Caspar disk space s.
 Doyen rib s.
 Harrington s.
 lamina s.
 Texas Scottish Rite Hospital
  eyebolt s.
spreading
 s. cortical depression theory
 s. depression
spring
 coiled s.
 compression s.
 s. finger
 Gruca-Weiss s.
 internal fixation s.
 s. mechanism
springing mydriasis
sprouting
 neuronal s.
spur
 Morand's s.
 traction s.
spurious
 s. meningocele
 s. torticollis
Spurling's maneuver
Spurr's epoxy resin
square-ended hook
SRT
 speech reception threshold
SSEP
 somatosensory evoked potential
  short-latency SSEP
SSI
 segmental spinal instrumentation
  anterior-posterior fusion
   with SSI
STA
 superficial temporal artery
stabilimeter
stability
 lumbar spine rotational s.
 temporal s.
stabilization
 anterior s.
 anterior internal s.
 anterior short-segment s.

 s. approach
 atlantoaxial s.
 atlanto-occipital s.
 cervical s.
 cervical spine s.
 cervicothoracic junction s.
 flexion-compression spine
  injury s.
 fracture s.
 iliac crest bone graft s.
 lower cervical spine s.
 lower cervical spine
  posterior s.
 lumbar spine s.
 occipitocervical s.
 odontoid fracture s.
 posterior s.
 posterior lower cervical
  spine s.
 sacral spine s.
 screw s.
 spinal s.
 spinal injury operative s.
 spinal osteotomy s.
 subluxation s.
 thoracolumbar spine s.
 TSRH s.
 TSRH crosslink s.
 wire s.
stable
 s. cervical spine injury
 s. xenon CT
staccato speech
Staderini's nucleus
staged
 s. bilateral stereotactic
  thalamotomy
 s. embolization
stagger
stagnant hypoxia
stain
 Perls' s.
staining
 specimen s.
stainless
 s. steel equipment
 s. steel plate
 s. steel screw
staircase phenomenon
stalk
 infundibular s.
 pituitary s.

STA-MCA
  superficial temporal artery to
    middle cerebral artery
    STA-MCA anastomosis
stammering
  s. of the bladder
stand
  Brown-Roberts-Wells floor s.
  Contraves s.
standard
  s. bone algorithm program
  s. retroperitoneal flank
    approach
  s. retroperitoneal flank
    incision
  s. thoracotomy
STA-PCA
  superficial temporal artery-
    posterior cerebral artery
    STA-PCA bypass
stapedial artery
Staphcillin
Staphylococcus aureus
staphyloma
staphyloplegia
stare
  postbasic s.
Starling's reflex
START
  stereotactic-assisted radiation
    therapy
StaRT
  stereotactic radiation therapy
    fractionated StaRT
startle
  s. epilepsy
  s. reaction
  s. reflex

STA-SCA
  superficial temporal artery-
    superior cerebellar artery
    STA-SCA bypass
stasis retinopathy
state
  absent s.
  anxiety s.
  apallic s.
  central excitatory s.
  convulsive s.
  dreamy s.
  hypercoagulable s.
  local excitatory s.
  oxidation s.'s
  permanent vegetative s.
  refractory s.
  twilight s.
  vegetative s.
static
  s. ataxia
  s. convulsion
  s. infantilism
  s. magnetic field
  s. reflex
  s. sense
  s. tremor
station test
statokinetic reflex
statotonic reflexes
status
  s. choreicus
  s. convulsivus
  s. cribrosus
  s. criticus
  s. dysmyelinisatus
  s. dysraphicus
  s. epilepticus
  s. hemicranicus
  s. lacunaris
  s. marmoratus

NOTES

status *(continued)*
s. nervosus
s. raptus
s. spongiosus
s. typhosus
s. vertiginosus
stauroplegia
steal
cerebral ischemia s.
s. index
intracerebral s.
s. phenomenon
subclavian s.
STEAM
stimulated spin echo sequence
Steele-Richardson-Olszewski
S.-R.-O. disease
S.-R.-O. syndrome
steep-dose gradient
steeple skull
Steffee
S. instrumentation
S. pedicle screw-plate
system
S. plate
S. plating
stege
Steinert's disease
Steinmann pin
Stelazine
stellate
s. cells of cerebral cortex
s. ganglion
s. skull fracture
stellectomy
stem
brain s.
infundibular s.
stenogyria
Stenosimeter
stenosis, pl. stenoses
aqueductal s.
cervical spinal s.
foraminal s.
lateral recess s.
lumbar spinal s.
spinal s.
thoracolumbar spinal
canal s.
stenostenosis
Stensen's duct
stepdown connector

steppage
s. gait
stercoralis
Strongyloides s.
Stereoadapter
Laitinen S.
stereoagnosis
stereoanesthesia
stereoelectroencephalography
stereoencephalometry
stereoencephalotomy
stereognosis
stereognostic
stereoguide collimator
stereomagnification
s. angiography
stereotactic, stereotaxic
s. anatomic target
localization
s. angiography
s. anteroposterior and
lateral metrizamide
ventriculography
s. aspiration
s. atlas
s. biopsy
s. brachytherapy
s. catheter drainage
s. cordotomy
s. craniotomy
s. focused-radiation therapy
s. frame
s. guidance
s. instrument
s. instrumentation
s. linear accelerator
radiotherapy
s. neurosurgery
s. operation
s. PET image
s. puncture
s. radiation therapy (StaRT)
s. radiosurgery
s. surgery
s. surgical ablation
s. thalamotomy
s. VIM thalamotomy
s. VL thalamotomy
**stereotactic-assisted radiation
therapy (START)**
stereotaxis
stereotaxy
functional s.

10-β

sterile abscess
Steritek ICP mini monitor
sternal
    s. occipital mandibular
      immobilization (SOMI)
    s. puncture
sternobrachial reflex
sternocleidomastoid
    s. muscle
    s. muscle weakness
sternohyoid muscle
sternomastoid muscle
sternothyroid muscle
sternotomy
sternum-splitting approach
sternutatory absence
steroid
stethoparalysis
stethospasm
Stevens-Johnson syndrome
Stewart-Holmes sign
Stewart-Morel syndrome
sticky platelet syndrome
stiff-man syndrome
stiff neck
stiffness
    axial s.
    fusion s.
    hemiparkinsonian s.
    torsional s.
Stilling's
    S. column
    S. gelatinous substance
    S. nucleus
    S. raphe
stimulated spin echo sequence
  (STEAM)
stimulation
    brain s.
    direct brain s. (DBS)
    dorsal column s.

    dorsal cord s. (DCS)
    electrical s.
    electrophysiological s.
    magnetoelectric s.
    percutaneous s.
    photic s.
    spinal cord s. (SCS)
    transcranial electrical s.
    transcutaneous electrical
     nerve s.
stimulator
    constant current s.
    EMG s.
    magnetic s.
    nerve s.
Stimulators
    SPF Spinal Fusion S.
stimulus, pl. stimuli
    adequate s.
    conditioned s.
    heterologous s.
    homologous s.
    inadequate s.
    liminal s.
    maximal s.
    s. sensitive myoclonus
    subliminal s.
    subthreshold s.
    supramaximal s.
    s. threshold
    threshold s.
    train-of-four s.
    unconditioned s.
STIR
    short inversion recovery imaging
    STIR sequence
stitch
    running s.
STM
    short-term memory

NOTES

stock
    bone s.
stocking anesthesia
Stoffel's operation
stoker's cramps
Stokes-Adams
    S.-A. disease
    S.-A. syndrome
Stokes' law
stomatitis
    aphthous s.
stomodeum
Stookey-Scarff operation
storage
strabismus
straight
    s. clip
    s. connector
    s. forceps
    s. gyrus
    s. knot-tying forceps
    s. leg raising test
    s. line bayonet forceps
    s. microscissors
    s. needle
    s. needle electrode
    s. nerve hook
    s. ring curette
    s. sinus
straight-in ventriculostomy
strain gauge
strangalesthesia
strap muscle
strata
stratum, gen. **strati**, pl. **strata**
    s. album profundum
    s. cerebrale retinae
    s. cinereum colliculi
      superioris
    s. ganglionare nervi optici
    s. ganglionare retinae
    s. gangliosum cerebelli
    s. granulosum cerebelli
    s. griseum colliculi
      superioris
    s. griseum medium
    s. griseum profundum
    s. griseum superficiale
    s. interolivare lemnisci
    s. lemnisci
    s. moleculare
    s. moleculare cerebelli

    s. moleculare retinae
    s. neuroepitheliale retinae
    s. neuronorum piriformium
    s. nucleare externum et
      internum retinae
    s. nucleare externum retinae
    s. nucleare internum retinae
    s. opticum
    s. pigmenti bulbi
    s. pigmenti retinae
    s. plexiforme externum et
      internum retinae
    s. zonale
Straus' sign
streak
    angioid s.'s
    fatty s.
    meningitic s.
    primitive s.
streaming
    intravascular s.
strength
    axial gripping s.
    bending s.
    bone-screw interface s.
    C-D instrumentation
      fixation s.
    Cotrel pedicle screw
      fixation s.
    field s.
    pedicle screw pullout s.
    pullout s.
    signal s.
    torsional gripping s.
strephosymbolia
Streptococcus
    S. pneumoniae
    S. pyogenes
    S. viridans
streptokinase
streptomycin
stress
    measured s.
    s. relaxation
    shear s.
    tensile s.
    s. ulcer
stress-relaxation
    intraoperative s.-r.
stretch
    s. receptors
    s. reflex

stretching
    soft tissue s.
stria, gen. and pl. **striae**
    acoustic striae
    auditory striae
    s. fornicis
    Gennari's s.
    striae lancisi
    lateral longitudinal s.
    s. longitudinalis lateralis
    s. longitudinalis medialis
    medial longitudinal s.
    striae medullares ventriculi
      quarti
    s. medullaris thalami
    medullary striae of the
      fourth ventricle
    medullary s. of the
      thalamus
    striae olfactoriae
    olfactory striae
    s. tecta
    terminal s.
    s. terminalis
    s. ventriculi tertii
striatal
striate
    s. area
    s. body
    s. cortex
    s. veins
striatocapsular infarction
striatonigral
    s. degeneration
striatopetal fiber
striatum
    corpus s.
string sign
strip
    sensory-motor s.
    Telfa s.

stripe
stripe of Gennari
stripout
    screw s.
stroboscope
stroke
    ischemic s.
    pure sensory s.
    retinal s.
    sensory-motor s.
    spinal s.
    s. syndrome
Strongyloides stercoralis
Strümpell-Marie disease
Strümpell's
    S. disease
    S. phenomenon
    S. reflex
Strümpell-Westphal disease
strut
    s. fusion technique
    s. grafting
Struthers' ligament
strychninism
Stuart-Power factor
stuck finger
study
    animal s.
    chromosome s.
    efficacy s.
    ICA-occluded stable Xe/CT
      CBF s.
    metrizamide contrast s.
    nerve conduction s.
    neural imaging s.
    radionuclide s.
    Xe/CT CBF s.
stump
    s. embolization syndrome
    s. hallucination
    s. neuralgia

NOTES

stun
stupefacient, stupefactive
stupor
　　benign s.
　　depressive s.
　　malignant s.
stuporous
Sturge-Kalischer-Weber syndrome
Sturge's disease
Sturge-Weber
　　S.-W. disease
　　S.-W. syndrome
stutter
stuttering
　　urinary s.
stylet, stylette
　　Frazier s.
styloradial reflex
subacute
　　s. combined degeneration of
　　the spinal cord
　　s. inclusion body
　　encephalitis
　　s. necrotizing myelitis
　　s. necrotizing myelopathy
　　s. sclerosing
　　leukoencephalitis
　　s. sclerosing panencephalitis
　　s. spongiform
　　encephalopathy
subarachnoid
　　s. cavity
　　s. hemorrhage (SAH)
　　s. lipoma
　　s. screw
　　s. seeding
　　s. space
subarachnoidal cisterns
subcalcarine
subcallosal
　　s. area
　　s. fasciculus
　　s. gyrus
subcapsular
subcaudate tractotomy
subchoroidal approach
subclavian
　　s. artery
　　s. loop
　　s. steal
　　s. steal syndrome
subclinical absence
subcollateral

subcommissural organ
subconjunctival hemorrhage
subconscious
subconsciousness
subcortex
subcortical
　　s. arteriosclerotic
　　encephalopathy
　　s. hemorrhage
subcranial
subcutaneous sacrococcygeal
　　myxopapillary ependymoma
subdelirium
subdural
　　s. abscess
　　s. cavity
　　s. grid
　　s. grid electrode
　　s. grid implantation
　　s. hematoma
　　s. hematorrhachis
　　s. hemorrhage
　　s. hygroma
　　s. ICP monitoring
　　s. space
　　s. strip electrode
　　s. tap
　　s. tumor
subdural-pleural shunt
subendymal, subependymal
subependymoma
subepicranium
subfalcial herniation
subfissure
subfolium
subfrontal approach
subfrontal-transbasal approach
subgaleal
　　s. drain
　　s. emphysema
　　s. hematoma
　　s. hemorrhage
subgrundation
subhyaloid hemorrhage
subicular
subiculum, pl. subicula
subintimal hemorrhage
subjective
　　s. sensation
　　s. vertigo
　　s. vision
sublabial midline rhinoseptal
　　approach

sublaminar
  s. fixation
  s. wire
  s. wiring
sublenticular limb of internal capsule
Sublimaze
subliminal
  s. stimulus
sublingual ganglion
subluxation
  atlantoaxial s.
  degenerative s.
  s. stabilization
  vertebral s.
submandibular ganglion
submaxillary ganglion
subnucleus caudalis
suboccipital
  s. approach
  s. decompression
  s. neuralgia
  s. neuritis
  s. Ommaya reservoir
  s. subtemporal approach
  s. transmeatal approach
subparietal sulcus
subperiosteal
  s. cyst
  s. dissection
  s. hematoma
subpial
substance
  s. abuse disorders
  anterior perforated s.
  basophil s.
  central gray s.
  chromophil s.
  gelatinous s.
  gray s.
  innominate s.

  medullary s.
  neurosecretory s.
  Nissl s.
  s. P
  posterior perforated s.
  reticular s.
  Rolando's gelatinous s.,
    Rolando's s.
  Schwann's white s.
  Stilling's gelatinous s.
  tigroid s.
  white s.
substantia, pl. substantiae
  s. alba
  s. basophilia
  s. cinerea
  s. ferruginea
  s. gelatinosa
  s. gelatinosa centralis
  s. grisea
  s. grisea centralis
  s. innominata
  s. intermedia centralis et
    lateralis
  s. medullaris
  s. nigra
  s. nigra disorder
  s. perforata anterior
  s. perforata posterior
  s. reticularis
substitute
  human dural s.
subsultus
  s. clonus
  s. tendinum
subtemporal
  s. approach
  s. decompression
  s. dissection
  s. intradural approach

NOTES

311

subtentorial
    s. lesion
subtest
    Logical Memory and Visual
      Reproduction s. (Russell's
      revised)
subtetanic
subthalamic
    s. nucleus
subthalamus
subthreshold stimulus
subtraction
    s. imaging
    s. technique
subvocal speech
succinate
    chloramphenicol sodium s.
    cortisol and sodium s.
    methylprednisolone and
      sodium s.
succinic semialdehyde
succinylcholine
sucker
    malleable s.
sucralfate
suction
    s. dissection
    Ferguson s.
    s. injury
    s. ophthalmodynamometry
    s. Regugauge regulator
    s. tube
suction-irrigator
    Brackmann s.-i.
sudanophilic leukodystrophy
Sudeck's
    S. atrophy
    S. syndrome
sudomotor fibers
Suetens-Gybels-Vandermeulen
  angiographic localizer
sufentanil
Sugita
    S. aneurysm clip
    S. clip
    S. cross-legged clip
    S. fork
    S. headholder
    S. multipurpose head frame
    S. retractor
Sugita-Ikakogyo clip
suicidal ideation
sulbactam

sulcal enlargement
sulci (*gen. and pl. of* sulcus)
sulcocommissural artery
sulcomarginal tract
sulcus, gen. and pl. sulci
    anterior parolfactory s.
    anterolateral s.
    basilar s.
    s. basilaris pontis
    calcarine s.
    s. calcarinus
    callosal s.
    s. callosomarginalis
    central s.
    s. centralis
    cerebellar sulci
    cerebral sulci
    cerebral s.
    sulci cerebri
    s. cinguli
    s. of cingulum
    s. circularis insulae
    circular s. of Reil
    collateral s.
    s. collateralis
    s. corporis callosi
    s. of corpus callosum
    cortical s.
    fimbriodentate s., s.
      fimbriodentatus
    s. frontalis inferior
    s. frontalis medius
    s. frontalis superior
    s. frontomarginalis
    s. hippocampi
    hypothalamic s.
    s. hypothalamicus
    inferior frontal s.
    inferior temporal s.
    s. intermedius anterior
    s. intermedius posterior
    interparietal s.
    s. intragracilis
    intraparietal s.
    s. intraparietalis
    intraparietal s. of Turner
    lateral cerebral s.
    s. lateralis anterior
    s. lateralis cerebri
    s. lateralis posterior
    lateral occipital s.
    s. limitans

s. limitans fossae
rhomboideae
limiting s. of Reil
limiting s. of rhomboid
fossa
lunate s.
s. lunatus cerebri
s. medialis cruris cerebri
median s. of fourth
ventricle
median frontal s.
s. medianus posterior
medullae oblongatae
s. medianus posterior
medullae spinalis
s. medianus ventriculi
quarti
middle frontal s.
middle temporal s.
Monro's s.
s. nervi oculomotorii
s. occipitalis lateralis
s. occipitalis superior
s. occipitalis transversus
occipitotemporal s.
s. occipitotemporalis
s. olfactorius
olfactory s.
orbital sulci
sulci orbitales
parieto-occipital s.
s. parieto-occipitalis
s. parolfactorius anterior
s. parolfactorius posterior
postcentral s.
s. postcentralis
posterior median s. of
medulla oblongata
posterior median s. of
spinal cord
posterior parolfactory s.

posterolateral s.
precentral s.
s. precentralis
rhinal s.
s. rhinalis
subparietal s.
s. subparietalis
superior frontal s.
superior occipital s.
superior temporal s.
sulci temporales transversi
s. temporalis inferior
s. temporalis medius
s. temporalis superior
transverse occipital s.
transverse temporal sulci
Turner's s.
s. ventralis
s. verticalis
sulfadiazine
sulfamethoxazole
sulfate
amikacin s.
bleomycin s.
ephedrine s.
gentamicin s.
guanethidine s.
metaproterenol s.
morphine s.
tobramycin s.
vinblastine s.
vincristine s.
sulfatide lipidosis
sulfatidosis
sulfinpyrazone
sulfosuccinate
dioctyl sodium s.
sulfoxide
dimethyl s. (DMSO)
sulindac
sumatriptan

NOTES

summation
    s. of stimuli
sunburst mechanism
Sundt
    S. AVM micro clip system
    S. booster clip
    S. clip
    S. cross-legged clip
    S. straddling clip
Sundt-Kees
    S.-K. clip
    S.-K. encircling patch clip
    S.-K. graft clip
    S.-K. Slimline clip
SUN microsystem
superconducting
    s. magnet
    0.5-T s. magnet
superconductivity
superconductor
    Type 2 s.
superficial
    s. middle cerebral vein
    s. origin
    s. reflex
    s. temporal artery (STA)
    s. temporal artery to middle cerebral artery (STA-MCA)
    s. temporal artery-posterior cerebral artery (STA-PCA)
    s. temporal artery to posterior cerebral artery bypass
    s. temporal artery-superior cerebellar artery (STA-SCA)
    s. temporal vein
superior
    s. alternating hemiplegia
    s. anastomotic vein
    s. cerebellar artery
    s. cerebellar artery syndrome
    s. cerebellar peduncle
    s. cerebral veins
    s. cervical ganglion
    s. cervical ganglionectomy
    s. choroid vein
    s. colliculus
    s. frontal convolution
    s. frontal gyrus
    s. frontal sulcus

    s. ganglion of glossopharyngeal nerve
    s. ganglion of the vagus nerve
    s. hemorrhagic polioencephalitis
    s. hypophyseal artery (SupHypArt)
    s. hypophyseal artery aneurysm
    s. intradural approach
    s. laryngeal artery
    s. laryngeal nerve
    s. laryngeal nerve external branch
    s. longitudinal fasciculus
    s. medullary velum
    s. mesenteric artery syndrome
    s. mesenteric ganglion
    s. oblique tendon sheath syndrome
    s. occipital gyrus
    s. occipital sulcus
    s. olivary nucleus
    s. olive
    s. ophthalmic vein
    s. orbital fissure
    s. paraplegia
    s. parietal gyrus
    s. parietal lobule
    s. part of vestibulocochlear nerve
    s. polioencephalitis
    s. pulmonary sulcus tumor
    s. quadrigeminal brachium
    s. root of cervical loop
    s. root of vestibulocochlear nerve
    s. sagittal sinus occlusion
    s. salivary nucleus
    s. semilunar lobule
    s. surface of cerebellar hemisphere
    s. temporal convolution
    s. temporal fissure
    s. temporal gyrus
    s. temporal sulcus
    s. thalamostriate vein
    s. thoracic pedicle screw
    s. thyroid artery
    s. thyroid vein

s. veins of cerebellar
hemisphere
s. vena cava syndrome
s. vestibular area
s. vestibular nucleus
supermotility
superolateral surface of cerebrum
superparamagnetic iron oxide
superparamagnetism
superposition
superselective angiography
SupHypArt
superior hypophyseal artery
supination reflex
supinator
s. jerk
s. longus reflex
s. reflex
supplementary motor cortex
support
external s.
suppressant
vestibular s.
suppression
bone marrow s.
vestibulo-ocular reflex s.
suppurative
s. cerebritis
s. encephalitis
supracallosal gyrus
supracerebellar
s. approach
supracerebral
supraclavicular approach
supraclinoid aneurysm
supraliminal
supramarginal
s. convolution
s. gyrus
supramaximal stimulus

supranuclear
s. lesion
s. palsy
s. paralysis
supraoptic
s. commissures
s. nucleus
supraopticohypophysial tract
supraorbital
s. nerve
s. neuralgia
s. pericranial flap
s. reflex
s. ridge
s. rim
supraorbital-pterional approach
suprapatellar reflex
suprapineal recess
suprascapular nerve
suprasellar
s. cistern
s. cyst
suprasylvian
supratentorial
s. approach
s. brain
s. glioma
s. lesion
s. primitive neuroectodermal
tumor
s. tumor
supraumbilical reflex
sural
s. nerve
s. nerve bridge graft
s. nerve cable graft
surface
s. coil
s. coil array
inferior s. of cerebellar
hemisphere

NOTES

surface *(continued)*
    s. landmark
    medial s. of cerebral
      hemisphere
    superior s. of cerebellar
      hemisphere
    superolateral s. of cerebrum
surgery
    adult scoliosis s.
    anterior cervical s.
    anterior cervical spine s.
    anterior cervicothoracic s.
    anterior cervicothoracic
      junction s.
    anterior lower cervical
      spine s.
    cervical decompression s.
    cervicothoracic junction s.
    computer-assisted
      stereotactic s. (CASS)
    coronary bypass s.
    craniofacial s.
    cytoreductive s.
    decompressive s.
    DREZ s.
    ECA-PCA bypass s.
    endoscopic sinus s.
    epilepsy s.
    extracranial-intracranial
      bypass s.
    hypotensive s.
    intradural tumor s.
    intraorbital s.
    laser s.
    lower posterior lumbar
      spine and sacrum s.
    nasal s.
    posterior cervical spine s.
    posterior lower cervical
      spine s.
    posterior lumbar interbody
      fusion s.
    posterior lumbar spine and
      sacrum s.
    posterior upper cervical
      spine s.
    resective s.
    stereotactic s., stereotaxic s.
    stereotaxic s.
    thoracic and thoracolumbar
      spine s.
    transsphenoidal s.
    vascular s.

surgical
    s. anatomy
    s. correction
    s. decompression
    s. dressing
    s. exposure
    s. microscope
    s. resection
    s. seeding
    s. technique
Surgicel
susceptibility
    s. agent
    s. effect
    magnetic s.
suspension
    Alksne's iron s.
    magnesium hydroxide s.
    penicillin G benzathine s.
Sustacal
sustentacular fibers of retina
suture
    American silk s.'s
    s. clamp
    cranial s.
    metopic s.
    nerve s.
    nylon s.
    Prolene s.
    retracting s.
    tacking s.
    tension s.
suturectomy
swallowing
    s. disorder
    s. reflex
swan
    s. neck deformity
    s. neck deformity reduction
Swan-Ganz catheter
sweating test
Swedish Gamma Knife group
swelled head
swelling
    brain s.
    Spielmeyer's acute s.
Swiftl scanner
swimer's view
Sydenham's
    S. chorea
    S. disease
syllabic speech

sylvian
    s. angle
    s. approach
    s. aqueduct
    s. dissection
    s. fissure
    s. hematoma
    s. line
    s. point
    s. seizure
    s. ventricle
Sylvius
    aqueduct of S.
symbolia
Symmetrel
symmetrical
    s. sacral plate
    s. thoracic vertebral plate
symmetric distal neuropathy
symmetry
    Hermetian s.
sympathectomy, sympathetectomy
    cervical perivascular s.
    chemical s.
    s. effect
    Leriche s.
    lumbar s.
    periarterial s.
    presacral s.
    Smithwick s.
    visceral s.
sympathetic
    s. ganglia
    s. hypertonia
    s. imbalance
    s. iridoplegia
    s. nerve
    s. nervous system
    s. part
    s. plexuses
    s. reflex dystrophy

    s. segment
    s. trunk
sympathetoblastoma
sympathicectomy
sympathicoblastoma
sympathicogonioma
sympathiconeuritis
sympathicopathy
sympathicotonia
sympathicotonic
sympathicotripsy
sympathoblastoma
sympathogonioma
symptom
    Epstein's s.
    Frenkel's s.
    Gordon's s.
    Haenel's s.
    Kerandel's s.
    Macewen's s.
    Romberg-Howship s.
    Romberg's s.
    Trendelenburg's s.
    Wartenberg's s.
symptomatic
    s. epilepsy
    s. headache
    s. impotence
    s. neuralgia
    s. paramyotonia
    s. root
    s. spondylolisthesis
    s. torticollis
synalgia
synalgic
synaphoceptors
synapse, pl. **synapses**
    axoaxonic s.
    axodendritic s.
    axosomatic s.

NOTES

synapse *(continued)*
    electrotonic s.
    pericorpuscular s.
synaptic
    s. boutons
    s. cleft
    s. endings
    s. terminals
    s. trough
    s. vesicles
synaptology
synaptophysin
synaptosome
syncheiria, synchiria
synchondrosis
synchrocyclotron operation
SynchroMed model 8611H
  prototype implantable pump
synchronous reflex
synchrony
    bilateral s.
synclonic spasm
synclonus
syncopal
syncope
    carotid sinus s.
    hysterical s.
    laryngeal s.
    local s.
    micturition s.
    postural s.
    vasovagal s.
syncopic
syndesmosis
syndrome
    acquired hepatocerebral s.
    acquired
      immunodeficiency s.
      (AIDS)
    acroparesthesia s.
    acute disconnection s.
    Adams-Stokes s.
    Adie's s.
    Adie's tonic pupil s.
    adiposogenital s.
    adult respiratory distress s.
      (ARDS)
    Aicardi's s.
    alcohol amnestic s.
    Alice in Wonderland s.
    amnestic s.
    Angelucci's s.
    anterior bulb s.

    anterior chiasmal s.
    anterior compartment s.
    anterior spinal artery s.
    antiphospholipid s.
    Anton's s.
    aortic arch s.
    apallic s.
    Apert's s.
    Arnold-Chiari s.
    auriculotemporal nerve s.
    Avellis' s.
    Babinski-Nageotte s.
    Balint's s.
    Bannayan s.
    Bardet-Biedl s.
    Barlow's s.
    basal cell nevus s.
    basilar artery thrombosis s.
    battered infant s.
    Benedikt's s.
    Bernard-Horner s.
    Bernhardt-Roth s.
    Beuren s.
    Biemond s.
    biopercular s.
    Bonnet-Dechaume-Blanc s.
    Bonnier's s.
    brachial-basilar
      insufficiency s.
    Briquet's s.
    Brissaud's s.
    Brown's s.
    Brown-Séquard's s.
    carotid sinus s.
    carpal tunnel s.
    cataract-oligophrenia s.
    cauda equina s.
    caudal regression s.
    cavernous sinus s.
    central cord s.
    cerebellar s.
    cerebellar hemisphere s.
    cerebellomedullary
      malformation s.
    cerebellopontine angle s.
    cerebrohepatorenal s.
    cervical compression s.
    cervical disk s.
    cervical fusion s.
    cervical rib s.
    cervical tension s.
    Cestan-Chenais s.
    Charcot-Weiss-Baker s.

cherry-red spot
  myoclonus s.
Chiari II s.
chiasma s.
Churg-Strauss s.
Claude's s.
cloverleaf skull s.
Cobb's s.
Cockayne's s.
Cogan's s.
Collet-Sicard s.
compartment s.
compression s.
costoclavicular s.
CREST s.
Crigler-Najjar s.
crocodile tears s.
cubital tunnel s.
Cushing's s.
DaCosta's s.
Dandy-Walker s.
deafferentation pain s.
deficit s.
Dejerine-Roussy s.
Dejerine's anterior bulb s.
de Morsier's s.
De Sanctis-Cacchione s.
dialysis encephalopathy s.
diencephalic s.
diencephalic s. of infancy
disconnection s.
disk s.
Doose s.
dorsal mesencephalic s.
dorsal midbrain s.
dorsomedial
  mesencephalic s.
Down's s.
dry eye s.
Duane's retraction s.
Duchenne's s.

Duncan's s.
dysarthria-clumsy hand s.
dysmnesic s.
Eagle s.
ectopic ACTH s.
effort s.
Ehlers-Danlos s.
Eisenlohr's s.
Ekbom s.
empty sella s.
encephalotrigeminal
  vascular s.
episodic s.
extrapyramidal s.
facet s.
Fahr's s.
failed back s.
failed back surgery s.
  (FBSS)
Fanconi's s.
Felty's s.
Figueira's s.
Fisher's s.
flashing pain s.
flat back s.
Flynn-Aird s.
Foix-Alajouanine s.
Foix's s.
Foster Kennedy s.
Foville's s.
Frey's s.
Fröhlich's s.
Froin's s.
frontal lobe s.
Garcin's s.
Gélineau's s.
general-adaptation s.
Gerstmann's s.
Gerstmann-Sträussler s.
Gilles de la Tourette's s.
Gorlin's s.

NOTES

syndrome *(continued)*
  Gowers' s.
  Gradenigo's s.
  Gubler's s.
  Guillain-Barré s.
  Gunn's s.
  gustatory sweating s.
  Hakim's s.
  Hallervorden-Spatz s.,
    Hallervorden s.
  happy puppet s.
  head-bobbing doll s.
  hemispheric disconnection s.
  Herrmann's s.
  Holmes-Adie s.
  Horner's s.
  Hunt's s.
  hyperabduction s.
  hyperkinetic s.
  hyperperfusion s.
  hypertrophied frenula s.
  hypokinetic s.
  hypophysial s.
  hypophysio-sphenoidal s.
  iliac crest s.
  s. of inappropriate
    antidiuretic hormone
    secretion
  s. of inappropriate secretion
    of antidiuretic hormone
    (SIADH)
  indifference to pain s.
  intermediolateral
    mesencephalic s.
  internal capsule s.
  inverse Anton's s.
  inversed jaw-winking s.
  Jahnke's s.
  jaw-winking s.
  Joubert's s.
  jugular foramen s.
  Kallmann's s.
  Kasabach-Merritt s.
  Kearns-Sayre s.
  Kennedy's s.
  Kiloh-Nevin s.
  Klippel-Feil s.
  Klippel-Trenaunay s.
  Klippel-Trenaunay-Weber s.
  Klumpke-Dejerine s.
  Klüver-Bucy s.
  Koerber-Salus-Elschnig s.
  Korsakoff's s.

  Krabbe's s.
  Labbé's neurocirculatory s.
  labyrinthine concussion s.
  Landau-Kleffner s.
  Landry s.
  Landry-Guillain-Barré s.
  lateral inferior pontine s.
  lateral medullary s.
  lateral superior pontine s.
  Laurence-Biedl s.
  Laurence-Moon s.
  Laurence-Moon-Bardet-
    Biedl s.
  Lawford's s.
  Leigh's s.
  Lennox-Gastaut s.,
    Lennox s.
  Leriche's s.
  Lesch-Nyhan s.
  lissencephalic s.
  locked-in s.
  loculation s.
  Louis-Bar s.
  lower motor neuron s.
  lumbar flat back s.
  Mad Hatter s.
  Maffucci's s.
  Magendie-Hertwig s.
  MAGIC s.
  Marcus Gunn s.
  Marfan's s.
  Marinesco-Garland s.
  Marinesco-Sjögren s.
  May-White s.
  medial inferior pontine s.
  medial medullary s.
  medial midpontine s.
  medial pontine s.
  medial superior pontine s.
  Meige s.
  MELAS s.
  Melkersson-Rosenthal s.
  Ménière's s.
  Menkes' s.
  Menkes' kinky hair s.
  MERRLA s.
  midline s.
  Millard-Gubler s.
  Miller-Dieker s.
  Milles' s.
  Möbius' s.
  Monakow's s.
  Morgagni-Adams-Stokes s.

Morgagni's s.
morning glory s.
Morquio's s.
multiple mucosal
  neuroma s.
myasthenic s.
myelopathy s.
myofascial s.
Naffziger s.
narcolepsy-cataplexy s.
Nelson's s.
neural crest s.
neurocutaneous s.
neuroleptic malignant s.
neuromusculoskeletal s.
Nothnagel's s.
ocular ischemic s.
Oden's s.
one-and-a-half s.
Oppenheim's s.
optic chiasmal s.
opticocerebral s.
opticopyramidal s.
optic tract s.
orbital apex s.
organic brain s. (OBS)
organic mental s. (OMS)
osmotic demyelination s.
overdrainage s.
paleostriatal s.
pallidal s.
Pancoast's s.
paramedian mesencephalic s.
paramedian pontine s.
paraneoplastic s.
parietal lobe s.
Parinaud's s.
Parsonage-Aldren-Turner s.
Parsonage-Turner s.
Pepper s.
Petit's s.

Pfeiffer's s.
Pick's s.
piriformis s.
postadrenalectomy s.
postconcussion s.
postconcussional s.
posterior fossa s.
posterior inferior cerebellar
  artery s.
posterior joint s.
postlaminectomy s.
postpartum pituitary
  necrosis s.
posttraumatic s.
posttraumatic chronic
  cord s.
posttraumatic neck s.
Pourfour du Petit's s.
premotor s.
pretectal s.
pronator teres s.
punchdrunk s.
Putnam-Dana s.
s. of the pyramid
radicular s.
radiculomedullary s.
Raeder's paratrigeminal s.
Ramsay Hunt s.
Raymond-Cestan s.
Raymond's s.
red man s.
red neck s.
Refsum's s.
Reichert-Mundinger s.
Reiter's s.
restless legs s.
Rett's s.
Reye's s.
Richards-Rundle s.
Riley-Day s.
Romano-Ward s.

NOTES

syndrome *(continued)*
    Romberg's s.
    rostral basilar artery s.
    Roussy-Lévy s.
    Russell's s.
    Saethre-Chotzen s.
    scalenus anterior s.
    Schirmer's s.
    Schmidt's s.
    Schmidt's vagoaccessory s.
    Schüller-Christian s.
    sciatic notch s.
    Sheehan's s.
    shoulder-girdle s.
    shoulder-hand s.
    Shy-Drager s.
    sick sinus s.
    Sjögren's s.
    slit-ventricle s.
    Sneddon's s.
    somnolence s.
    Sotos s.
    Spens' s.
    sphenocavernous s.
    split brain s.
    split notochord s.
    Steele-Richardson-
      Olszewski s.
    Stevens-Johnson s.
    Stewart-Morel s.
    sticky platelet s.
    stiff-man s.
    Stokes-Adams s.
    stroke s.
    stump embolization s.
    Sturge-Kalischer-Weber s.
    Sturge-Weber s.
    subclavian steal s.
    Sudeck's s.
    superior cerebellar artery s.
    superior mesenteric artery s.
    superior oblique tendon
      sheath s.
    superior vena cava s.
    Tapia's s.
    tarsal tunnel s.
    tegmental s.
    Terson's s.
    tethered cord s.
    tethered spinal cord s.
    thalamic s.
    thyrohypophysial s.
    tight filum terminale s.
    Tolosa-Hunt s.
    top of the basilar s.
    Torré's s.
    Torsten Sjögren's s.
    Tourette's s.
    toxic shock s.
    trapped ventricle s.
    s. of the trephined
    triangular s.
    trisomy 21 s.
    Trousseau's s.
    Turcot's s.
    Unverricht-Lundborg s.
    vagoaccessory s.
    vasovagal s.
    ventral medial
      mesencephalic s.
    Vernet's s.
    very low-density s.
    vibration s.
    Villaret's s.
    Vogt s.
    von Hippel-Lindau s.
    Wallenberg's s.
    Warburg s.
    Waring blender s.
    Weber-Leyden s.
    Weber's s.
    Wernicke-Korsakoff s.
    Wernicke's s.
    West's s.
    Wilson's s.
    Wyburn-Mason s.
    X-linked
      lymphoproliferative s.
    Zellweger's s.
synencephalocele
synergic control
synesthesia
    s. algica
    auditory s.
synesthesialgia
synkinesis
synostosis
    coronal s.
    metopic s.
    tribasilar s.
synovial cyst
synovitis
syntactical aphasia
Synthes guide pin
synthesis
    Fourier s.

Synthroid
syphilis
    meningovascular s.
syphilitic meningoencephalitis
Syracuse
    S. anterior I-plate
    S. anterior I-plate insertion
syringeal
syringe grip
syringes (*pl. of* syrinx)
syringobulbia
syringocele
syringocisternostomy
syringocystadenoma
syringoencephalomyelia
syringohydromyelia
syringoid
syringomeningocele
syringomyelia
    secondary post-traumatic s.
syringomyelic
    s. dissociation
    s. hemorrhage
syringomyelocele
syringomyelomeningocele
syringomyelus
syringoperitoneal shunt
syringopontia
syringosubarachnoid shunt
syrinx, pl. syringes
    s. shunt
system
    angiographic reference s.
    (ARS)
    Anspach 65K
    instrument s.'s
    Anspach 65K neuro s.
    anterior Kostuik-Harrington
    distraction s.
    arc-centered guidance s.
    arc-quadrant stereotactic s.

arc radius s.
association s.
autonomic nervous s.
bilateral variable screw
    placement s.
Brown-Roberts-Wells arc s.
Bruker Biospec s.
Budde halo retractor s.
Budde surgical s.
bulbosacral s.
CASS whole brain
    mapping s.
central nervous s. (CNS)
cerebrospinal s.
Codman neurological
    headrest s.
COMPASS arc-quadrant
    stereotactic s.
COMPASS stereotactic s.
computer-controlled
    neurological stimulation s.
Cosman-Roberts-Wells
    stereotactic s.
Cotrel-Dubousset
    distraction s.
Cotrel-Dubousset screw-
    rod s.
cranial osteosynthesis s.
craniosacral s.
CRW s.
CRW arc s.
CUSA CEM s.
data acquisition s.
Dingman oral retraction s.
double-pore vent s.
Edwards modular s.
endocrine s.
Epstein's staging s.
esthesiodic s.
exterofective s.
extrapyramidal motor s.

NOTES

system *(continued)*
feedback s.
F.L. Fischer modular
stereotaxy s.
fluoroptic thermometry s.
gamma efferent s.
gamma motor s.
GE 9800 CT s.
Greenberg retracting s.
Haid universal bone
plate s.
halo retractor s.
Harrington rod and hook s.
Hematome s.
high-force Sundt clip s.
high-resolution brain
SPECT s.
hypothalamohypophysial
portal s.
immune s.
internal fixation plate-
screw s.
interofective s.
involuntary nervous s.
Isola spinal implant s.
isolated granulomatous
angiitis of the central
nervous s. (GANS)
Kelly stereotactic s.
Kostuik-Harrington
distraction s.
Ladd fiberoptic s.
LDD delivery s.
Leibinger titanium mini-
Würzburg implant s.
Leksell Micro-Stereotactic s.
limbic s.
LINAC s.
    linear accelerator system
LINAC-based
radiosurgical s.
linear accelerator s. (LINAC
system)
Lorenz 1 mm micro
osteosynthesis s.
Magerl s.
Magerl hook-plate s.
Magerl plate-screw s.
Malis CMC-III
electrosurgical s.
Mayfield headrest s.
Mayfield surgical s.
metameric nervous s.

microcatheter s.
Micro-Plus titanium
plating s.
Midas Rex
instrumentation s.
Midas Rex power s.
Mini Würzburg implant s.
Moe s.
nervous s.
NEUROVIEW integrated
visualization s.
Nicolet Viking II
electrophysiologic s.
nonspecific s.
oculomotor s.
parasympathetic nervous s.
Patil stereotactic s. II
pedal s.
Pelorus surgical s.
peripheral nervous s.
phased-array color-flow
ultrasound s.
Phoenix fifth ventricle s.
polar coordinate s.
posterior rod s.
pressoreceptor s.
projection s.
Puno-Winter-Byrd s.
reticular activating s. (RAS)
Rogozinski spinal rod s.
Secor s.
Sentinel s.
Shiley catheter distention s.
Simmons plating s.
somesthetic s.
Songer cable s.
Spetzler s.
Steffee pedicle screw-plate s.
Sundt AVM micro clip s.
sympathetic nervous s.
Talairach s.
Talairach stereotactic s.
Texas Scottish Rite Hospital
cross-link s.
Texas Scottish Rite Hospital
screw-rod s.
thoracolumbar s.
thoracolumbosacroiliac
implant s.
TSRH universal spinal
instrumentation s.
unilateral variable screw
placement s.

variable screw placement s.
vegetative nervous s.
venous s.
vertebrobasilar s.
vestibular s.
visceral nervous s.
Wiltse s.
Würzburg implant s.
ZD stereotactic s.
Zeiss OPMI CS-NC2
  surgical microscope s.

systema
  s. nervosum
  s. nervosum autonomicum
  s. nervosum centrale
  s. nervosum periphericum
systematic vertigo
systemic
  s. lupus erythematosus
    (SLE)
  s. myelitis
  s. sclerosis

NOTES

T1

    T1 relaxation
    T1 weighting

T2

    T2 relaxation
    T2 relaxation rate
    T2 shortening
    T2 weighting

T11-L5 thoracolumbar burst fracture

T12-L1 fracture-dislocation reduction

T8-L3 thoracolumbar burst fracture

tabes

    t. diabetica
    t. dorsalis
    t. ergotica
    peripheral t.
    t. spasmodica
    t. spinalis

tabetic

    t. arthropathy
    t. crisis
    t. cuirass
    t. dissociation

tabetiform

tabic

tabid

table

    American Sterilizer operating t.
    American Sterilizer operating room t.

tablet

    Koala Pad graphics t.

taboparesis

tache

    t. cérébrale
    t. méningéale
    t. spinale

tachycardia

tacking suture

tactile

    t. agnosia
    t. anesthesia
    t. anomia
    t. corpuscle
    t. disk
    t. hyperesthesia
    t. image

    t. meniscus
    t. sense
    t. transfer deficit

taction

tactometer

tactor

tactual

Taenia solium

Tagamet

tail

    t. of caudate nucleus
    t. of dentate gyrus
    dural t.

tailor's

    t. cramp
    t. spasm

Takayasu's

    T. arteritis
    T. disease

Talairach

    T. stereotactic frame
    T. stereotactic system
    T. system
    T. whole brain mapping

talc

talipes

    t. spasmodicus

Talma's disease

Talwin

tamoxifen

tamp

    Richards t.

tampon

    Merocel t.

Tanacetum parthenium

tanate

    pitressin t.

tandem

    t. clipping technique
    t. connectors

tangent screen examination

tangle

    neurofibrillary t.

tannate

    vasopressin t.

Tantalum

    T. cranioplasty
    T. mesh

tanycyte

tap
- heel t.
- shunt t.
- spinal t.
- subdural t.

tape
- merceline t.

tapered
- t. blade
- t. brain spatula

tapetum, pl. **tapeta**
- t. nigrum
- t. oculi

tapeworm

Tapia's
- T. syndrome
- T. vagohypoglossal palsy

tapir mouth

tardive
- t. dyskinesia
- t. oral dyskinesia

tardy epilepsy

target
- t. acquisition
- brain t.
- t. localization

targeting
- multiple t.

targetry
- angiographic t.

Tarin's
- T. space
- T. tenia
- T. valve

Tarlov's cyst

tarsal
- t. tunnel
- t. tunnel syndrome

tarsophalangeal reflex

tarsorrhaphy
- bilateral temporary t.
- lateral t.

tartrate
- ergotamine t.
- levallorphan t.
- metoprolol t.

taste
- after-t.
- t. blindness
- t. cells
- color t.
- t. disorder

tattoo
- facial t.

tautomeric
- t. fibers

Taylor retractor

Tay-Sachs disease

Tc
- technetium

^{99m}Tc
- ^{99m}technetium
- technetium-99m
  - ^{99m}Tc HMPAO SPECT
  - ^{99m}Tc HMPAO T/C ratio

Tc-99m HMPAO cerebral perfusion SPECT imaging

TCCS
- transcranial color-coded real-time sonography

TCD
- transcranial Doppler sonography
- transcranial Doppler ultrasound
  - TCD pulsatility index
  - TCD recanalization

TCDB
- Traumatic Coma Data Bank

^{99m}Tc-hexamethylpropyleneamine oxime (^{99m}Tc-HMPAO)

^{99m}Tc-HMPAO
- ^{99m}Tc-hexamethylpropyleneamine oxime
  - ^{99m}Tc-HMPAO leukocyte scintigram
  - ^{99m}Tc-HMPAO leukocyte scintigraphy
  - ^{99m}Tc-HMPAO SPECT imaging

T:C ratio

TE
- echo time

Te
- tellurium

tear
- intraoperative dural t.

teardrop
- t. dissector
- t. fracture

technetium (Tc)

^{99m}technetium (^{99m}Tc)

technetium-99m (^{99m}Tc)

technique
- angiographic road-mapping t.

Barbour t.
Brooks t.
carotid preservation t.
cervical screw insertion t.
cervical spondylotic
  myelopathy fusion t.
Cloward t.
Cobb t.
composite addition t.
continuous-wave t.
contoured anterior spinal
  plate t.
decortication t.
destructive interference t.
Dolenc t.
double-rod t.
Drake's tandem clipping t.
drilling t.
Drummond's spinous
  wiring t.
endovascular t.
facet excision t.
fat-suppression t.
finger fracture t.
fixation t.
Flamm's t.
flow detection t.
Fourier transform t.
fusion t.
Gallie t.
Gallie wiring t.
Håkanson's t.
Harriluque t.
Hartel t.
Hunt-Early t.
immunoelectrotransfer
  blot t.
interspinous segmental
  spinal instrumentation t.
intravenous oxygen-15 water
  bolus t.

Jacobs locking hook spinal
  rod t.
Lamaze t.
Leksell t.
Luque instrumentation
  concave t.
Luque instrumentation
  convex t.
Luque sublaminar wiring t.
macroelectrode t.
mandibular swing t.
midface degloving t.
Mille Pattes t.
operative t.
posterolateral
  costotransversectomy t.
preservation t.
recombinant DNA t.
reduction t.
Roy-Camille t.
screw insertion t.
Seldinger t.
Seldinger retrograde
  wire/intubation t.
sling/wrapping t.
Smith-Robinson t.
Spiller-Frazier t.
spinal fusion t.
strut fusion t.
subtraction t.
surgical t.
tandem clipping t.
thoracolumbar spondylosis
  surgical t.
time-of-flight t.
triple-wire t.
wire removal t.
^{133}Xe intravenous
  injection t.
tecta (*pl. of* tectum)
tectal glioma

NOTES

tectobulbar tract
tectopontine tract
tectospinal
    t. decussation
    t. tract
tectum, pl. tecta
    t. mesencephali
Teflon
    T. felt
    T. liner
    T. tube graft
tegmen, gen. tegminis, pl. tegmina
    t. cruris
    t. ventriculi quarti
tegmenta (pl. of tegmentum)
tegmental
    t. decussations
    t. fields of Forel
    t. syndrome
tegmentotomy
tegmentum, pl. tegmenta
    t. mesencephali
    mesencephalic t.
    midbrain t.
    t. of pons
    pontine t.
    t. rhombencephali
    t. of rhombencephalon
tegmina (pl. of tegmen)
tegminis (gen. of tegmen)
Tegopen
Tegretol
teichopsia
tela, gen. and pl. telae
    t. choroidea
    t. choroidea inferior
    t. choroidea superior
    t. choroidea ventriculi
      quarti
    t. choroidea ventriculi tertii
    choroid t. of fourth
      ventricle
    choroid t. of third ventricle
    t. vasculosa
telalgia
telangiectasia
    ataxia t.
    capillary t.
    cephalo-oculocutaneous t.
    hereditary hemorrhagic t.
telangiectasis, pl. telangiectases

telangiectatic
    t. angiomatosis
    t. glioma
telencephalic
    t. flexure
    t. vein
    t. ventriculofugal artery
    t. vesicle
telencephalization
telencephalon
teleopsia
teleradiotherapy unit
telergy
TeleSensor
    Cosman T.
teletactor
televised
    t. radiofluoroscopic control
    t. radiofluoroscopy
Telfa strip
tellurium (Te)
telodendron
temperature
    t. sense
    t. spot
template
    Marchac forehead t.
temporal
    t. arteritis
    t. artery
    t. bone
    t. cortex
    t. fossa
    t. horn
    t. lobe
    t. lobectomy
    t. lobe epilepsy
    t. lobe radiation
    t. lobe retraction
    t. pole
    t. retraction
    t. stability
temporal-cerebral arterial
    anastomosis
temporary clip
temporofrontal tract
temporomandibular
    t. joint
    t. joint dislocation
temporopontine
    t. tract
tender
    t. lines

t. points
t. zones
tenderness
scalp t.
tendineus
annulus t.
tendo Achillis reflex
tendon reflex
tenia, pl. teniae
teniae acusticae
t. choroidea
t. fimbriae
t. fornicis
t. of the fornix
t. of fourth ventricle
t. hippocampi
medullary teniae
t. semicircularis
Tarin's t.
t. tecta
t. telae
t. terminalis
t. thalami
thalamic t.
t. ventriculi quarti
t. ventriculi tertii
teniola
t. corporis callosi
tenosynovectomy
tensile stress
Tensilon test
tension
t. headache
oxygen t.
t. pneumocephalus
t. suture
tenth cranial nerve
tentorial
t. angle
t. apex meningioma
t. herniation

t. incisura
t. leaf meningioma
t. plexus
t. pressure
t. ring
t. sinus
t. traversal
tentorium, pl. tentoria
t. cerebelli
t. of hypophysis
tephromalacia
tephrylometer
teratogen
teratoma
malignant t.
sacrococcygeal t.
terebrant, terebrating
terebration
teres major muscle
terminal
axon t.'s
t. boutons
t. filum
t. ganglion
t. myelocystocele
t. nerve corpuscles
t. nuclei
t. plate
t. stria
synaptic t.'s
t. thread
t. vein
t. ventricle
t. ventriculostomy
terminale
filum t.
terminalis
primitive lamina t.
ventriculus t.
terminatio, pl. terminationes

NOTES

terminatio *(continued)*
    terminationes nervorum
      liberae
terminationes
Terson's syndrome
tesla
Tessier osteotomy
Test
    California Verbal
      Learning T.
    Fused Rhymed Dichotic
      Words T.
    Maudsley Mentation T.
      (MaMT)
    Wisconsin Card Solving T.
test
    air conduction t.
    Alcock's t.
    Allen's t.
    balloon occlusion t.
    Bielschowsky head tilt t.
    Binet t.
    blood t.
    bromocriptine t.
    caloric t.
    cardiac function t.
    CO_2-withdrawal seizure t.
    C-reactive protein t.
    dexamethasone
      suppression t.
    Dix-Hallpike t.
    edrophonium chloride t.
    excitability t.
    finger-nose t.
    finger-to-finger t.
    Fisher's exact t.
    Goldscheider's t.
    Hallpike t.
    head-dropping t.
    heel-tap t.
    Hendler t.
    Hirschberg t.
    Hollander t.
    hyperventilation t.
    insulin hypoglycemia t.
    internal carotid balloon t.
    Janet's t.
    Jolly t.
    Katzman t.
    Kernig t.
    Krimsky t.
    labyrinthine fistula t.
    Lasègue's t.

    leg-raising t.
    lidocaine t.
    Matas' t.
    metyrapone t.
    Naffziger's t.
    neostigmine t.
    neuropsychological t.
    oculocephalic t.
    Pachon's t.
    palmomental t.
    Patrick's t.
    Phalen's t.
    Prostigmin t.
    Queckenstedt t.
    Queckenstedt-Stookey t.
    Rinne t.
    Romberg t.
    Schirmer t.
    Schlichter t.
    Schwabach t.
    station t.
    straight leg raising t.
    sweating t.
    Tensilon t.
    Wada t.
    Weber t.
testing
    Amsler grid t.
    biomechanical t.
    conduction t.
    confrontation t.
    Diamox challenge t.
    electrodiagnostic t.
    intra-arterial Amytal t.
    intracarotid sodium Amytal
      memory t.
    provocative t.
testis, pl. **testes**
    irritable t.
testosterone enanthate
tetania
    t. epidemica
    t. gastrica
    t. gravidarum
    t. neonatorum
    t. parathyreopriva
    t. rheumatica
tetanic
    t. contraction
    t. convulsion
tetaniform
tetanigenous
tetanilla

tetanism
tetanization
tetanize
tetanode
tetanoid
    t. chorea
    t. paraplegia
tetanometer
tetanomotor
tetanus
    t. anticus
    apyretic t.
    benign t.
    cephalic t.
    cerebral t.
    t. completus
    t. dorsalis
    drug t.
    extensor t.
    flexor t.
    generalized t.
    head t.
    hydrophobic t.
    imitative t.
    intermittent t.
    local t.
    t. neonatorum
    t. posticus
    Ritter's opening t.
    Rose's cephalic t.
    toxic t.
    t. toxoid
    traumatic t.
tetany
    t. of alkalosis
    duration t. (DT)
    epidemic t.
    gastric t.
    hyperventilation t.
    hypoparathyroid t.
    infantile t.

    latent t.
    manifest t.
    neonatal t.
    parathyroid t.
    parathyroprival t.
    postoperative t.
    rheumatic t.
tethered
    t. cord syndrome
    t. spinal cord
    t. spinal cord syndrome
tethering
tetrabenazine
tetracaine
tetracycline
tetrad
    narcoleptic t.
tetraparesis
tetraplegia
tetraplegic
Texas Scottish Rite Hospital (TSRH)
    TSRH Scottish Rite Hospital corkscrew device
    TSRH Scottish Rite Hospital crosslink
    TSRH Scottish Rite Hospital cross-link system
    TSRH Scottish Rite Hospital eyebolt spreader
    TSRH Scottish Rite Hospital hook
    TSRH Scottish Rite Hospital hook holder
    TSRH Scottish Rite Hospital hook inserter
    TSRH Scottish Rite Hospital l-bolt
    TSRH Scottish Rite Hospital mini-corkscrew device

NOTES

Texas Scottish Rite Hospital
(continued)
  TSRH Scottish Rite
    Hospital pedicle screw
  TSRH Scottish Rite
    Hospital rod fixation
  TSRH Scottish Rite
    Hospital screw
  TSRH Scottish Rite
    Hospital screw-rod system
  TSRH Scottish Rite
    Hospital trial hook
  TSRH Scottish Rite
    Hospital wrench
text blindness
6TG
  6-thioguanine
thalamectomy
thalamencephalic
thalamencephalon
thalami (*pl. of* thalamus)
thalamic
  t. aphasia
  t. astrocytoma
  t. circulation
  t. glioma
  t. gustatory nucleus
  t. syndrome
  t. tenia
thalamic-subthalamic hemorrhage
thalamocaudate arteriovenous
  malformation
thalamocortical
thalamostriate
  t. veins
thalamotomy
  gamma t.
  staged bilateral
    stereotactic t.
  stereotactic t.
  stereotactic VIM t.
  stereotactic VL t.
  Vim t.
  VL t.
thalamus, pl. **thalami**
thallium-201 (^{201}Tl)
T-handled
  T-h. bone awl
  T-h. Jacob's chuck
  T-h. nut wrench
  T-h. screw wrench

Thane's method
theca, pl. **thecae**
  t. vertebralis
thecal sac compression
thecoperitoneal Pudenz-Schulte
  shunt
thematic paraphasia
thenar eminence
theophylamine
theophylline
theory
  Burn and Rand t.
  decision t.
  flow t.
  gate-control t.
  injury-healing t.
  mass action t.
  McLone and Knepper
    etiological t.
  mnemic t.
  relaxation t.
  Semon-Hering t.
  spreading cortical
    depression t.
  vasogenic t.
  Wolff vasogenic t.
  Wollaston's t.
therapeutic
  t. embolism
  t. embolization
  t. malaria
Therapeutic Intervention Scoring
  System
therapy
  adjuvant t.
  adjuvant whole-brain
    radiation t.
  anticoagulation t.
  anticonvulsant t.
  antifibrinolytic t.
  antimigraine t.
  antiplatelet t.
  Bragg peak proton beam t.
  electrotherapeutic sleep t.
  endovascular t.
  focused radiation t.
  gene t.
  immunosuppressive t.
  multimodal adjuvant t.
  oxygen t.
  photoradiation t.
  radiation t.
  reflex t.

stereotactic-assisted
radiation t. (START)
stereotactic focused-
radiation t.
stereotactic radiation t.
(StaRT)
thrombolytic t.
transvenous t.
ultrasonic t.
whole brain radiation t.
(WBRT)
thermal
t. anesthesia
t. blanket
t. rhizotomy
t. sense
thermalgesia
thermalgia
thermanalgesia
thermanesthesia
thermesthesia
thermesthesiometer
thermic
t. anesthesia
t. sense
Thermistor needle
thermoalgesia
thermoanalgesia
thermoanesthesia
thermocoagulation
radiofrequency t.
thermocouple
copper-constantan t.
thermoesthesia
thermoesthesiometer
thermography
thermohyperalgesia
thermohyperesthesia
thermohypesthesia
thermohypoesthesia
thermorhizotomy

theta
t. rhythm
t. wave
thiabendazole
thiamylal
thiazide
thickening
hyaline t.
thickness
lumbosacral junction
cortical t.
thigh
driver's t.
Heilbronner's t.
**thigh-high alternating compression
air boots**
thigmesthesia
**thin-layer agarose gel
electrophoresis**
thin-section image
6-thioguanine (6TG)
thiopental
t. sodium
thioridazine
thiothixene
third
t. cranial nerve
t. nerve avulsion
t. nerve palsy
t. temporal convolution
t. ventricle
t. ventricular
hemangioblastoma
t. ventriculostomy
third-generation cephalosporin
Thomsen's disease
thoracic
t. curve scoliosis
t. discectomy
t. disk herniation
t. duct injury

NOTES

thoracic *(continued)*
    t. ganglia
    t. hypokyphosis
    t. interspace
    t. kyphosis
    t. meningioma
    t. nerve
    t. nucleus
    t. outlet
    t. pedicle
    t. pedicle marker
    t. spinal fusion
    t. spine
    t. spine biopsy
    t. spine decompression
    t. spine fracture
    t. spine kyphotic deformity
    t. spine lordosis
    t. spine pedicle diameter
    t. spine scoliotic deformity
    t. spine vertebral
    osteosynthesis
    t. and thoracolumbar spine
    surgery
    t. vertebra
thoracoabdominal approach
thoracolumbar
    t. burst fracture
    t. curve
    t. degenerative disease
    t. fracture
    t. idiopathic scoliosis
    t. junction
    t. junction surgical exposure
    t. kyphoscoliosis
    t. kyphosis
    t. pedicle screw
    t. retroperitoneal approach
    t. scoliosis
    t. spinal canal stenosis
    t. spinal injury
    t. spine
    t. spine anterior exposure
    t. spine decompression
    t. spine flexion-distraction
    injury
    t. spine fracture-dislocation
    t. spine scoliosis
    t. spine stabilization
    t. spine vertebral
    osteosynthesis
    t. spondylosis

    t. spondylosis surgical
    technique
    t. standing orthosis
    t. system
    t. trauma
    t. vertebra
thoracolumbosacral
    t. orthosis (TLSO)
    t. plate
thoracolumbosacroiliac implant
  system
thoracostomy
thoracotomy
    left-sided t.
    right-sided t.
    standard t.
Thorazine
thorn
    dendritic t.'s
thread
    polyene t.
    terminal t.
three-column
    t.-c. cervical spine injury
    t.-c. concept
three-dimensional (3-D)
    t.-d. analysis
    t.-d. fast low-angle shot
    imaging
    t.-d. Fourier transform
    (3DFT)
    t.-d. Fourier transform
    gradient-echo imaging
    t.-d. imaging
    t.-d. neuroimaging
    t.-d. reconstruction
    t.-d. SPECT phantom
three-point bending moment
threshold
    absolute t.
    t. of consciousness
    convulsant t.
    differential t.
    t. differential
    double-point t.
    pain t.
    relational t.
    signal-to-noise t.
    speech reception t. (SRT)
    stimulus t.
    t. stimulus
throat pain

thrombin
    topical t.
Thrombinar
thromboangiitis obliterans
thrombocythemia
thrombocytosis
thromboembolectomy
Thrombogen
thrombogenic
    t. coils
    t. ferrous mixture
thrombolysis
thrombolytic therapy
thrombophlebitis
thromboplastin
    plasma t.
thrombosed giant vertebral artery
  aneurysm
thrombosis, pl. thromboses
    cavernous sinus t.
    cerebral t.
    iliofemoral t.
    septic t.
    wire t.
Thrombostat
thrombotic
    t. apoplexy
    t. hydrocephalus
    t. thrombocytopenic purpura
Thromboxane AZ
thumbprinting appearance
thumb reflex
Thypinone
thyroglobulin
thyrohypophysial syndrome
thyroid
    t. cartilage
    desiccated t.
    t. gland
    t. orbitopathy
thyroid-stimulating hormone (TSH)

thyrotoxic
    t. coma
    t. encephalopathy
thyrotroph cell
thyrotropin
thyrotropin-producing adenoma
thyrotropin-releasing hormone
thyroxine
Thytropar
^{201}TI
TIA
    transient ischemic attack
tibial
    t. nerve
    t. phenomenon
tic
    convulsive t.
    t. douloureux
    facial t.
    glossopharyngeal t.
    habit t.
    local t.
    mimic t.
    psychic t.
    rotatory t.
    spasmodic t.
ticarcillin
tick-borne
    t.-b. encephalitis (Central
      European subtype)
    t.-b. encephalitis (Eastern
      subtype)
tickling
tick paralysis
ticlopidine hydrochloride
Tiedmann rongeur
Tigan
tight
    t. brain
    t. filum terminale syndrome
tigretier

NOTES

tigroid
  t. bodies
  t. substance
tigrolysis
TIL
  tumor-infiltrating lymphocytes
tile plate facet replacement
tilting
  t. of images
  t. of visual images
time
  biologic t.
  bleeding t.
  central somatosensory
    conduction t. (CSCT)
  correlation t.
  echo t. (TE)
  inertia t.
  interhemispheric
    propagation t.
  long pulse repetition t.
  long pulse repetition
    time/long echo t.
  prothrombin t. (PT)
  proton relaxation t.
  pulse repetition t.
  reaction t.
  recognition t.
  relaxation t.
  scan t.
  t. sense
  short pulse repetition t.
  short pulse repetition
    time/echo t.
  short pulse repetition
    time/short echo t.
time-of-flight
  t.-o.-f. effect
  t.-o.-f. technique
timing of decompression
timolol maleate
Tinel's sign
tingle
tingling
tinnitus
tip
  forceps t.
  Frazier suction t.
  Japanese suction t.
  multipore suction t.
  t. of posterior horn
  slotted suction t.
tirilazad

tissue
  t. culture flask
  t. fibrin sealant
  t. forceps
  t. magnetic susceptibility
    artifact
  t. plane dissector
  t. plasminogen activator
  t. respiration
  t. transplantation
  t. welding
tissue-plasminogen activator
titanium
  t. micro mesh
  t. mini burr hole covering
  t. plate
titillation
titubation
^{201}Tl
  thallium-201
    ^{201}Tl chloride
    ^{201}Tl scintigraphy
    ^{201}Tl SPECT
TLSO
  thoracolumbosacral orthosis
tobramycin
  t. sulfate
tocopherol
Todd's
  T. paralysis
  T. postepileptic paralysis
toe
  t. clonus
  t. phenomenon
  t. reflex
toe-drop
Tofranil
tolazamide
tolbutamide
tolerance
  pain t.
tolfenamic acid
Tolinase
Tolosa-Hunt syndrome
tomogram
tomograph
  CTI/Siemens 933 t.
  PC-2048B positron
    emission t.
  Tomomatic 64 single
    photon emission
    computed t.
Tomographic 64

tomography
    computed t. (CT)
    cranial computed t. (CCT)
    dynamic single photon
      emission computed t.
    emission computed t.
    infusion computed t.
    plain t.
    positron emission t. (PET)
    preoperative t.
    single photon emission
      computed t. (SPECT)
    xenon-enhanced computed t.
      (Xe-CT)
Tomomatic 64 single photon
  emission computed tomograph
tonaphasia
tone
    muscle t.
tongs
    Gardner-Wells t.
tongue
    t. of cerebellum
    t. phenomenon
tongue-in-groove operation
tonic
    t. control
    t. convulsion
    t. epilepsy
    t. pupil
    t. reflex
    t. spasm
tonic-clonic seizure
tonicoclonic
tonoclonic
    t. spasm
tonometry
tonsil
    cerebellar t.
tonsilla, pl. tonsillae
    t. cerebelli

tonsillar herniation
tooth spasms
topagnosis
topalgia
top of the basilar syndrome
topectomy
top-entry (open body) hook
topesthesia
tophus
topical
    t. clonidine
    t. thrombin
topoanesthesia
topognosis, topognosia
toponarcosis
toposcope
topothermesthesiometer
torch
    saline t.
torcular
    t. herophili
    t. meningioma
Torkildsen shunt
Torkildsen's ventriculocisternostomy
tornado epilepsy
torpent
torpid
torpidity
torpor
torque
    unwanted screw t.
torr
Torré's syndrome
torsion
    t. dystonia
    t. neurosis
    t. spasm
torsional
    t. gripping strength
    t. nystagmus
    t. stiffness

NOTES

torsionometer
Torsten Sjögren's syndrome
torticollar
torticollis
  benign paroxysmal t.
  dermatogenic t.
  dystonic t.
  fixed t.
  intermittent t.
  labyrinthine t.
  ocular t.
  psychogenic t.
  rheumatic t.
  spasmodic t.
  t. spastica
  spurious t.
  symptomatic t.
toruloma
total
  t. aphasia
  t. hypophysectomy
  t. parenteral nutrition
touch
  t. corpuscle
Tourette's
  T. disease
  T. syndrome
tourniquet
  Drake t.
towel clip
tower skull
toxic
  t. delirium
  t. dementia
  t. epidermal necrolysis
  t. hydrocephalus
  t. neuritis
  t. shock syndrome
  t. tetanus
toxicity
  drug t.
toxin
  botulinum A t.
toxoid
  tetanus t.
Toxoplasma
toxoplasmosis
  intramedullary t.
trace
  t. conditioned reflex
  memory t.
tracer
trachea

tracheal injury
trachelagra
trachelism, trachelismus
trachelocyrtosis
trachelodynia
trachelokyphosis
trachelology
tracheostomy
Tracker
  T. catheter
  T. infusion catheter
  T. microcatheter
Tracrium
tract
  anterior corticospinal t.
  anterior pyramidal t.
  anterior spinocerebellar t.
  anterior spinothalamic t.
  Arnold's t.
  association t.
  auditory t.
  Burdach's t.
  central tegmental t.
  cerebellorubral t.
  cerebellothalamic t.
  Collier's t.
  comma t. of Schultze
  corticobulbar t.
  corticopontine t.
  corticospinal t.
  crossed pyramidal t.
  cuneocerebellar t.
  deiterospinal t.
  dentatothalamic t.
  descending t. of trigeminal
    nerve
  direct pyramidal t.
  dorsal spinocerebellar t.
  dorsolateral t.
  fastigiobulbar t.
  Flechsig's t.
  frontopontine t.
  frontotemporal t.
  geniculocalcarine t.
  genitourinary t.
  t. of Goll
  Gowers' t.
  habenulointerpeduncular t.
  Hoche's t.
  hypothalamohypophysial t.
  lateral corticospinal t.
  lateral pyramidal t.
  lateral spinothalamic t.

Lissauer's t.
Loewenthal's t.
mamillothalamic t.
Marchi's t.
mesencephalic t. of
  trigeminal nerve
Monakow's t.
t. of Münzer and Wiener
nerve t.
occipitocollicular t.
occipitopontine t.
occipitotectal t.
olfactory t.
olivocerebellar t.
olivospinal t.
optic t.
parietopontine t.
posterior spinocerebellar t.
prepyramidal t.
pyramidal t.
reticulospinal t.
rubrobulbar t.
rubroreticular t.
rubrospinal t.
t. of Schütz
sensory t.
septomarginal t.
solitary t.
spinal t.
spinal dermal sinus t.
spinal t. of trigeminal nerve
spinocerebellar t.'s
spino-olivary t.
spinotectal t.
spinothalamic t.
spiral foraminous t.
Spitzka's marginal t.
sulcomarginal t.
supraopticohypophysial t.
tectobulbar t.
tectopontine t.

tectospinal t.
temporofrontal t.
temporopontine t.
tuberoinfundibular t.
Türck's t.
urinary t.
ventral spinocerebellar t.
ventral spinothalamic t.
vestibulospinal t.
Waldeyer's t.
traction
  Ace Trippi-Wells tong
    cervical t.
  Ace universal tong
    cervical t.
  t. anchor
  axial t.
  bipolar vertebral t.
  device for transverse t.
    (DTT)
  t. spur
  transverse t.
tractotomy
  anterolateral t.
  bulbar t.
  bulbar cephalic pain t.
  intramedullary t.
  mesencephalic t.
  pontine t.
  pyramidal t.
  Schwartz t.
  Sjöqvist t.
  spinal t.
  spinothalamic t.
  subcaudate t.
  trigeminal t.
  Walker t.
tractus, gen. and pl. **tractus**
  t. centralis tegmenti
  t. cerebellorubralis
  t. cerebellothalamicus

NOTES

tractus *(continued)*
   t. corticobulbaris
   t. corticopontini
   t. corticospinalis
   t. corticospinalis anterior
   t. corticospinalis lateralis
   t. descendens nervi trigemini
   t. dorsolateralis
   t. fastigiobulbaris
   t. frontopontinus
   t. habenulopeduncularis
   t. mesencephalicus nervi trigemini
   t. occipitopontinus
   t. olfactorius
   t. olivocerebellaris
   t. opticus
   t. parietopontinus
   t. pyramidalis
   t. pyramidalis anterior
   t. pyramidalis lateralis
   t. reticulospinalis
   t. rubrospinalis
   t. solitarius
   t. spinalis nervi trigemini
   t. spinocerebellaris anterior
   t. spinocerebellaris posterior
   t. spinotectalis
   t. spinothalamicus
   t. spinothalamicus anterior
   t. spinothalamicus lateralis
   t. spiralis foraminosus
   t. spiralis foraminulosus
   t. supraopticohypophysialis
   t. tectobulbaris
   t. tectopontinus
   t. tectospinalis
   t. tegmentalis centralis
   t. temporopontinus
   t. tuberoinfundibularis
   t. vestibulospinalis
trained reflex
train-of-four stimulus
tram track sign
trance
   death t.
tranexamic acid
transantral
   t. ethmoidal approach
   t. ethmoidal orbital decompression

transarterial platinum coil embolization
transarticular screw
transcallosal transventricular approach
transcavernous
   t. approach
   t. transpetrous apex approach
transcerebellar hemispheric approach
transcochlear approach
transcortical
   t. aphasia
   t. approach
   t. apraxia
   t. sensory aphasia
   t. transventricular approach
transcranial
   t. approach
   t. B-mode ultrasound
   t. color-coded real-time sonography (TCCS)
   t. Doppler
   t. Doppler sonography (TCD)
   t. Doppler ultrasonography
   t. Doppler ultrasound (TCD)
   t. electrical stimulation
   t. frontal-temporal-orbital approach
   t. real-time color Doppler imaging
   t. supraorbital approach
transcubital approach
transcutaneous electrical nerve stimulation
transducer
   t. cell
   Combitrans t.
   force t.
transducer-tipped catheter
transduction
   pain t.
transesophageal echocardiography
transfemoral catheter
transfer
   deficit
   energy t. (LET)
transferred sensation
transferrin
   anti-human t.

transfontanel Doppler ultrasound
transform
    Fourier t.
    isotrophic three-dimensional
      Fourier t.
    multidimensional Fourier t.
    three-dimensional Fourier t.
      (3DFT)
    two-dimensional Fourier t.
      (2DFT)
transforming growth factor beta
transfrontal approach
transfusion
    albumin t.
    autologous t.
    autologous blood t.
    fetal t.
transient
    t. ischemic attack (TIA)
    t. monocular visual loss
    t. signal abnormality
transilient
transillumination
transinsular
transisthmian
transitional
    t. convolution
    t. gyrus
    t. vertebra
translabyrinthine
    t. approach
    t. and suboccipital approach
translation
    coronal plane deformity
      sagittal t.
translational
    t. fracture
    t. position
transluminal angioplasty
transmandibular-glossopharyngeal
  approach

transmission
    duplex t.
    neurohumoral t.
    neuromuscular t.
transmitter
    radiofrequency t.
transneuronal atrophy
transoral
    t. approach
    t. root
transorbital
    t. leukotomy
    t. lobotomy
transosseous venography
transpalatal approach
transparent septum
transpedicular
    t. approach
    t. fixation
    t. fixation effective pedicle
      diameter
    t. fixation system design
    t. screw
    t. screw-rod fixation
    t. spinal instrumentation
transperitoneal approach
transplantation
    adrenal medulla t.
    brain t.
    tissue t.
transport
    axoplasmic t.
transposition
    seventh cranial nerve t.
    vertebral artery t.
transsinus approach
transsphenoidal
    t. approach
    t. encephalocele
    t. evacuation
    t. hypophysectomy

NOTES

transsphenoidal *(continued)*
    t. removal
    t. surgery
transsylvian approach
transsynaptic
    t. chromatolysis
    t. degeneration
transtentorial
    t. approach
    t. herniation
transthalamic
transthoracic
    t. approach
    t. discectomy
    t. vertebral body resection
transtorcular
    t. approach
    t. embolization
    t. occlusion
transvenous
    t. approach
    t. therapy
transverse
    t. connector
    t. crest
    t. fibers of pons
    t. fissure of cerebellum
    t. fissure of cerebrum
    t. fixation
    t. fixator application
    t. fornix
    t. gradient coil
    t. magnetization
    t. magnetization phase
    t. myelitis
    t. occipital sulcus
    t. pedicle angle
    t. pedicle diameter
    t. relaxation
    t. relaxation rate
    t. rhombencephalic flexure
    t. septum
    t. temporal convolutions
    t. temporal gyri
    t. temporal sulci
    t. traction
transversectomy
Tranxene
tranylcypromine
trapezius muscle
trapezoid
    t. body
trapped ventricle syndrome

Trasylol
Traube-Hering-Mayer wave
trauma
    abdominal t.
    cervical t.
    cervical spine t.
    cranial t.
    head t.
    intestinal t.
    lumbar spine t.
    maxillofacial t.
    nonpenetrating t.
    penetrating t.
    thoracolumbar t.
Traumacal
traumasthenia
traumatic
    t. anesthesia
    t. aneurysm
    t. brain injury
    t. cervical discopathy
    t. cervical disk herniation
    t. disorder
    t. displacement
    t. encephalopathy
    t. hematoma
    t. meningocele
    t. neurasthenia
    t. neuritis
    t. neuroma
    t. neurosis
    t. progressive
    encephalopathy
    t. pseudomeningocele
    t. psychosis
    t. tetanus
Traumatic Coma Data Bank
  (TCDB)
Travasorb
traversal
    tentorial t.
treatment
    compression rod t.
    distraction/compression
    scoliosis t.
    dual compression scoliosis t.
    endovascular t.
    hypervolemic t.
    insulin coma t.
    micro-operative t.
    neuromuscular scoliosis t.
    neuromuscular scoliosis
    orthotic t.

poliomyelitis t.
prophylactic t.
spinal deformity t.
trefoil tendon deformation
trembling
    t. palsy
tremogram
tremograph
tremor
    action t.
    alternating t.
    arsenical t.
    t. artuum
    benign essential t.
    cerebellar t.
    coarse t.
    continuous t.
    essential t.
    familial t.
    fibrillary t.
    fine t.
    flapping t.
    heredofamilial t.
    intention t.
    kinetic t.
    mercurial t.
    metallic t.
    t. opiophagorum
    passive t.
    persistent t.
    postural t.
    t. potatorum
    progressive cerebellar t.
    saturnine t.
    senile t.
    static t.
    t. tendinum
    volitional t.
tremorgram
tremulous
Trendelenburg position

Trendelenburg's symptom
trepan
trepanation
trephination
trephine
trephined
    syndrome of the t.
trepidant
trepidation
Treponema pallidum
triad
    Charcot's t.
trial
    lower hook t.
    upper hook t.
triamcinolone
    t. acetonide
triangle
    t. of fillet
    Glasscock's t.
    Gombault's t.
    Mullan's t.
    opticocarotid t.
    paramedian t.
    Parkinson's t.
    Philippe's t.
    Reil's t.
triangular
    t. base transverse bar
      configuration
    t. lamella
    t. recess
    t. syndrome
triangulated pedicle screw
Triavil
tribasilar synostosis
triceps
    t. reflex
    t. surae reflex
trichalgia
trichilemmoma

NOTES

trichinosis
trichodynia
trichoepithelioma
trichoesthesia
trichofolliculoma
trichosis
    t. sensitiva
tricortical iliac crest bone graft
tricyclic antidepressant
Tridione
triethiodide
    gallamine t.
trifacial
    t. nerve
    t. neuralgia
trifluoperazine hydrochloride
trifurcation
trigeminal
    t. crest
    t. decompression
    t. ganglion
    t. lemniscus
    t. nerve
    t. nerve neurinoma
    t. neuralgia
    t. neurinoma
    t. neuroma
    t. neuropathy
    t. nucleus caudalis lesioning
    t. rhizotomy
    t. root
    t. tractotomy
trigeminofacial reflex
trigeminus
trigger
    t. area
    t. finger
    t. point
    t. zone
trigona (pl. of trigonum)
trigone
    t. of auditory nerve
    collateral t.
    t. of fillet
    t. of habenula
    t. of hypoglossal nerve
    t. of lateral ventricle
    Müller's t.
    olfactory t.
    t. of vagus nerve
trigonocephaly
trigonum, pl. trigona
    t. acustici

    t. cerebrale
    t. collaterale
    t. habenulae
    t. hypoglossi
    t. lemnisci
    t. nervi hypoglossi
    t. nervi vagi
    t. olfactorium
    t. ventriculi
trihexoside
    ceramide t.
trihexosyl ceramide
trihexyphenidyl
    t. hydrochloride
Trilafon
trimethadione
trimethaphan
trimethobenzamide hydrochloride
trimethoprim
trimethoprim-sulfamethoxazole
trinitrate
    glyceryl t.
triphosphate
    adenosine t. (ATP)
triplegia
triple-wire technique
trismic
trismoid
trismus
    t. capistratus
    t. dolorificus
    t. nascentium, t. neonatorum
    t. sardonicus
trisomy 21 syndrome
triton tumor
trochanter reflex
trochlear
    t. nerve
    t. nerve neoplasm
    t. nerve palsy
    t. nerve paresis
    t. nucleus
Trolard
    vein of T.
Trolard's vein
Trömner's reflex
trophesic
trophesy
trophic
    t. change
    t. gangrene
trophicity
trophism

trophodermatoneurosis
trophoneurosis
    facial t.
    lingual t.
    muscular t.
    Romberg's t.
trophoneurotic
    t. atrophy
    t. leprosy
trophotropic zone of Hess
tropical spastic paraparesis
trough
    synaptic t.
Trousseau's
    T. point
    T. sign
    T. spot
    T. syndrome
true
    t. anosmia
truncation artifact
truncus, gen. and pl. **trunci**
    t. corporis callosi
trunk
    t. of corpus callosum
    meningohypohyseal t.
    sympathetic t.
trypanosome fever
trypanosomiasis
    acute t.
    African t.
    chronic t.
    East African t.
    Gambian t.
    Rhodesian t.
    West African t.
tryptophan
TSH
    thyroid-stimulating hormone

T-shaped
    T-s. Edwards-Barbaro
    syringeal shunt
    T-s. incision
TSRH
    Texas Scottish Rite Hospital
    TSRH buttressed laminar
    hook
    TSRH circular laminar
    hook
    TSRH crosslink stabilization
    TSRH double-rod construct
    TSRH implant
    TSRH instrumentation
    TSRH pedicle hook
    TSRH pedicle screw-laminar
    claw construct
    TSRH plate
    TSRH stabilization
    TSRH universal spinal
    instrumentation system
T-tube shunt
tube
    Adson suction t.
    blunt suction t.
    Dandy suction t.
    endotracheal t.
    flow regulated suction t.
    Frazier suction t.
    Hardy suction t.
    malleable multipore
    suction t.
    medullary t.
    nasogastric t.
    neural t.
    Nishizaki-Wakabayashi
    suction t.
    Rhoton-Merz suction t.
    Spetzler's Microvac
    suction t.
    suction t.

NOTES

tube *(continued)*
    tympanostomy t.
    Yankauer suction t.
    Yankauer-type suction t.
tuber, pl. **tubera**
    t. anterius
    ashen t.
    t. cinereum
    t. corporis callosi
    t. dorsale
    gray t.
    subependymal t.
    t. valvulae
    t. vermis
tuberal nuclei
tubercle
    acoustic t.
    amygdaloid t.
    anterior t. of thalamus
    ashen t.
    t. of cuneate nucleus
    gracile t.
    gray t.
    mamillary t. of
      hypothalamus
    t. of nucleus gracilis
    olfactory t.
    Rolando's t.
    t. of saddle
    wedge-shaped t.
tubercula (*pl. of* tuberculum)
tuberculoma
tuberculosis
    cerebral t.
    Mycobacterium t.
    spinal t.
tuberculous
    t. abscess
    t. meningitis
    t. spondylitis
tuberculum, pl. **tubercula**
    t. anterius thalami
    t. cinereum
    t. hypoglossi
    t. nuclei cuneati
    t. nuclei gracilis
    t. olfactorium
    t. sellae
tuberoinfundibular tract
tuberothalamic infarction
tuberous sclerosis
tubi (*pl. of* tubus)
tubular necrosis

tubulization
tubus, pl. **tubi**
    t. medullaris
tuck position
tufted cell
tulip pedicle screw
tumor
    acoustic nerve sheath t.
    adhesio interthalamica t.
    aortic body t.
    t. bed
    benign lymphoepithelial
      parotid t.
    bone t.
    brain t.
    t. bulk
    carotid body t.
    cartilaginous t.
    cavernous sinus t.
    cerebellopontine angle t.
    chemoreceptor t.
    chondromatous t.
    chromaffin t.
    convexity metastatic t.
    dermoid t.
    diffuse intrinsic brainstem t.
    eighth nerve t.
    epidermoid t.
    epidural t.
    Erdheim t.
    extradural t.
    germ cell t.
    giant cell t.
    giant glomus t.
    glomus jugulare t.
    granular cell t.
    inclusion t.
    interdural t.
    intracavernous t.
    intracranial t.
    intradural t.
    intraorbital granular cell t.
    intraventricular t.
    invasive t.
    leptomeningeal t.
    Lindau's t.
    lumbar t.
    lymphoepithelial parotid t.
    lymphomatous t.
    malignant germ cell t.
    t. marker
    medullary t.

melanotic
  neuroectodermal t.
meningeal t.
metastatic t.
metastatic brain t.
metastatic spinal t.
t. metastatic to spine
mixed germ cell t.
t. necrosis
Nelson t.
nerve sheath t.
neuroectodermal t.
neuroepithelial t.
neuronal t.
occipital lobe t.
orbital t.
Pancoast t.
parachiasmal epidermoid t.
parasellar t.
parotid t.
pearl t.
pediatric supratentorial
  hemispheric t.
peripheral nerve sheath t.
petroclival t.
pineal t.
pineal cell t.
pontine angle t.
potato t. of neck
Pott's puffy t.
primary t.
primitive neuroectodermal t.
Rathke's pouch t.
recurrent t.
t. resection
sand t.
sarcomatous t.
sellar t.
small-bowel carcinoid t.
spinal t.
spindle-cell t.

subdural t.
subependymal t.
superior pulmonary sulcus t.
supratentorial t.
supratentorial primitive
  neuroectodermal t.
triton t.
turban t.
vertebral body t.
visual system t.
tumor:cerebellum ratio (T:C ratio)
tumor-infiltrating lymphocytes
  (TIL)
tumorous involvement
tunnel
  t. cells
  cubital t.
  tarsal t.
  t. vision
tunneled ventriculostomy
Tuohy needle
turban tumor
turbidity
turbulence
turcica
  sella t.
Türck's
  T. bundle
  T. column
  T. degeneration
  T. tract
Turcot's syndrome
turnbuckle jack
Turner's sulcus
turricephaly
tussive absence
tutamen, pl. **tutamina**
  tutamina cerebri
Tutoplast
  T. allograft
  T. Dura

NOTES

T1-weighted
    T.-w. image
    T.-w. inversion recovery
    scan
    T.-w. MR image
    T.-w. spin echo
    T.-w. spin-echo image
T2-weighted
    T.-w. image
    T.-w. MR image
    T.-w. spin echo
    T.-w. spin-echo image
twelfth cranial nerve
twilight
    t. state
twinge
twist drill
twitch
    Cogan's lid t.
two
    rule of t.
two-column cervical spine injury
two-component microgrip precision control suction unit

two-dimensional
    t.-d. Fourier transform
    (2DFT)
    t.-d. Fourier transform
    gradient-echo imaging
    t.-d. imaging
    t.-d. mapping
two-stage procedure
tying forceps
Tylenol
Tylox
tympanic
    t. ganglion
    t. intumescence
tympanometry
tympanostomy tube
tympanum
type II curve pattern
Type 2 superconductor
typical absence
typist's cramp
tyramine

unit *(continued)*
  Leksell stereotactic
    gamma u.
  Malis electrocoagulation u.
  motor u.
  Radionics bipolar
    coagulation u.
  Sheffield gamma u.
  Signa 1.5 Tesla u.
  201-source cobalt-60
    gamma u.
  u. spinal rod
  stereotaxic gamma u.
  teleradiotherapy u.
  two-component microgrip
    precision control
    suction u.
  valve u.
  ZD-Neurosurgical
    localizing u.
uniting
  u. canal
  u. duct
universal instrumentation
unmedullated
unmyelinated
  u. fibers
unruptured aneurysm
unspecified aneurysm
unstable cervical spine injury
Unverricht-Lundborg syndrome
Unverricht's disease
unwanted screw torque
upper
  u. abdominal periosteal
    reflex
  u. cervical spine anterior
    construct
  u. cervical spine anterior
    exposure
  u. cervical spine fusion
  u. cervical spine posterior
    construct

  u. cervical spine procedure
  u. hook trial
  u. motor neuron
  u. motor neuron lesion
  u. thoracic spine
upward gaze paresis
urea
uremic polyneuropathy
ureter injury
ureterolysis
urethrism, urethrismus
urethritis
urethrospasm
urge incontinence
urgency incontinence
uric acid
urinary
  u. reflex
  u. sphincter
  u. stuttering
  u. tract
Uristix
  Dextrostix U.
urocrisis, urocrisia
urokinase
urticaria
  giant u., u. gigans, u.
    gigantea
  u. tuberosa
urticate
urtication
U-shaped scalp flap
uterine curette
utricle
utricular
  u. reflexes
  u. spot
utriculosaccular duct
utriculus, pl. **utriculi**
uveitis
uvula, pl. **uvuli**
  u. cerebelli
  u. vermis

vaccine
diphtheria, tetanus toxoids, and pertussis v. (DTP)
vacuum
v. disk
v. headache
vadum
vagal
v. attack
v. part of accessory nerve
vagale
glomus v.
vagectomy
vagina, gen. and pl. **vaginae**
v. cellulosa
vaginate
vagoaccessory syndrome
vagoglossopharyngeal
v. neuralgia
vagolysis
vagolytic
vagomimetic
vagotomy
vagotonia
vagotonic
vagotropic
vagovagal
vagus
v. area
v. nerve
v. neuropathy
Valentin's
V. corpuscles
V. ganglion
Valium
vallecula, pl. **valleculae**
v. cerebelli
v. sylvii
Valleix's points
vallis
valproate
valproic acid
Valsalva maneuver
value
C-reactive protein v.
Valve
Low Profile V.
valve
ball-in-cone v.
Delta v.

Denver v.
Hakim v.
Heyer-Pudenz v.
Holter v.
Holter-Hausner v.
Mishler v.
Orbis-Sigma v.
v. patency
Phoenix ancillary v.
Phoenix cruciform v.
prosthetic heart v.
Pudenz v.
Tarin's v.
v. unit
Vieussens' v.
valvula, pl. **valvulae**
v. semilunaris tarini
van
v. Bogaert-Canavan disease
v. Bogaert's disease
v. der Kolk's law
Vancocin
vancomycin
vane-type motor
vaporized
variable
v. screw placement (VSP)
v. screw placement system
v. screw placement system instrumentation
v. screw placement system-instrumented lumbar spine
v. screw placement system-plated patient
vari-angled clip holder
variant
anatomical v.
primitive trigeminal artery v.
varicella encephalitis
varicella-zoster virus
varices (*pl. of* varix)
orbital v.
Varidase
VARIMIC 900 microscope
varix, pl. **varices**
vas, gen. **vasis**,
gen. and pl. **vasorum**, pl. **vasa**
vasa recta

vascular
v. circle of optic nerve
v. decompression
v. dementia
v. erosion
v. groove
v. headache
v. injury
v. malformation
v. occlusion
v. patch graft
v. perforations
v. surgery
vasculitis, pl. vasculitides
hypersensitivity v.
leukocytoclastic vasculitides
mesenteric v.
radiation v.
retinal v.
septic venous v.
vasculomotor
vasculomyelinopathy
Vaseline gauze packing
vasis (*gen. of* vas)
vasoconstriction
vasoconstrictor
vasodilation
vasodilator
vasodilator-stimulated rCBF single photon emission computed tomographic measurement
vasogenic
v. shock
v. theory
vasomotor
v. absence
v. ataxia
v. epilepsy
v. imbalance
v. rhinitis
v. spasm
vasoneuropathy
vasoneurosis
vasopressin
v. tannate
vasopressor reflex
vasoreactivity
cerebral v.
vasoreflex
vasorum (*gen. and pl. of* vas)
vasosensory
vasospasm
angiographic v.

arterial v.
cerebral v.
vasostimulant
vasovagal
v. attack
v. epilepsy
v. syncope
v. syndrome
Vater-Pacini corpuscles
Vater's corpuscles
vault
cranial v.
VCR
vincristine
VDS
ventral derotation spondylodesis
vector
v. field
M v.
magnetic field v.
nuclear magnetization v.
v. phase
vecuronium bromide
VEE
Venezuelan equine encephalomyelitis
vegetation
vegetative
v. nervous system
v. state
veil
aqueduct v.
vein
anterior cerebral v.
anterior jugular v.
anterior v. of septum pellucidum
basal v. of Rosenthal
brachiocephalic v.
Browning's v.
carotid v.
v.'s of cerebellum, cerebellar v.'s
cerebral v.'s
cervical intersegmental v.
choroid v.
v. of corpus striatum
cortical v.
deep cerebral v.'s
deep middle cerebral v.
diencephalic v.
diploic v.
draining v.

emissary v.
v.'s of Galen
v. of Galen
v. of Galen aneurysm
v. of Galen malformation
great cerebral v.
great v. of Galen
inferior anastomotic v.
inferior v.'s of cerebellar
  hemisphere
inferior cerebral v.'s
inferior choroid v.
inferior thalamostriate v.'s
innominate v.
internal cerebral v.'s
internal jugular v.
jugular v.
jugulocephalic v.
v. of Labbé
Labbé's v.
lingual v.
linguofacial v.
maxillary v.
meningeal v.
meningorachidian v.
mesencephalic v.
myelencephalic v.
ophthalmic v.
orbital v.
posterior callosal v.
posterior v. of septum
  pellucidum
precentral cerebellar v.
Rosenthal's v.
saphenous v.
v. of septum pellucidum
striate v.'s
superficial middle
  cerebral v.
superficial temporal v.
superior anastomotic v.

superior v.'s of cerebellar
  hemisphere
superior cerebral v.'s
superior choroid v.
superior ophthalmic v.
superior thalamostriate v.
superior thyroid v.
telencephalic v.
terminal v.
thalamostriate v.'s
v. of Trolard
Trolard's v.
vela (*pl. of* velum)
Velban
vellicate
vellication
vellus
  v. olivae inferioris
velocity
  average v.
  blood v.
  flow v.
  nerve conduction v. (NCV)
  v. profile
  spectral v.
  spin v.
velum, pl. **vela**
  anterior medullary v.
  inferior medullary v.
  v. interpositum
  v. medullare inferius
  v. medullare superius
  posterior medullary v.
  v. semilunare
  superior medullary v.
  v. tarini
  v. terminale
  v. transversum
  v. triangulare
vena, gen. and pl. **venae**
  v. anastomotica inferior

NOTES

vena *(continued)*
- v. anastomotica superior
- v. basalis
- v. cava injury
- venae cerebelli
- venae cerebelli inferiores
- venae cerebelli superiores
- v. cerebri anterior
- venae cerebri inferiores
- venae cerebri internae
- v. cerebri magna
- v. cerebri media profunda
- v. cerebri media superficialis
- venae cerebri profundae
- venae cerebri superficiales
- venae cerebri superiores
- v. choroidea inferior
- v. choroidea superior
- venae hemispherii cerebelli inferiores
- venae hemispherii cerebelli superiores
- v. petrosa
- venae pontis
- v. precentralis cerebelli
- v. septi pellucidi anterior
- v. septi pellucidi posterior
- venae striatae
- v. terminalis
- venae thalamostriatae inferiores
- v. thalamostriata superior
- v. vermis inferior
- v. vermis superior

Venezuelan equine encephalomyelitis (VEE)

venography
- digital subtraction v.
- transosseous v.
- vertebral v.

venorespiratory reflex

venous
- v. aneurysm
- v. angioma
- v. angle
- v. embolism
- v. hypertension
- v. lake
- v. occlusive disease
- v. outflow obstruction
- v. sinus
- v. stasis retinopathy
- v. system

ventilation
- assisted v.
- high-frequency percussive v. (HFPV)

ventilator
- v. alarm

Ventolin

ventral
- v. anterior nucleus of thalamus
- v. column of spinal cord
- v. derotation spondylodesis (VDS)
- v. horn
- v. intermediate nucleus of thalamus
- v. lateral nucleus of thalamus
- v. medial mesencephalic syndrome
- v. nucleus of thalamus
- v. nucleus of trapezoid body
- v. part of the pons
- v. plate of neural tube
- v. pontine infarction
- v. posterior intermediate nucleus of thalamus
- v. posterior lateral nucleus of thalamus
- v. posterior nucleus of thalamus
- v. posterolateral nucleus of thalamus
- v. posteromedial nucleus of thalamus
- v. root
- v. spinocerebellar tract
- v. spinothalamic tract
- v. tegmental decussation
- v. thalamic peduncle
- v. tier thalamic nuclei

ventralis
- v. intermedius (VIM)
- v. lateralis (VL)

ventricle
- Arantius' v.
- cerebral v.'s
- v. of cerebral hemisphere
- v. of diencephalon
- Duncan's v.

fifth v.
fourth v.
lateral v.
v. of rhombencephalon
sixth v.
sylvian v.
terminal v.
third v.
Verga's v.
Vieussens' v.
Wenzel's v.
ventricular
v. drainage
v. ependyma
v. fibrillation
v. fluid
v. layer
v. needle
v. Ommaya reservoir
v. peritoneal shunting
v. puncture
v. wall
ventriculi (*pl. of* ventriculus)
ventriculitis
ventriculoamniotic shunting
ventriculoatrial shunt
ventriculocisternostomy
Torkildsen's v.
ventriculofugal artery
ventriculogram
iohexol CT v.
ventriculography
air v.
cerebral v.
stereotactic anteroposterior
and lateral metrizamide v.
water-soluble contrast v.
ventriculomastoidostomy
ventriculomegaly
ventriculoperitoneal (VP)

v. shunt
v. shunting
ventriculopuncture
ventriculoscopy
ventriculostomy
straight-in v.
terminal v.
third v.
tunneled v.
ventriculosubarachnoid
ventriculotomy
ventriculus, pl. ventriculi
v. lateralis
v. quartus
v. quintus
v. terminalis
v. tertius
ventrobasal nucleus
ventro-intermedius
nucleus v.-i.
ventrolateral (VL)
v. nuclear complex
ventromedial nucleus of hypothalamus
ventroposterolateral (VPL)
VER
visual evoked response
verapamil
verbal agraphia
vergae
cavum v.
Verga's ventricle
vergence movement
vermian
v. atrophy
v. split
vermis, pl. vermes
Vermont
V. spinal fixator
V. spinal fixator articulation
vernal encephalitis

NOTES

Vernet's syndrome
Verneuil's neuroma
Verocay bodies
versatility
    attachment v.
vertebra, pl. vertebrae
    atlas v.
    axis v.
    block v.
    butterfly v.
    cervical v.
    coronal cleft v.
    inferior v.
    lumbar v.
    lumbosacral v.
    thoracic v.
    thoracolumbar v.
    transitional v.
vertebral
    v. angiogram
    v. angiography
    v. artery
    v. artery injury
    v. artery occlusion
    v. artery transposition
    v. body anterior cortex
    v. body anterior cortex
      penetration
    v. body corpectomy
    v. body decompression
    v. body tumor
    v. cervical instability
    v. collapse
    v. column
    v. corpectomy
    v. dissection
    v. end-plate enhancement
    v. exposure
    v. fascia
    v. fracture
    v. fusion
    v. ganglion
    v. hemangioma
    v. level
    v. osteosynthesis
    v. osteosynthesis fusion rate
    v. part
    v. plate
    v. plate application
    v. pulp
    v. resection
    v. subluxation
    v. venography

vertebrectomy
    cervical v.
    cervical spondylotic
      myelopathy v.
vertebrobasilar
    v. aneurysm
    v. artery
    v. infarction
    v. insufficiency
    v. system
vertical
    v. gaze
    v. gaze paresis
    v. midline incision
    v. pedicle diameter
    v. vertigo
vertiginous
vertigo
    benign paroxysmal v.
    Charcot's v.
    chronic v.
    endemic paralytic v.
    epidemic v.
    galvanic v.
    gastric v.
    height v.
    horizontal v.
    laryngeal v.
    lateral v.
    mechanical v.
    nocturnal v.
    objective v.
    organic v.
    paralyzing v.
    positional v.
    postural v.
    rotary v.
    sham-movement v.
    subjective v.
    systematic v.
    vertical v.
    voltaic v.
very low-density syndrome
Vesalius
    canal of V.
    foramen of V.
vesical reflex
vesicle
    cerebral v.
    encephalic v.
    forebrain v.
    hindbrain v.
    midbrain v.

ocular v.
optic v.
primary brain v.
synaptic v.'s
telencephalic v.
vesicospinal
vesicula, gen. and pl. **vesiculae**
v. ophthalmica
vessel
blood v.
cerebral blood v.
collateral v.
nutrient v.
vest
Bremer AirFlo v.
halo v.
vestibular
v. area
v. crest
v. disorder
v. fissure of cochlea
v. function
v. ganglion
v. hair cells
v. labyrinth
v. membrane
v. nerve
v. nerve section
v. neurectomy
v. nuclei
v. organ
v. part of vestibulocochlear
nerve
v. root of vestibulocochlear
nerve
v. suppressant
v. system
vestibulocerebellar ataxia
vestibulocerebellum
vestibulocochlear
v. nerve

v. neuropathy
v. organ
vestibulo-equilibratory control
vestibulo-ocular
v.-o. reflex
v.-o. reflex suppression
vestibulospinal
v. reflex
v. tract
**V-groove hollow-ground connection
design**
vibration syndrome
vibratory sensibility
Vicq
V. d'Azyr's bundle
V. d'Azyr's centrum
semiovale
V. d'Azyr's foramen
Vicryl
victim
multiple trauma v.
vidarabine
videocassette recording
video/EEG monitoring
videotape assessment
Vieussens'
V. ansa
V. centrum
V. ganglion
V. loop
V. valve
V. ventricle
view
field of v.
swimmer's v.
Waters' v.
vigil
coma v.
vigilambulism
vigilance
Viking II nerve monitoring device

NOTES

Villaret's syndrome
villus, pl. villi
    arachnoid v.
    arachnoid villi
VIM
    ventralis intermedius
Vim thalamotomy
vinblastine sulfate
vincristine (VCR)
    v. sulfate
vinculum, pl. vincula
    vincula lingulae cerebelli
violinist's cramp
viral
    v. infection
    v. rhinitis
Virchow-Robin space
Virchow's
    V. disease
    V. psammoma
viridans
    Streptococcus v.
virus
    v. encephalomyelitis
    human immunodeficiency v.
    (HIV)
    varicella-zoster v.
visceral
    v. anesthesia
    v. brain
    v. disorder
    v. epilepsy
    v. motor neuron
    v. nervous system
    v. pain
    v. sense
    v. sympathectomy
viscerogenic
    v. reflex
visceromotor reflex
viscerosensory
    v. reflex
viscosity
    blood v.
vision
    color v.
    double v.
    facial v.
    subjective v.
    tunnel v.
Vista American Health 0.5 Tesla
  MRI scanner
Vistaril

visual
    v. acuity loss
    v. agnosia
    v. alexia
    v. allesthesia
    v. aphasia
    v. area
    v. blurring
    v. change
    v. claudication
    v. cortex
    v. evoked potential
    v. evoked response (VER)
    v. field defect
    v. field deficit
    v. fixation
    v. image inversion
    v. image movement
    disorder
    v. inattention
    v. loss
    v. orbicularis reflex
    v. receptor cells
    v. system tumor
visual-spatial agnosia
visuoauditory
visuognosis
visuomotor
visuopsychic
visuosensory
visuospatial
    v. disorientation
vital
    v. center
    v. knot
    v. node
Vitallium
    V. equipment
    V. plate
vitamin
    v. B_{12}
    v. B_{12} neuropathy
    v. K
vitrectomy
vitreous
    v. disease
    v. hemorrhage
    primary v.
vitritis
VL
    ventralis lateralis
    ventrolateral
    VL thalamotomy

vocal
    v. amusia
    v. cords
Vogt-Spielmeyer disease
Vogt syndrome
Voigt's lines
volitional tremor
Volkmann's contracture
voltaic vertigo
volume
    blood v.
    caudate v.
    cerebellar v.
    cerebrospinal fluid v.
    v. expansion
    v. regulation
    v. segmentation
volumetric infusion pump
voluntary mutism
vomiting
    cyclic v.
    v. reflex
von
    v. Economo's disease
    v. Economo's encephalitis
    v. Graefe's sign
    v. Graefe strabismus hook
    v. Hippel-Lindau disease
    v. Hippel-Lindau syndrome
    v. Recklinghausen's disease
    v. Recklinghausen's
      neurofibromatosis
voxel
VP
    ventriculoperitoneal
    VP shunt
VP-16
VPL
    ventroposterolateral
    VPL pallidotomy
VSP
    variable screw placement
    VSP plate instrumentation
Vulpian's
    V. atrophy
    V. effect

NOTES

Wackenheim's clivus canal line
Wada test
waddle
wafer
        polyanhydride biodegradable
        polymer w.
waiter's cramp
wakefulness disorder
waking numbness
Waldenstrom
        macroglobulinemia of W.
Waldeyer's
        W. tract
        W. zonal layer
Walker tractotomy
walking
        chromosome w.
wall
        ventricular w.
Wallenberg's syndrome
wallerian
        w. degeneration
        w. law
Walther's ganglion
wand
        3-dimensional
        reconstruction w.
wandering cell
waning discharge
Warburg syndrome
Wardrop's method
warfarin
        w. sodium
Waring blender syndrome
Wartenberg's symptom
washer
        plate-spacer w.
wasting
        nitrogen w.
        w. palsy
        w. paralysis
watchmaker's cramp
water intoxication
watershed
        w. infarction
        w. region
water-soluble
        w.-s. contrast myelography
        w.-s. contrast
        ventriculography

Waters' view
watertight closure
wave
        alpha w.
        w. analyzer
        beta w.
        brain w.
        delta w.
        flat top w.'s
        Hering-Traube w.'s
        random w.'s
        theta w.
        Traube-Hering-Mayer w.
        ultrasonic w.'s
waveform
        signal voltage w.
waveshape
wax
        bone w.
        Horsley's bone w.
WBRT
        whole brain radiation therapy
weakness
        abduction w.
        adduction w.
        arm w.
        eye muscle w.
        pharyngeal w.
        sternocleidomastoid
        muscle w.
Weber-Leyden syndrome
Weber's
        W. sign
        W. syndrome
Weber test
Webster needle holder
Wechsler
        W. Adult Intelligence Scale
        W. Adult Intelligence Scale,
        Revised
        W. Intelligence Scale for
        Children, Revised (WISC-
        R)
        W. Memory Scale
Weck clip
Wedensky facilitation
wedge-compression fracture
wedge-shaped
        w.-s. fasciculus
        w.-s. tubercle

WEE
    western equine
    encephalomyelitis
Wegener's granulomatosis
weight
    w. gain
    w. loss
weighting
    proton density w.
    T1 w.
    T2 w.
Weingrow's reflex
Weiss' sign
Weitlaner retractor
welding
    tissue w.
Wells stereotaxic apparatus
Wenzel's ventricle
Werdnig-Hoffmann disease
Wernekinck's
    W. commissure
    W. decussation
Wernicke-Korsakoff
    W.-K. encephalopathy
    W.-K. syndrome
Wernicke's
    W. aphasia
    W. area
    W. center
    W. disease
    W. encephalopathy
    W. field
    W. radiation
    W. reaction
    W. region
    W. sign
    W. syndrome
    W. zone
West
    W. African sleeping sickness
    W. African trypanosomiasis
Westco Neurostat-Mark II
Westergren method
westermani
    Pargonimus w.
**western equine encephalomyelitis
    (WEE)**
Westphal-Erb sign
Westphal-Piltz phenomenon
Westphal's
    W. disease
    W. phenomenon

W. pseudosclerosis
W. pupillary reflex
W. sign
Westphal-Strümpell pseudosclerosis
West's syndrome
wet beriberi
Wever-Bray phenomenon
whiplash
    w. injury
white
    w. commissure
    w. iritis
    w. matter
    w. matter disease
    w. substance
whole-body cooling
**whole brain radiation therapy
    (WBRT)**
whole-spine MRI
wick
    Silastic w.
wide area network
Wilbrand's knee injury
Wilder's law of initial value
Wilde's cords
Willis
    circle of W.
Willis' centrum nervosum
Wilson's
    W. disease
    W. syndrome
Wiltberger's fusion
Wiltse
    W. system
    W. system aluminum
        master rod
    W. system cross-bracing
    W. system double-rod
        construct
    W. system H construct
    W. system single-rod
        construct
    W. system spinal rod
windage
wind contusion
window
    acoustic bone w.
    CT bone w.'s
wing
    ashen w.
    gray w.

w. plate
sphenoid w.
Winkelman's disease
winking spasm
wink reflex
Winston-Lutz method
Wintrobe method
wire
w. contour preparation
w. extrusion
Kirschner w.
Mullan's w.
w. osteosynthesis
w. passage
w. penetration depth
w. removal technique
spinous process w.
w. stabilization
sublaminar w.
w. thrombosis
wiring
facet w.
facet fracture
stabilization w.
facet subluxation
stabilization w.
posterior interspinous w.
spinous process w.
sublaminar w.
Wisconsin Card Solving Test
WISC-R
Wechsler Intelligence Scale for
Children, Revised
withdrawal reflex
Wohlfart-Kugelberg-Welander
disease
Wolff vasogenic theory

Wolf-Orton bodies
wolfram needle electrode
Wollaston's theory
Wolman's disease
woodcutter's encephalitis
Woodson dural separator
word
w. blindness
w. deafness
wound
gunshot w.
wrap
cotton w.
wrench
Texas Scottish Rite
Hospital w.
T-handled nut w.
T-handled screw w.
Wrisberg
nerve of W.
Wrisberg's
W. ganglia
W. nerve
wrist
w. clonus
w. clonus reflex
wrist-drop
writer's cramp
writing
w. disorder
w. hand
wrong-way deviation
wryneck
wry neck
Würzburg implant system
Wyburn-Mason syndrome

NOTES

xanthine
    x. oxidase inhibitor
xanthochromia
xanthomatosis
    cerebrotendinous x.
xanthosarcoma
X chromosome
Xe
    xenon
^{133}Xe
    xenon-133
        ^{133}Xe intravenous injection
        technique
Xe-CT
    xenon-enhanced computed
    tomography
Xe/CT CBF study
xenon (Xe)
    x. CT measurement
    x. CT scanning
    x. method
xenon-133 (^{133}Xe)

xenon-enhanced
    x.-e. computed tomography
    (Xe-CT)
    x.-e. CT
XeScan
    Linde X.
x gradient
xiphodynia
xiphoidalgia
XKnife
X-linked
    X.-l. lymphoproliferative
    syndrome
    X.-l. spastic paraparesis
Xomed nerve integrity monitor-2
Xomed-Treace nerve integrity
  monitor-2
x-ray
    intraoperative x.-r.
Xylocaine
xyrospasm

Y-9179
Yale brace
Yankauer suction tube
Yankauer-type suction tube
Yasargil
    Y. clip
    Y. craniotomy
    Y. cross-legged clip
    Y. flat serrated ring forceps
    Y. retractor

Yasargil-Aesculap
    Y.-A. instrument
    Y.-A. spring clip
Yasargil-Leyla brain retractor
yellow
    y. ligament
    y. spot
y **gradient**
yttrium-90